Speech Correction

PRENTICE-HALL INTERNATIONAL, INC., *London*
PRENTICE-HALL OF AUSTRALIA, PTY., LTD., *Sydney*
PRENTICE-HALL OF CANADA, LTD., *Toronto*
PRENTICE-HALL FRANCE, S.A.R.L., *Paris*
PRENTICE-HALL OF JAPAN, INC., *Tokyo*
PRENTICE-HALL DE MEXICO, S.A., *Mexico City*

CHARLES VAN RIPER

Director, Speech and Hearing Clinic
Western Michigan University

Speech Correction
Principles and Methods

FOURTH EDITION

Prentice-Hall, Inc., *Englewood Cliffs, N.J.*

Fourth printing.....March, 1965

Library of Congress Catalog Card No.: 63-17080

Printed in the United States of America

8 2 9 5 1 - C

Preface to the Fourth Edition

The first edition of this book came out in 1939, perhaps a bit earlier than some of its readers. In preparing for the present revision, the author took a long look at that first volume and its successors to attempt to discover the secret of their persistence on the bookshelves of his colleagues and their students. It was a difficult task—perhaps because the flaws in any book always glare accusingly at the one who gave them birth. If he found anything to explain the text's survival (and he is far from certain about this) it was that the pages always seemed to smell of the therapy vineyard in which the author has labored hard and long. These were not texts in scientific speech pathology for those who wear the long black beard. They were tools designed for the hands of those who wanted to help the person who could not talk normally.

In this revision, the author has not so much revised as rewritten the text. He hopes that his constant experimenting with new approaches in actual therapy with all types of speech disorders has enabled this new book not only to reflect current practices but also to pioneer new ones. Most of all, he hopes that it too will be put to work in the vineyard.

C. Van Riper

Table of Contents

Appendices

List of Figures

Speech Correction

CHAPTER ONE

✻ Defective Speech: An Introduction

This is a book about people troubled by the way
they speak, about children and adults who stutter
or lisp or use a falsetto voice or possess some other kind of a speech
disorder. Most of us speak almost as easily and as automatically as
we breathe. This world of ours is a verbal world; our hours tick by
in talk. Nothing is more common, more obvious than speaking, yet
it is always difficult to scrutinize the obvious, to look at the common
and familiar experiences of life with strange eyes. But this is what
we must do if we are to understand the problems of those with
tangled tongues, those who cannot talk as we do.

Speech Is a Motor Act. So let us look with strange eyes at this act
of speaking. It is first of all a motor act. Muscles must move; mouths
must open; vocal cords must vibrate; tongues must make contacts
and shape contours. All this is obvious but it becomes important
when we hear the flutter in the voice of a man with a paralyzed
vocal cord, when we watch a cleft-palate child squeezing his nostrils
in a vain effort to reduce the abnormality of his snorted *s* sounds.
We cannot escape this view of speech as a motor act when we
watch the child with cerebral palsy jerking and writhing as he half
swallows his cry for "Mama!" Speaking involves some of the most
complicated coordinations ever attempted by man. One old German
scholar wrote a whole monograph describing the muscular coordinations involved in the utterance of the single syllable "pop," and
in his preface he apologized for its incompleteness. If we are to
understand the difficulties of a child who has never learned how
to produce a normal *r* sound we cannot escape this view of speech

1

as a motor act. If he says something like *wabbit* for *rabbit,* he will
have to learn to move his tongue and mouth in a different way.

~~*Speech as Sound.*~~   But speech is more than a motor act; it is also
an acoustic event. It is something that can be heard both by the
listener and the speaker. This too seems obvious. Yet let us look a
little deeper to understand. Many a child who cannot articulate his
speech sounds correctly can recognize in another person's speech
the same errors that he cannot hear in his own. One successful
speech therapist of our acquaintance does most of her work with
such a child, not face to face, but sitting behind him with her
mouth just above his hair. Why? "It's because I want to create a
sound field as similar as possible to the child's," she explained. "His
mouth is two inches under his ears; mine is two inches above and
we are both facing in the same direction. When I sit across the
table from him he can't hear the difference between my voice and
his as well as when I am behind him."

We cannot understand the child with a speech disorder without
understanding this view of speech as something to be heard both
by the child and by others. Wendell Johnson has said that stuttering does not begin in the child's mouth but in the parent's ear.
What he means by this is that an overanxious mother may interpret
her child's normal hesitations as being abnormal, thereby making
the child so anxious about them that he begins to struggle and
avoid. Or let us listen just once to the child whose deafness has
never let him hear himself. The voice is odd; the speech sounds are
distorted; the rhythm is faulty; the sentences are strange. Often he
cannot make himself understood without resorting to gesture. Or
perhaps you have heard your own voice emerging from the tape
recorder, sounding totally unlike the one you think is yours, though
other voices on the same tape sound familiar. We have heard adults
with voices so harsh and nasal they could have been used for filing
a saw, who never had realized what irritation constantly emerged
from their mouths. One of them threw a chair at the tape recorder
that gave back what he had just put into it. There are mysteries in
this business of self-hearing which must be unraveled before we
can help a child to speak normally and rejoin the human race.

But there are other ways of viewing speech. We can view it in
terms of its functions. These sound and movement features are important but we cannot overlook the role of speech in the formula-

tion of thought, in communication, in emotional expression, in social control, and in the identification of the self. These sound like dull abstractions but they are not. No one can possibly understand defective speech without taking these functions of speech into account.

Speech in Thinking. Let us consider, then, the role of speech in the formulation of thought. Psychologists have long wrestled with the definition of thinking and as yet have not been able to agree on one. At one time, the early behaviorists felt that thinking was merely sub-audible speech, that and nothing else. Various researchers have shown that this proposition is not true. Some thinking seems to have no verbal coding. Einstein claims to have thought in the visual symbols of his mathematics. Artists report aesthetic experiences which require contours and colors and lines for their formulation. Musicians compose with tones and postures. Perhaps the closest we can come to grips with the nature of thinking is to

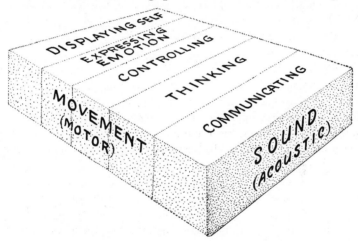

FIGURE 1. *Aspects and Functions of Speech*

view it as covert symbolic behavior. It is covert because it is hidden, invisible, and private. It is symbolic since experience is somehow coded and transformed and translated into representative symbols. Finally, these symbols are bits of behavior.

Much thinking consists of covert speech behavior. Little children often think aloud in self-talk but we find others who have been delayed in their speech development who can think "up" only by a tiny lifting of the head. We think in "body English" as well as with inner speech, but verbal symbols are so much more convenient and usable than gestures or postures when it comes to remembering, perceiving, or predicting that the human race has long ago given a strong emphasis to this inner speech as one of the chief tools of thinking. Let us say it again, not all thinking is inner speech but much of it is, and we must take this into account if we wish to help the person who cannot speak normally.

Perhaps a few examples may make this matter clear. One of the common problems faced by speech therapists in the public schools is that they are often able to teach their children with defective sounds to produce them perfectly in the therapy room only to find that when the children return to the classroom or playground they speak as poorly as before. Much of this difficulty in transfer is due to the fact that these children are still thinking with defective inner speech. They may be able to say *school* or *six* when the speech therapist is there to remind them of the standard utterance but if they still think *thkool* and *thikth* these will be the words they will utter in the hot flow of communication.

Children are not parrots or myna birds although some parents almost seem to feel that they must be taught to talk in the same fashion. We worked with a six-year-old whose only speech accomplishment was that he could mechanically count to ten in parrot fashion. He had no concept of number, and his only other utterances were grunts and squeals. He was not mentally retarded; he could work out complicated form board puzzles and he seemed to understand the speech of others without difficulty. But he formulated his ideas and communicated with his parents in a language of gesture and posture. Once, he was even able to tell us, by pretending to sleep, then dancing around, then blowing out imaginary candles, that the day before he had been to a birthday party. Some people can understand Spanish without being able to speak it. Some can even speak Spanish without being able to think in that language but they cannot speak it well if they must so translate. The child with defective speech must learn to think with normal speech. We cannot ignore this fact if we desire to help such a child.

We shall refer to this function of speech as a part of thinking often in this book, so let us give here some other glimpses of its importance. Severe stutterers often report that certain words have become so feared as a result of the abnormality, frustration, and penalty that they cannot think of them save in a distorted way. For one stutterer, his own name, Charles, was for thirty years a broken word with a monstrous *CH*, followed by a long aching gap of silence, and then a weak *arles*. As he learned to speak again this word has come together and is a unit, but for years he never thought of his own name except in this stuttering fashion. It is for this reason that in the chapter on stuttering we recommend that stutterers talk aloud to themselves and verbalize their thoughts when alone.

Again, when we discuss the problem of aphasia, the disorder that results from a stroke or brain injury, we will describe how the therapist must verbalize for the patient his thoughts at the moment they occur. These patients show a bewildering variety of symptoms— confusion, jargon, muteness, inability to read or write or even comprehend. Their language processes are jumbled, confused. We can help many of them but we can do so only by relating speech to thought.

If you could have seen us today working with a five-year-old boy, a twin, with no intelligible speech, you would understand the importance of viewing speech as a form of thinking. First of all we did some self-talk, describing in very short sentences and phrases what we were seeing and doing as we opened a box and began to put a toy tractor together. We thought *aloud* in very simple language, giving a play-by-play description of all of our actions and perceptions. Then we gave the boy another box with another toy to assemble. As he did so, we verbalized *for* him in the same fashion *his* thoughts. We tried to time our parallel talk so that it would coincide with his behavior and his thinking. When he tried to put a round peg in a square hole and failed, we said: "Put in hole . . . no go in . . . where more stick? . . . over there . . . I put this one in . . . OK . . . push hard . . . turn over . . . sharp there . . . finger hurt . . . throw down . . . look in box . . ." We were providing for him the verbal coding he lacked. We were building a foundation for speech. We did not ask him to talk, to repeat after us sounds meaningless to him. There is more to speech than "Polly-wants-a-cracker." Speech involves thinking and thinking involves speech.

Speech as Communication. All of us recognize the utility of speech in the transmission of information, in the sending and receiving of messages. The air is full of these winged words. One would expect then that most speech correction would be found in the context of communication. Unfortunately this is not often the case. If you will watch the usual mother teaching her child to talk, demanding that he say this and say that, asking him to repeat phrases after her, you will understand that most of us have had to learn to speak the hard way. Most speech therapists marvel not that there are so many persons with speech defects but so few. And yet even speech therapists often fall into the same trap. It is so easy to think of words as words rather than as thoughts or messages, to view words only as sounds or coordinations rather than as carriers of communication. Again we find the problem of "carry-over" in public school speech correction. The lisping child who can easily rattle through a hundred *s* words in the speech room will, in the share-and-tell period of the classroom, say something like this: "My thithter found a thalamander yetherday. He wath about tho long and she found him in the grath by the back thepth. He wiggoth."

In the disorder of stuttering we find a dramatic example of the importance of speech as communication. Most stutterers can talk to themselves without difficulty, with almost complete fluency. And yet, the moment they have a listener who must understand the message they begin to send, the speech breaks down and repetition, fixation, or contortion appears. No one can help a stutterer regain his fluency except in the context of communication.

Let us take a brief glimpse at some speech therapy structured in terms of communication. The teacher has a glass of water before her and she is blindfolded. Three children with lisps sit before her watching. "Remember now," she cautions, "*Think* is not the same as *sink, ssssink.* SSSink means to go down into the water. Now, I've got something in my hand and I want you to tell me if it will ssssink or float when I put it in the water. Remember, I can't see it so you'll have to tell me which it does. Jimmy, what's this I have in my hand?"

"It's a penny." The teacher puts it into the water.

"It thinkth." Jimmy was thinking *thinkth;* he was also comunicating.

"Pennies can't think; only people think."

"SSSSink," cried another child. "It sink."

"Yeth," said Jimmy, "It sssink. It don't float."

One experience of this sort is worth a thousand correct repetitions of isolated words in the conquest of a speech defect. Speech therapy cannot be carried out in a vacuum. The ebb and flow of communication, the give and take of messages, these are the opportunities for learning to speak as others do. We shall return to this theme often in this book.

Speech as Social Control. We must not overlook another function of speech, its function as a tool to manipulate others. The baby learns this very early. There is a magic to this speech act. The child cries, "Mama!" and lo! there she is. "Moh miuk!" he demands, and more milk is provided forthwith. This is the abracadabra and open sesame of Aladdin with his lamp. Say the right things and you are king of the castle. This is a marvelous discovery, this realization that the mouth can reach further and do more than the hands. Alas, some little children never learn it or learn it only weakly. In speech therapy we often have to return to this early discovery if we would help our children with the tangled tongues. No parental applause for parrot speech is half so reinforcing as the realization that speaking enables a person to control his environment, to boss other people around.

How do we use this feature of speech in helping the person who cannot talk? Today we were working with a strange deep-eyed little boy who could do little but grunt or cry. We played silently with him until he relaxed and joined us. Then we began to make noises as we shot a gun or moved a truck, and so did he. In fact once he said bugga-bugga-bugga. We played this follow-the-leader game for a time and then moved over to a large jack-in-the-box. We cupped a hand and said to the box, "Bugga-bugga!" It was a command, and by pressing the secret button, Jack jumped out. The little boy screamed with delight and helped us put Jack back where he belonged. We did it again and again, and soon the boy was giving the magical command of "Bugga-bugga!" without ever being asked to do so. This was all we did in that therapy session but it was enough. The boy had had a crucial experience: he had learned that speech need not be painful, that speech was magical, that by speaking he could control something outside himself. Every journey begins with one step.

Later on with this boy we shall make sure that many of his first words and phrases will be commands. When he commands "Oh doh" we shall open the door without delay. We can help him learn the standard ways of articulating the speech sounds later, but first we must give him the motivation he will need if he is ever to speak as we do. Throughout his life he will find pleasure in manipulating his environment by means of his mouth. He will ask questions, thereby demanding answers. He will warn and beg, protest and insist, with words. He will make friends, win his mate, and earn his living, partly by the action of his mouth. Some children do not know that this magical power exists and so they do not talk or find no pleasure in talking. Speech as a social control function is important.

Speech as Emotional Expression. An old theory used to explain the origin of speech in the human race states that primitive man first began to talk when his snarls of rage, grunts of contempt, or cries of fright were heard by another hairy ancestor of ours and interpreted with meaning. There are other speculations equally interesting and equally untestable but we can be sure, just by cocking our ears, that one of the functions of speech is the expression of emotion.

Speech has been called the barometer of the soul. Certainly it reflects how the speaker is feeling about himself and others. Many of the disorders of speech are produced or affected by emotional conflicts. One of our cases stopped talking at the age of five when his father punished him severely after he had confessed setting fire to a barn. Three years later he was still mute and it took a long and patient course of treatment before he began to talk again. A minister came to us from South Carolina with the complaint that his voice failed him and faded into a whisper as soon as he had said a few words from the pulpit. It turned out that unconsciously he was afraid he might preach strongly against segregation. The hysterical loss of voice saved him. We have also known baby talkers who resisted fiercely any attempt to improve their speech because they liked being infantile. Some people have nasal voices because they are nasty people and full of complaints.

Stutterers build up fears of sounds and words and different speaking situations. One stutterer may speak well over the phone because he knows his listener cannot see his facial contortions. Another may dread this same situation because he imagines his listener is laughing. When we work with aphasics, those who have lost their speech due to brain injury, we must work very carefully, constantly scanning their frustration tolerances, their anxieties, so that we will not overload their fragile integrative capacities. And yet we have known instances in which such an aphasic under extreme emotion could say something very well, something he could not say under ordinary circumstances. There are many accounts of such patients being able to yell "Fire!" in an emergency when they could never say it otherwise. No one who attempts to help any of these people with defective speech can ignore this emotional aspect of the problem. We do not deal with incorrectly spoken words; we deal with human beings in trouble. Emotional problems can cause speech disorders; speech disorders can produce emotional problems. All the basic features of speech—the voice, the articulation, the rhythm, and the language —reflect and are affected by emotion.

Speech as Self-expression. A final way of looking at this act of speaking is to view it as the identification and exhibition of the *self*. Much of our talking is what we might term "cock-a-doodle-doo" speech. It is a form of crowing, of calling attention to ourselves, of making sure that our listeners do not ignore our existence. If you will listen with strange ears to the conversations of those about you, this function of speech will become very vivid. You will hear the prevalence of the perpendicular pronoun, "I." Only a fraction of our speech consists of sending messages back and forth; the larger share is ego centered. In this cluttered world of ours, each man is essentially alone—it's a frightening thing to be alone. So he talks to create the necessary illusion that he exists, that he is important and a member of the clan. Many a child cries at bedtime or nags ceaselessly for a drink or to go to the bathroom or for another dolly because in silence and darkness, she suddenly seems to disappear, to vanish. To close one's eyes and to hear nothing is for some little children to cease to exist. So they use their barbaric little yawps to reassure themselves that they are there, that they are important to other people too. This need to assert one's self, to parade one's existence, is a pretty basic need in our culture. Much of our speech is motivated by that need.

We find many ways in which this need for self-expression must be considered in speech correction. Last week one of our student speech therapists came barreling into our office with triumph on her face. "Johnny said 'I.' He said 'I won't do it!' He didn't say '*Johnny* won't do it' or '*Me* won't do it!' " We agreed that this small

bit of behavior was of great significance. John was seven. Three
weeks before this experience, his speech output had been both
small and unintelligible. He was almost a non-talker. In this short
time, he had made marked progress, discovered the magical use of
speech as a tool to command others, and now had found its importance in asserting the *self*. It was worth a bit of whooping!

Another example we can cite to illustrate our point concerns the
person with an abnormal voice. Speech therapists know that one of
the chief obstacles that they will confront in teaching a new and
better voice is that the person will find that his new voice almost
seems to turn him into a stranger. One such person, a husky athlete,
who came to us with a tiny high-pitched falsetto voice, was so
shocked to hear the deep bass voice we taught him that at first he
could not bear to use it. His friends stared when he spoke; his wife
was disturbed by it. "I almost feel as though suddenly I had a new
face," he said. "I know it's a better face but it doesn't seem like me!"

Again, most people who stutter severely have certain words which
they fear more than others. These "Jonah words," as they call them,
usually seem to produce longer and more severe abnormality. Stutterers avoid these feared words if they can do so, using synonyms
or other phrasing to escape their evil power. It has been our experience that the stutterer's own name is almost always one of the
chief "Jonah words." For most of us, our own name is about the
easiest utterance available. Television interviewers or personnel
men in employment offices often attempt to put the stranger at ease
by asking for his name and address. For the stutterer these two
questions spell catastrophe.

Why? We would explain it in this way. One's own name and
address are loaded with self-identification, with the person's self-
concept. When that self-identification is not a pleasant thing, speech
becomes exposure.

Some psychologists once performed an experiment in which they
asked their subjects to answer this sudden question differently three
times. "What are you?" Most of the normally speaking male subjects gave as their first answer "a man." A common second answer
was "a college student" or "an athlete," and so on. But when they
asked the stutterers to answer the question, the majority said, "I am
a stutterer," as their first choice. Feeling this way, it is easy to see

why they would have more stuttering on their name or other personal data.

These little glimpses of speech therapy may help you to realize that the correction of defective speech involves much more than drills or tongue-twisters. Indeed, it is a fascinating field, this exploration of the disorders of speech. For speech is the peculiarly *human* function and its disorders reflect all the complex troubles of humanity.

PROJECTS

Each of the following items illustrates one of the important points of the preceding chapter.

1. Allport, a famous psychologist, once asked this question: "Why are the very early memories so impermanent? Why is it so hard to remember events that happened during your first and second years?" "One answer," said Allport, "is that infantile experiences are not _____ and hence cannot be held as concepts in consciousness." If you can't fill in the blank from your reading of this chapter, you can find the answer in Allport's book, *Personality: A Psychological Interpretation.* New York: Holt, Rinehart & Winslow, Inc., 1937.

2. We differ not only in handedness but also in tonguedness. Researchers have found, by observing tongue-click movements, that tonguedness (right versus left clicking) corresponds to handedness in 70 per cent of 193 cases. Make a similar investigation in 10 of your acquaintances and in addition ask them to say *lalalalalalala* using tongue tappings to the right, then to the left of the mouth. Which direction is done more easily? What has this to do with the material in this chapter?

3. Perform an experiment for half a day in which you attempt to inhibit all use of the pronoun "I" and describe your own need for egocentric speech.

4. Listen to the speech of other people for a half-day and record as verbatim as possible all instances of speech as emotional expression.

5. *Think* the following sequence of numbers, first as you normally would, then again with your mouth wide open and your tongue protruded: 11, 12, 13, 14, 15, 16, 17, 18, 19, 20. Which of the two trials takes longer? Why?

6. Make tape recordings of a short passage read by several male and several female speakers, then play the appropriate recording back to

each of them. Ask each subject if his or her voice sounds higher or lower in pitch when recorded. Is there any sex difference?

7. Call three numbers selected at random from the telephone directory and say, "I wonder if you can tell if the cubba mo will meet at you owf today." Repeat it as asked, and report the reactions.

8. What other two consonant sounds have the same tongue contact as the *t*? What other consonant sound has the same tongue contact as the *v*?

9. Is it possible to whisper an isolated prolonged *zzz* sound? What aspect of speech is illustrated by these experiences?

10. Does the pitch of your own voice seem higher or lower when you read aloud normally than when you plug your ears tightly with your fingers?

11. How much of the Lord's Prayer consists of the social control type of speech? Analyze it phrase by phrase.

12. Research has shown that when congenitally deaf people dream they often move their fingers constantly. Why?

13. What does Piaget say about egocentric speech in children? Go to the library.

14. Why was Donald so silent? Read Chapter 32 in Travis, L. E. (ed.). *Handbook of Speech Pathology.* New York: Appleton-Century-Crofts, 1957.

15. Which aspect of speech is illustrated by the tale of Hector and Rector in Chapter 4 of Van Riper's *Your Child's Speech Problem.* New York: Harper & Row, Publishers, 1961.

16. Summarize the findings of this article: Ames, L. B. "The Sense of Self of Nursery Children as Manifested by their Verbal Behavior," *Journal Genetic Psychology.* Volume 81, 1952, 193-232.

17. Interview some staff member of the speech department concerning the problem of stage fright, its causes and its appearance, and relate this to the material in this chapter.

18. What does your tongue do to make an *rrr* sound as in the word *run*? If you cannot tell by self-observation, read the account in Chapter 12 of Van Riper and Irwin. *Voice and Articulation.* Englewood Cliffs, N.J.: Prentice-Hall, Inc., 1958.

19. Summarize the first chapter of Backus and Beasley's *Speech Therapy with Children.* Boston: Houghton-Mifflin, 1951.

20. Summarize Chapter 7 in Van Riper and Butler's *Speech in the Elementary Classroom.* New York: Harper and Brothers, 1955.

21. Summarize Chapter 19 in Brown's *Introduction to Speech.* Boston: Houghton-Mifflin Company, 1955.

22. How is communication impaired in the aphasic? Read this article: W. Alonzo Hall. "Return from Silence—A Personal Experience,"

Journal *Speech and Hearing Disorders*, Volume 26, 1961, pages 174-177.

23. Summarize this article: Hahn, E. "Communication in the Therapy Session," *Journal Speech and Hearing Disorders*, Volume 25, 1960, pages 18-23.

24. Summarize this article: Low, G., Crerar, M., and Lassers, L. "Communication Centered Speech Therapy," *Journal Speech and Hearing Disorders*, Volume 24, 1959, pages 361-368.

25. In what ways does the following article emphasize the role of emotion in speech? Bangs, J. L., and Freidinger, A. "Diagnosis and Treatment of a Case of Hysterical Aphonia in a Fourteen Year Old Girl," *Journal Speech and Hearing Disorders*, Volume 14, 1949, 313-317.

26. In what ways does the case described by the author of the following article illustrate the material in this chapter? Rose, J. A. "Dynamics and Treatment of Speech Disorders," *American Journal of Orthopsychiatry*, Volume 16, 1943, pages 284-289.

27. MACTESE is an acronym for the subjects treated in this chapter. Create another pronounceable acronym of the same sort.

28. Summarize the following article: Hahn, E. "Indications for Direct, Non-direct, and Indirect Methods in Speech Correction," *Journal Speech and Hearing Disorders*, Volume 26, 1961, 230-236.

CHAPTER TWO

The Disorders of Speech

Spasmophemia, rhotacism, uranoscolalia, lambda-cism, rhinolalia, sigmatism, idioglossia, and brady-lalia. Do not worry. We do not intend to inflict such a heavy burden of polysyllabic jaw-breakers upon your tender memory. Translated, in sequence, these terms refer to stuttering, defective *r* sounds, cleft-palate speech, defective *l* sounds, excessive nasality, lisping, delayed speech characterized by jargon, and speech which is uttered too slowly. And there are others, for this is not a complete list by any means. We start this chapter with this esoteric chanting only to make the point that there are many speech disorders. We must learn how to identify them.

A few letters may help to vivify the need for such identifying information.

> Dear Sir: I am a country schoolteacher in a two-room school. In my room there is a little boy in the third grade with a kind of funny voice. I mean he doesn't talk like other children. He can't say some of the words right that he knows just as well as I do. I have tried to correct him on the word "scissors" which is hard for him but he just can't get it out right. Is this stammering or just baby talk and how can I cure him? Please send me some tongue exercises or something. He is a sweet little child and needs some help.

Here is another:

> I want you should help me. My boy he dont talk right. He gets tan-geled up in his nose and it sounds funny. When can I bring him.

And another:

14

I have a bad habit in talking that makes my talk so other people cant understand me although I know what I'm saying. They yell at me as if I'm deaf and dumb but I can hear good. I just can't talk good.

One more:

I have an impediment or something in my mouth. Sometimes I talk all right but not always. I open my mouth and the words won't come out right.

These examples should demonstrate not only the necessity for further investigation and analysis but also the need for information as to the common patterns of abnormal speech. In this chapter we present the symptom pictures of the various speech disorders. Once we know these we can hope to begin our differential diagnosis.

But first we must face another problem well known to the physician too: "Does this person actually have anything wrong with him?" There are thousands upon thousands of variations in normal speech. If there were not, we could never recognize our friends by their voices. Even the same person seldom says the same word twice in identical fashion. When is a speech difference a speech defect? How do we judge?

These questions are not academic. Misdiagnosis has caused untold misery. A mother who did not know that few children master their *str* and *spl* blends before the age of five, grew anxious about her three-year-old's mistakes on those sounds, and then she corrected him so frequently, made so many visits to elocution teachers, faith healers, and physicians, and punished him so severely that finally the child stopped talking altogether and remained mute for three years. Another child with delayed speech was misdiagnosed as being deaf and feeble-minded. We found her, at sixteen, using sign language and unable to understand except when she lip-read, this despite the fact that her audiogram revealed normal hearing and a performance test a normal IQ. Many a normal child has been turned into a severe stutterer by having the normal hesitations and repetitions of early speech labeled and penalized as stuttering until finally he came to accept the label and began to avoid speech or to struggle with his utterance. Many a child has been treated as a lisper when his *s* and *z* sounds were well within the limits tolerated by anyone except the hypercritical parent or teacher who committed the crime.

So let us define a speech defect.

Definition: Speech is defective when it deviates so far from the speech of other people that it calls attention to itself, interferes with communication, or causes its possessor to be maladjusted.

We can condense this definition into three adjectives. Speech is defective when it is *conspicuous, unintelligible, or unpleasant.* The first adjective refers to the fact that abnormal speech is different enough to be noted. It varies too far from the norm. A child of three who says "wabbit" for "rabbit" has no speech defect, but the adult of fifty who uses that pronunciation would have one because it would be a real deviation from the pronunciation of other adults. If you said *deze, doze* and *dem* for *these, those* and *them* in a hobo jungle, none of the other vagrants would notice. If you used the same sounds in a talk to a P.T.A. meeting a good many ears would prickle. Many of us force the airstream down too broad a tongue groove to produce the high-pitched *s* sound characteristic of our English speech. Because we do so does not necessarily mean that we have lateral lisps. Only when our *s* is so slushy and low in pitch that it calls attention to itself can we be said to have that type of speech defect.

How wide a variation is required before we should be concerned about a speech difference? Only the cultural norms can answer this question. Among the Pilagra Indians no attention is ever paid to baby talk or peculiar speech until the child is at least seven years of age. Many Indian tribes do not even have a word for stuttering although many of their membership no doubt have hesitant speech. According to the famous anthropologist Sapir, who worked among the Nootka, repetitive and hesitant speech seems to be more common than fluent rhythmic speech in this tribe of Indians. One would have to stutter badly indeed to have a speech defect in such a culture. In England the dropping of an *h* or the flatting of a vowel would cause instant social penalty in upper class society where the same behavior would be quite unnoticeable in Australia. Excessive assimilation nasality would not be noticed by a Tennessee mountaineer when the same voice quality in an Eastern girls' school would send its owner to the speech clinic. A speech defect, then, is one which is so different from the normal speech of the social group that it is highly conspicuous. The individual who refers a case to the speech therapist should evaluate its context accordingly.

The second part of the definition refers to intelligibility. When a speech difference interferes with communication it tends to be labeled as defective.

When you listen, not to what a stranger says, but to his peculiar voice or hesitations or distorted consonants, communication is broken. If his face suddenly jumps around as he struggles to utter an ordinary word, all communicative content is lost in amusement or amazement. Many stutterers habitually lower their eyes to escape the shock of observing the expression of incredulity and surprise on the faces of their auditors. Cleft-palate adults have been known to pretend to be deaf and dumb and to beg for a pencil so that their communication could be accomplished without interruption.

If, as one of our eighteen-year-old cases illustrated, you heard someone reciting "Poh koh an tebbuh yee adoh ow pohpadduh baw poh uhpah dih kawinaw a new naytuh" you might find it very hard to understand him—unless you knew he was saying the first lines of Lincoln's Gettysburg Address. Speech is defective when it is difficult to understand, when its intelligibility is poor.

That communication is impaired when a person loses his voice (aphonia) is obvious. The person whose larynx has been removed is pretty helpless until he learns to swallow air and speak on the expelled burp. But even then, the monotone is difficult to listen to or to understand. The cleft-palate child's teacher finds great difficulty in fathoming what he is trying to recite. A falsetto voice distracts attention from what is being said. The more conspicuous the vocal abnormality, the more unintelligible the speech becomes.

Many a stutterer has had to ask for a paper and pencil in order to make his simplest wants known. The words emerge from such contortions and broken garblings of utterance that frequently both the stutterer and the listener give up.

A speech defect, then, is one which calls attention to itself and interferes with communication.

The final part of our definition deals with the maladjustment and emotional handicap which the speech defective adds to his disability. Sometimes this maladjustment is the dominant feature of the disorder. We worked with a woman who claimed to have stuttered actually only once in her life—during a high-school graduation speech. Her speech was certainly not fluent since it was marked by numerous hesitations, pauses, and avoidances of certain words. She was badly handicapped socially and vocationally. Her listeners were constantly puzzled and confused by her peculiar speech behavior. And yet she had actually "stuttered" only once. This case, of course, is an extreme instance of the importance of maladjustment in producing a speech defect. Usually, the abnormality of rhythm, voice, or articulation is sufficiently bizarre to provoke so many social penalties that maladjustment is almost inevitable.

We can understand the nature of defective speech by viewing it also in terms of its various aspects as outlined in our last chapter. For example, to illustrate the motor aspect of speech, we work with individuals who have what are known as cosmetic lisps. These persons produce *s* and *z* sounds which are perfectly correct acoustically, but they protrude their tongues so conspicuously when they make these sounds that listeners think the sounds are wrong. The child who says "I am thick" when he means "I am sick," illustrates the *acoustic* and *communicative* contributions to the unintelligibility part of our definition. When the person has aphasia resulting from a "stroke" his inability to *think* of the words he needs will make his speech attempts conspicuous and frustrating both to his listeners and himself. The stutterer who can speak perfectly when he talks only to himself may show horrible contortions and garbled utterance when he has to say something loaded with *emotion* to someone else. Few persons with speech disorders become officers in the armed services, because of their difficulty in giving commands. They are impaired in their ability to *control* others either because their commands are misunderstood or too conspicuously unpleasant to get the respect required. Finally, a severe speech defect, because it provokes rejection and other penalties due to its communicative unpleasantness, causes a loss in self-esteem, in ego strength. Thus, in all its various aspects and functions, speech is defective when it calls attention to itself, interferes with communication, or causes its possessor to be maladjusted.

CLASSIFICATION OF SPEECH DISORDERS

There are many ways in which we could classify the various speech disorders, but if we look at the behavior itself we find that they seem to fall into four major categories: *articulation, time* (or

rhythm), *voice*, and *symbolization* (language). This fourfold classification, it should be understood, refers to the *outstanding* features
of the behavior shown. Thus even though his stuttering causes certain sounds to be distorted, we place the stutterer in the second
category because the major feature of his disorder is the broken
timing of his utterance. The person with aphasia often shows articulation errors, broken rhythm, inability to produce voice, but the
outstanding feature of aphasia is the inability to handle symbolic

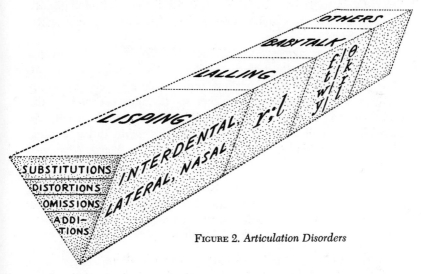

FIGURE 2. *Articulation Disorders*

meanings and language. Therefore, we would place aphasia under
disorders of symbolization or language. Certain individuals show
more than one of these disorders. A child with severe cerebral palsy,
for example, may show all four.

Articulation

Under disorders of articulation we include all those disorders
characterized by the substitution, omission, addition, and distortion
of the speech sounds. There are many somewhat synonymous and
overlapping terms in common use for these disorders, among which
we can name *baby talk* (infantile perseveration), a disorder with
no organic basis but characterized by stereotyped substitutions sim-

ilar to those used by the normal child in the early stages of speech development; *lalling,* characterized by defective *r, l, t, d,* or *s* sounds, and largely due to inactivity or sluggishness of the tongue tip; *lisping,* a disorder of the sibilant sounds, especially *s* and *z,* characterized by the substitution of the *th* (θ; ð) consonants (a lingual or frontal lisp), a mushy *sh* (ʃ) or *zh* (ʒ) sound (a lateral lisp), *t* or *d* (occluded lisp), or the nasal snort resulting from the attempt to make an *s* or *z* through the nose (nasal lisp); *delayed speech,* characterized by a narrow repertoire of consonants and unintelligibility; and *oral inaccuracy,* which is a wastebasket term for any mild articulatory defect.

Actually these names do not denote different types of disorders. They are not mutually exclusive. Lallers often lisp, and lispers talk baby talk, and all of them show oral inaccuracy. The important features of all articulatory disorders are the presence of defective and incorrect sounds. The forty-year-old farmer who wept when he heard his voice on a recording of a children's rhyme did so because of the defective and incorrect sounds he had produced. A six year old said this:

> Tinko Tinko itto tah,
> How I wondah wheh you ah,
> Up abuh duh woh soh high
> Yike a diamon' in duh kye.

As the above selection indicates, most articulatory cases have more than one error and are not always consistent in their substitutions, omissions, insertions, or distortions. This is not always the case, however. Thum lingual lithperth merely thubthitute a *th* for the *eth* thound. Otherzh shkwirt the air shtream over the shide of the tongue and are shed to have a lateral lishp. Others thnort the thnound (nasal lisp). Many children have been known to buy an "ite tream toda" or an all day "tucker."

It would be impossible to portray the acoustic characteristics of some of the distortions used by articulatory cases even if we used the phonetic alphabet. Seldom does an adult substitute a true *w* for the *r* as he attempts such a phrase as "around the rock." He usually produces a sound "something like a *w* and something like the velar *r* made with the back of the tongue elevated and the tip depressed." In some lateral lisping, the sound produced is more of a salivary unvoiced *l* instead of the *s*, a sloppy slurping sound which disgusts not only its hearers but its speaker too.

Many of the omissions heard in articulation cases are merely weakly stressed consonants. In a noisy room, an eighteen-year-old boy in describing a winter scene would seem to say, "The 'ky and 'no in wintuh." The missing sounds, however, were evident in quiet surroundings and were perfectly formed, but their duration was so brief that any noise seemed to mask their presence. Many cases, however, do entirely omit sounds they cannot produce.

Additions of linking sounds are frequently found in blends ("the buhlue-guhreen color of spuhruce trees"), and when a child adds *ee* to every final *r* sound, as one of our cases did, the peculiarity is very noticeable.

To many persons, articulatory defects seem relatively unimportant. But severe articulation cases find the demands of modern life very difficult. We knew a woman who could not produce the *s*, *l*, and *r* sounds and yet who had to buy a railroad ticket to Robeline, Louisiana. She did it with pencil and paper. A man with the same difficulty became a farmer's hired hand after he graduated from college rather than suffer the penalties of a more verbal existence. Many children are said to outgrow their defective consonant sounds. Actually, they overcome them through blundering methods of self-help, and far too many of them never manage the feat. One man, aged sixty-five, asked us bitterly when we thought he would outgrow his baby talk.

In several cases, communication is almost impossible. Mothers cannot understand their own children. The delayed-speech case, deprived of normal verbal outlets for his emotion, becomes a behavior problem. Try, for instance, to translate the following nursery rhymes as transcribed from phonograph recordings:

> Ha ta buh, Hah ta buh,
> Wuhnuh peh, two uh peh,
> Ha ta buh.

> Tippo Tymuh meh a pyemuh,
> Doh too peh,
> Ted Tippo Tymuh to duh pyemuh
> Yeh me tee oo weh.

One of the old names for a very severe articulation disorder was *idioglossia*. The term refers to self-language. When the number of articulatory errors is large, the speech becomes an unintelligible jargon. Mothers of children with this disorder tell us that they try in vain to make themselves understood. One child said, "Mighty no pidgaduh" over and over again, and not until he took his mother to the kitchen did she finally come to realize that he was saying "My ice cream (mm eye tee) is not in (no) the refrigerator (pidgaduh)." These children think in this jargon, in this mutilated English of idioglossia.

Many children who are severely handicapped by unintelligible speech also find it very difficult to express their emotions except by screaming or acting out their conflicts. Most of us relieve ourselves of our emotional evils by using others as our verbal handkerchiefs or wastebaskets. We talk it out. But when a child runs to his mother crying "Wobbuh toh ma tietihtoh" and she cannot understand that Robert stole his tricycle, all he can do is to fling himself into a tantrum. The same frustration results from his inability to use speech for self-exhibition. Often penalized or frustrated when he tries to talk, he soon finds it better to keep quiet, to use gestures, or to get attention in other ways. Many people tend to regard articulatory errors as being cute or relatively unimportant. Some of the most handicapped people we have ever known were those who could not speak clearly enough to be understood.

Disorders of Time or Rhythm

One of the dimensions of speech is *time*. We speak sequentially. Sound follows sound; syllable follows syllable. When speech is defective in the timing of its utterance we speak of disorders of time or rhythm. This rhythmic characteristic of speech is, of course, not evenly spaced or regular except in sing-song or some types of chanting. Nevertheless, the syllables of a sentence are definitely patterned in time. The sounds of a word, the words of a phrase, must fit into a set pattern if speech is to be normal. Again we find a range of permissible variation. Some of us speak very rapidly; others very slowly. Some of us are remarkably fluent and some of us have speech which is full of um's and er's, hesitations and repetitions. Only when the timing of our sounds and syllables is so far off the standard that our speech is conspicuous, unpleasant, or unintelligible do we have a disorder of rhythm. In stuttering we have such a disorder.

Stuttering. In considering this disorder, let us observe its various aspects. Speaking in terms of its motor and acoustic features, the stutterer shows breaks in the usual time sequence of utterance. The usual flow is interrupted. There are conspicuous oscillations and fixations, repetitions and prolongations of sounds and syllables. There are gaps of silence which call attention to themselves. If you ask a stutterer a question, the answer may not be forthcoming at the proper time. The stutterer's speech sometimes seems to have holes in it. Some sounds are held too long. Syllables seem to echo themselves repeatedly and compulsively. Odd contortions and struggles occur which interfere with communication. The stutterer may show marked signs of fear or embarrassment. He fits our definition because his speech behavior deviates from the speech of other people in such a way that it attracts attention. All of us hesitate and repeat ourselves but the stutterer hesitates and repeats himself differently than we do and more often.

One of the prime features of stuttering is that it seems to be more of a communicative disorder than one of speech. Most stutterers can sing without difficulty. Most of them speak perfectly when alone. Usually, it is only when they are talking to a listener that the difficulty becomes apparent. Stuttering varies with emotional stress and increases in situations invested with fear or shame. When very secure and relaxed, stutterers often are very fluent. In very severe cases, even the thinking processes seem to be affected—but only when they are thinking aloud, and again in the presence of a listener. This is probably due to the emotional stress under which they speak.

Stuttering takes many forms; it presents many faces. The only consistent behavior is the repetition and prolongation of syllables, sounds, or speech postures. It changes as it develops, for stuttering usually grows and gets worse if untreated. We distinguish four stages in the development of stuttering, and these will be discussed later in the chapters on this disorder. Here we wish to distinguish only between the first and last of these four stages, between *primary* stuttering and *secondary* stuttering. They differ markedly in the type of behaviors shown and we treat them differently.

Primary Stuttering. In this, the first stage of the disorder, the child's speech is broken by an excessive amount of repetitions of syllables and sounds or, less frequently, by the prolongation of a sound. He does not seem to be aware of his difficulty. He does not struggle or avoid speaking. He does not seem to be embarrassed at

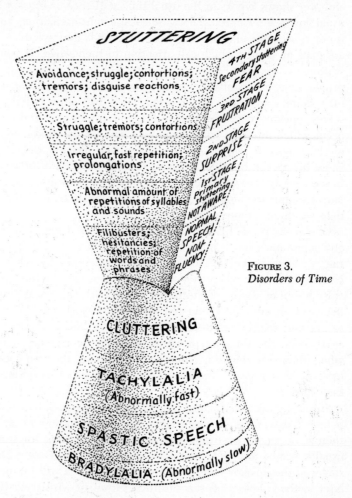

FIGURE 3.
Disorders of Time

all. Indeed he seems almost totally unconscious of his repetitive utterance. He just bubbles along, trying his best to communicate. An excerpt from a parent's letter may illustrate this primary stuttering:

I would appreciate some advice about my daughter. She is almost three years old, and has always been precocious in speech. Four weeks ago she recovered from a severe attack of whooping cough and it was immediately after that when she began to show some trouble with her speech. One morning she came downstairs and asked for orange juice, and it sounded like this: "Wh-wh-wh-wh-where's my orange juice?" Since then she has repeated one or two words in almost every sentence, sometimes repeating twice, and sometimes eight or nine times. It doesn't seem to bother her but I'm worried about it as it gets a lot worse when she asks questions or when she is tired, and I'm afraid other children will start laughing at her. One of her playmates has already imitated her several times. No one else in our family has any trouble talking. What do you think we should do? Up to now we have just been ignoring it and hoping it will go away.

Unfortunately, stuttering does not always remain in its primary form. The child begins to react to his broken communication by surprise and then frustration. The former effortless repetitions and prolongations become irregular, faster, and more tense. As the child becomes aware of his stuttering and frustrated by it, he begins to struggle. Finally, he becomes afraid of certain speaking situations and of certain words and sounds. Once this occurs, stuttering tends to become self-perpetuating, self-reinforcing. The more he fears, the more he stutters, and the more he stutters, the more he fears. He becomes caught in a vicious circle. When this stage is reached we call the disorder *secondary stuttering*.

Secondary Stuttering. Secondary stuttering occurs in many forms, since different individuals react to their speech interruptions in different ways. One German authority carefully described ninety-two different varieties of stuttering (each christened with beautiful Greek and Latin verbiage), and we are sure that there must be many more. Stutterers have been known to grunt or spit or pound themselves or protrude their tongues or speak on inhalation or waltz or jump or merely stare glassily when in the throes of what they call a "spasm" or a "block." The late Irvin S. Cobb described a certain Captain Joe Fowler who manifested his stuttering through the use of profanity. Captain Joe was able to speak very well under ordinary circumstances, but when he got angry or excited, his speech stopped entirely, and he was able to get started again only through the use of a stereotyped bit of cursing. Some of the imitations of stuttering heard in the movies and on the radio may seem grotesque, yet the reality may be even more unusual.

Some stutterers develop an almost complete inability to make a direct speech attempt upon a feared word. They approach it, back away, say "a-a-a-a" or "um-um-um," go back to the beginning of the sentence and try again and again, until finally they give up communication altogether. Many stutterers become so adept at substituting synonyms for their difficult words, and disguising the interruptions which do occur, that they are able to pose as normal speakers. We have known seven severe stutterers whose spouses first discovered their speech impediments after the wedding ceremony. Stutterers have preached and taught school and become successful traveling salesmen without ever betraying their infirmity, but they are not happy individuals. The nervous strain and vigilance necessary to avoid and disguise their symptoms often create stresses so severe as to produce profound emotional breakdowns.

Cluttering.   Another disorder in which the time sequence is disturbed is called cluttering. It is frequently confused with stuttering because it too shows many repetitions. However, the major features of cluttering are first, the excessive speed of speaking; second, the disorganized sentence structure; and third, the slurred or omitted syllables and sounds. The clutterer can speak perfectly when he speaks very slowly, but it's almost impossible for him to do so except for short periods. They truly have "tangled tongues." The speech is cluttered speech; it is disorganized, pell-mell speech, sputtered speech. The true clutterer has no seeming awareness of his excessive speed or garbled utterance. He is always surprised when others cannot understand him. He has no fears or shames. He does not struggle or avoid. Some clutterers become stutterers as well; most do not. Clutterers speak by spurts and their speech organs pile up like keys on a typewriter when a novice stenographer tries for more speed than her skill permits. An old text in speech correction has this description: ". . . a torrent of half articulated words, following each other like peas running out of a spout"; but the torrent is also irregularly interrupted in its flow. People constantly ask the clutterer to repeat. They are empathically irritated by his uneven volleys of hasty syllables. They find themselves interrupting during his panting pauses and then in turn being interrupted by a new overwhelming rush of jumbled words.

Voice-Disorders (Dysphonias)

Another dimension of speech involves the tones of the human voice. Speech is made up of noises and tones. In articulation we add noises and modify the tones. But the tones themselves may be defective; they may vary too far from the norm to be acceptable. When we scrutinize the tones of speech we find that they themselves have three sub-dimensions. The *loudness* of the speech tones is one of these sub-dimensions; *pitch* is another; and voice *quality* is the third. In each of these we may find abnormality and there are voices which may be defective in all three dimensions.

Disorders of Pitch. The normal range of pitch variations depends upon sex, age, and several other factors. The voices of men are generally lower in average pitch than those of women. A deep-voiced male would have no voice disorder; the woman who speaks with a bass voice is conspicuous. A six-year-old boy with a high-pitched treble voice would incur no penalty from society; a thirty-year-old man would find raised eyebrows if he began to speak in such tones. Under conditions of great excitement, many of us have voices which crack or show pitch breaks. But when an adult shows these same pitch breaks upward into the falsetto when he orders a hamburger or says goodbye, we suspect the abnormal. Again, there are times when it is appropriate to speak with a minimum of inflection but a person who consistently talks on a monopitch will find his listener either irritated or asleep. In deciding whether a person has a pitch disorder we must always use the normal yardstick.

The above discussion has anticipated our listing of the pitch disorders. They are as follows: *too-high pitch, too-low pitch, monotone* or *monopitch, pitch breaks,* and *stereotyped inflections.*

The following description was uttered by a two-hundred-pound football player in his high, piping, shrill child's voice:

> Yes, I was one of those boy sopranos and my music teacher loved me. I soloed in all the cantatas and programs and sang in the choir and glee clubs and they never let my voice change. I socked a guy the other day who wise-cracked about it, but I'm still a boy soprano at twenty-two. I'm getting so I'm afraid to open my mouth. Strangers start looking for a Charlie McCarthy somewhere. I got to get over it, and quick. Why, I can't even swear but some guy who's been saying the same words looks shocked.

A high-pitched voice in a male is definitely a handicap, communicative, economic, and social.

When a woman's voice is pitched very low and carries a certain type of male inflection, it certainly calls attention to itself and causes

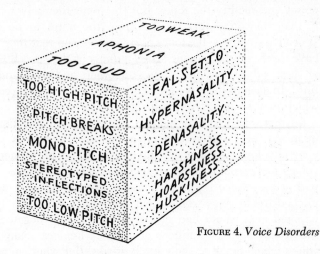

FIGURE 4. *Voice Disorders*

maladjustment. The following sentence, spoken by a casual acquaintance and overheard by the girl to whom it referred, practically wrecked her entire security: "Every time I hear her talk I look around to see if it's the bearded lady of the circus."

On every campus some professor possesses that enemy of education, a monotonous voice. A true monotone is comparatively rare, yet it dominates any conversation by its difference. To hear a person laugh on a single note is enough to stir the scalp. Questions asked in a true monotone seem curiously devoid of life. Fortunately most cases of monotonous voice are not so extreme. Many of them could be described as the "poker voice"—even as a face without expression is termed a "poker face." Inflections are present, but for fear of revealing insecurity or inadequacy they are reduced to a minimum.

By stereotyped inflections we refer to the voice which calls attention to itself through its pitch patterning. The sing-song voice, the voice that ends every phrase or sentence with a falling inflection, the "schoolma'am's voice" with its emphatic dogmatic inflections, are all types of variation which, *when extreme,* may be considered speech defects.

Pitch Breaks may be upward or downward, usually the former. The adolescent boy, learning to use his adult voice, often experiences them. Often they can be very traumatizing. To have your voice suddenly flip-flop upward into a falsetto or child's voice is to lose control of the self. When you want to speak you don't wish to yodel. Often individuals who fear this experience use a monopitch or too low or too high a pitch level to keep the flip-flopping from occurring. Pitch breaks wreck communication; they define the speaker as one who cannot control himself or who is very emotional. They often interfere with the person's ability to think on his feet since he must forever be monitoring his voice. They may sound funny to others but we have not found them so.

Disorders of Voice Intensity. Almost in parallel with the disorders of pitch are those of intensity. We have *too loud* a voice, *too weak* or soft a voice, no voice at all (*aphonia*), peculiar *stereotyped patterns of loudness* or emphasis, and voices which are *tremulous,* as in old age or in certain forms of cerebral palsy.

The intensity disorders need little illustration. Many of us have experienced *aphonia,* after prolonged abuse of voice through screaming or when laryngitis has caused us to "lose" our voice. People who earn their living by their mouths—among them, singers, train announcers, clergymen, and schoolteachers—are subject to aphonia, hysterical or otherwise. Most very soft or weak voices are due to insecurity or hearing loss. The extremely loud—to the point of irritation—voices are often due to personality problems or defective hearing. The *strident* voice combines excessive intensity with a harsh voice quality to pierce the ears and rasp the sensibilities of its victims. One of the most difficult voices to correct is that which is marked by sudden bursts of loudness or by the "trailing off into nothingness" at the end of each phrase. Both irritate their listeners.

It is obvious that a voice which is too soft or weak will handicap the person when he must speak under conditions of masking noise or to large audiences. Anyone who has lost his voice for a period of days will tell you that his existence changed markedly during that time. Aphonia may be due to organic reasons such as growths on the vocal folds or to emotional causes. Hearing loss may produce either too loud a voice or one too soft or one which blasts at inappropriate times. So can anger. The ears of others gauge our personalities by scanning our voices. One of the items they scan is our vocal intensity since often it indicates how we feel about ourselves.

Disorders of Voice Quality. The normal range of voice qualities is immense. There are almost as many different voices as faces in this world of ours. The quality of the voice depends on the patterning of the overtones and their variable intensities. The differing sizes and shapes of the many resonating cavities within different human heads account for the uniqueness which permits us to identify each other by listening to these tones. Indeed it almost seems incredible that we can do so since each of us is capable of producing voices of many differing qualities. We can speak nasally or harshly or huskily almost at will. Why we settle upon the voices we finally use habitually is often a mystery. Some of us adopt the voices of those with whom we identify most closely. Others use the voice which best reflects the way we feel about ourselves and others. Most of us seem unaware of these voice qualities of ours and are surprised when we hear them played back from a tape recorder. Some of us are shocked.

Among those who are shocked are those whose voices are *hypernasal, denasal, strident* (harsh), *falsetto, breathy* (husky), or *hoarse*. Those are the abnormal voice qualities sufficiently distinct to be labeled.

That the disorders of voice quality are difficult to describe is indicated not only by the names which we listed earlier in our classification but also by the names we omitted. Voices have been called *thick, thin, heavy, sweet, round, brilliant, hard, metallic,* and *rich,* as well as *poor*. The terms we have used are not much better, but at least they do not confuse auditory perceptions with those of taste or touch. The science of experimental phonetics has not yet been able to provide a better classification for variations in timbre.

The quality of *excessive nasality* (hypernasality, rhinolalia *aperta*) is easily recognized. Its possessor not only seems to speak his *m, n,* and ŋ sounds through his nose, but also many of the vowels and voiced continuants such as *r, v,* and *z*. When combined with certain inflection patterns it has been described as a "whining" voice. In certain sections of the country a variety of hypernasality is dialectal and of course in this setting it would not be a speech defect. In *assimilation nasality* only the sounds preceding or following the *m*, *n* and *z* sounds are excessively nasalized, but these can occur frequently enough to provoke audience irritation.

In *hyponasality* (denasality, adenoidal voice, rhinolalia clausa) the speaker does not or cannot utter the nasal sounds through the nose. The voice quality is deadened and muffled, as though its owner had a perpetual cold or post-nasal drip. The *m* resembles a blend of *m* and *b* spoken simultaneously, and the other nasals have similar cognates. Often habituated during the presence of adenoidal growths in early life, it persists long after the adenoids have been removed. People listening to denasal voices find themselves swallowing and clearing their throats and consumed by the urge to get out of range.

Other voice-quality disorders are occasionally noted by the teacher doing speech correction in the public school. Many boys' voices become husky and hoarse during the two or three years prior to voice change and become clear again after that event. Overstrain due to prolonged yelling, screeching, or shouting can cause this quality in any of us. Perhaps the *strident, hoarse, husky,* and *breathy* qualities of voice indicate a two-factor continuum involving (1) breath expenditure and (2) muscular strain. The strident voice shows a preponderance of tension in the muscles that squeeze the pharynx while the breathy voice represents a minimum of strain and a maximum of breath expenditure.

The words *throaty* and *pectoral* as adjectives to describe voice quality are probably identical save for the sex of the persons concerned. Throaty voices in the female are paralleled by the voice of hollow booming pectoral timbre in the male. Both involve lower pitch levels, rounded mouth openings, and retracted chins. Pectoral voice has been called the "rain-barrel voice." There are echoes in it. It reverberates like song in the bathtub. It was formerly much used by preachers and politicians and by undertakers and insecure high-school teachers. These terms, *throaty* and *pectoral* or *guttural*, are not terms commonly employed by speech therapists, perhaps because they probably are low-pitched falsetto voices. Usually *falsettos* are high in pitch and are produced by a complicated and different type of vocal cord vibration than that normally used. An adult who can speak only in *his* falsetto voice (for all of us have them) is truly handicapped.

Symbolization Disorders

The problem of *dysphasia* (the general term for all disorders of symbolic formulation and expression) is rarely met in public-school speech correction. Occasionally it occurs in mild form as a pronounced reading, writing, and speaking disability. In the speech clinic we often are required to help aphasics, and the end of World War II required the services of a good many speech correctionists to teach those who had received head and brain injuries. Children who have had meningitis or jaundice, and some adults who have

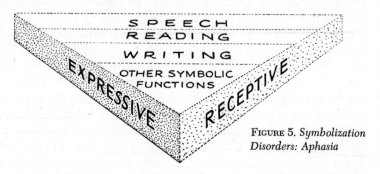

S P E E C H

R E A D I N G

W R I T I N G

EXPRESSIVE   OTHER SYMBOLIC FUNCTIONS   RECEPTIVE

FIGURE 5. *Symbolization Disorders: Aphasia*

suffered a paralytic stroke, often demonstrate the symptoms of aphasia. Such persons find it difficult to use or comprehend linguistic symbols, whether they be written or spoken. In the motoexpressive type of aphasia, the case may say "bum-bum-bum" for "cigarette," and "bum" for "shoe." Another aphasic may grope for words in attempting to say "pencil" but say "eraser" or "pen" or "stick" instead. Yet he knows his errors the instant they are spoken. In the receptive type of aphasia the difficulty lies in the perception. R. V. McKnight describes her own aphasic reaction to the word "your" as follows:

> I mentally heard it but it had no meaning. I felt that it was related to the word "you" but I could not figure out the relationship between the two. I continued to puzzle over this until the speaker had finished his lecture and sat down. . . . More generally when I do not recognize the meaning I do not recognize the sound. The word is a jumble of letters.

Children who have such difficulties are often mistakenly diagnosed as hard of hearing or feeble-minded. Some cases of delayed onset or slow development of speech are probably due to aphasia.

The child with *delayed speech* may, or may not, belong in the category of symbolization disorders. Injuries to the brain have often, in young children, interrupted speech development or retarded it. The differential diagnosis of "congenital aphasia" is always difficult, as we shall see in later chapters. It is also certain that many children who are mute or speak in an unintelligible jargon or gibberish have been called "brain-injured" when they were entirely normal individuals who just had not been taught to talk. Some parents learn their child's language instead of teaching them the adult tongue. Delayed speech often approximates the pattern of a very severe articulation disorder and some cases, so diagnosed, probably belong in this category.

Multiple Speech Disorders

We have been discussing the four major types of speech disorders, those of rhythm, articulation, voice, and symbolization, as though they were always distinctive entities. It is obvious that a given speaker might have deficiencies in more than one of these dimensions of speech. We have said that lallers may lisp; they may also possess an infantile voice. Clutterers certainly often have both a disorder of rhythm and one of slurred articulation. The aphasic often misarticulates certain of his speech sounds. It is always necessary to scan each one of our cases in terms of all four of these dimensions if we are to decide our point of attack upon the problem. Illustrating this need are certain disorders which almost always have multiple features of abnormality.

Cleft-palate Speech. People whose speech has been affected by their cleft lips or palates often show articulation errors such as nasally emitted consonants. Their voices usually are hypernasal though some denasality also often occurs. Finally, the rhythm of the speech may be faltering and labored due to the nasal leakage of air which makes it difficult to utter phrases or sentences on a single breath. They pause to breathe at the wrong times.

Foreign Accent is another disorder which involves both articulation and voice. Speakers of a foreign tongue use sound substitutions and distortions, and they also use inflection patterns unfamiliar to our ears. The rising inflection at the conclusion of the phrase as spoken by a Scandinavian speaking English may serve as an illustration. In treating such a disorder we organize our therapy so as to attack both phases of the problem.

Deaf and Hard-of-hearing Speech. These individuals also show multiple disorders. The congenitally deaf are deficient in language and symbolization; their voices are oddly abnormal in pitch, intensity, and quality; their rhythms are unusual; they make many articulation errors. Depending upon the degree of involvement, those persons who are hard of hearing may also show similar disabilities.

Cerebral Palsy. This handicapping problem is due to a brain injury which affects the coordination of the muscles. Some of the cere-

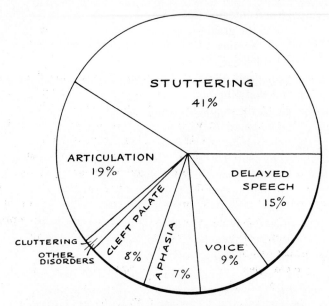

FIGURE 6. *Percentage of Different Types of Cases Referred to WMU Speech Clinic During the Years 1950-1960 (Hearing Cases Are Not Shown)*

bral palsied find it difficult or even impossible to walk or feed themselves. Some of them find speaking very hard. We have worked with cerebral palsied children who had aphonia, pitch breaks, weak voices, tremulous voices. As though those were not enough, they also found it almost impossible to twist their tongues into the proper postures necessary to produce many of the speech sounds. Some of them gasped and faltered in their flow of speech. Some were aphasic as well. A few of them spoke perfectly.

We hope that we have made it clear that speech has four dimensions and that abnormality may be found in any one or any combination of the four.

Frequency of Occurrence

The relative frequency of the different speech defects is difficult to determine with accuracy. There have been hundreds of surveys, each yielding percentages, but we can be sure that the defects of articulation are in the great majority. Every survey has demonstrated this fact. One of the most thorough of all the surveys, that by Mills and Streit,[1] in which each child in the elementary grades was examined individually and all those diagnosed were doubly and triply checked, found that 10 per cent of the school population had some speech defect. Of these speech defective children, 45 per cent were seriously handicapped. Articulation disorders characterized 7 per cent of all school children, voice disorders 1.5 per cent and rhythm disorders 1.5 per cent. This coincides roughly with the results of the White House Conference report of 1931.

A more recent survey of 87,288 children in New England [2] showed that 7.8 per cent were handicapped in speech. The proportions of speech and hearing children were as follows: articulation, 50 per cent; voice, 6.6 per cent; stuttering, 10.9 per cent; hard of hearing, 15.4 per cent; deaf, 8.4 per cent; delayed speech, 4.4 per cent; cleft palate, 1.2 per cent; cerebral palsy, 1.2 per cent; aphasia, 0.5 per cent; and miscellaneous, 1.6 per cent.

Using the *estimates* given in the report submitted by the American Speech and Hearing Association Committee for the 1950 White House Conference we have the following figures, which the report states "are the lowest estimates which can be scientifically de-

[1] A. W. Mills and H. Streit. "Report of a Speech Survey, Holyoke, Massachusetts," *Journal of Speech Disorders*, 1942, Volume 7, page 161-167.

[2] Wilbert Pronovost. "A Survey of Services for the Speech and Hearing Handicapped in New England," *Journal of Speech Disorders*, 1951, Volume 16, pages 148-156.

fended." Six per cent of the total population has some variety of speech defect. Four per cent of the total population has an articulation disorder. Seven individuals in each thousand are stutterers. Five out of every thousand have a voice disorder; five more have delayed speech; two more have speech disorders due to brain injuries; and one in each thousand has a cleft-palate speech problem.

When these percentages are applied to the 1951 population, we have the following numbers of individuals handicapped in speech:

ESTIMATES OF NUMBER OF SPEECH DEFECTS[3]

Type of Disorder	In the Total Population	In School Population
Functional Articulation	6,139,600	1,324,840
Stuttering	1,074,430	231,847
Voice Disorders	767,450	165,605
Retarded Speech Development	767,450	165,605
Cerebral Speech Disorders	306,930	66,242
Cleft-palate Speech	153,490	33,121

The frequency of occurrence is, however, not the true measure of the seriousness of the problem. Although their relative numbers are small, cases of stuttering, cleft palate, cerebral palsy, and hearing disabilities present great difficulties in treatment. Generally speaking, the articulatory cases respond most easily and quickly to therapy, but there are many exceptions to this rule. Our culture tends to judge articulation and voice defects as being less handicapping than the other speech disorders, but in the final analysis the speech defective individual himself is the only one who can make this evaluation. A tiny lisp may become invested with so much emotion that it may dominate an entire lifetime. The third part of our definition of a speech defect must always be considered.

CASE DESCRIPTIONS

The following references were chosen with some care so as to provide a wide variety of description of actual cases. By reading some of them, the student will find illustrations of the textual material in this chapter.

[3] Bernard Spilka and M. D. Steer. "Incidence of Speech and Hearing Deficiency in the General Population and Schools of the U.S., 1951," Purdue Speech and Hearing Clinic *Research Staff Report No. 2.*

By reading many of them, the prospective speech therapist can gain vicariously some of the experience that usually comes only from years of work.

1. Adams, H. M., and P. J. Glasner. "Emotional Involvements in some Forms of Mutism," *Journal Speech and Hearing Disorders,* Volume 19, 1954, pages 59-69.

2. Aikins, A. "Casting Out a Stuttering Devil," *Journal Abnormal Psychology,* Volume 18, 1923, pages 137-152.

3. Bangs, J., and L. Friedinger. "A Case of Hysterical Aphonia in an Adult," *Journal Speech and Hearing Disorders,* Volume 15, 1950, pages 316-323.

4. —————. "Diagnosis and Treatment of a Case of Hysterical Aphonia in a Thirteen-year-old Girl," *Journal Speech and Hearing Disorders,* Volume 14, 1949, pages 312-317.

5. Beder, A. E. "Cleft-palate Children," *Hygeia,* Volume 24, 1946, pages 834-835.

6. Bender, J. F., "A Case of Delayed Speech," *Journal Speech Disorders,* Volume 5, 1940, 363-364.

7. Berger, C. C. "Subjective Observations on Cerebral Palsy," *Journal Speech Disorders,* Volume 10, 1945, pages 397-402.

8. Blackman, R. S., and R. Battin. "Case Study of Delayed Language," *Journal Speech and Hearing Disorders,* Volume 22, 1957, pages 381-384.

9. Blank, J. P. "My Adventure in Freed Speech," *Reader's Digest,* May, 1948, pages 7-9.

10. Burton, A., and E. Harris. *"Case Histories in Clinical and Abnormal Psychology,"* Harper & Row, Publishers, 1945, pages 597-611.

11. Carlson, S. M. "Case Histories," *Journal Speech Disorders,* Volume 5, 1940, pages 368-370.

12. Carrow, M. A. "Case Study of Delayed Language," *Journal Speech and Hearing Disorders,* Volume 22, 1957, pages 381-384.

13. Celler, J. "Helpless, Not Hopeless," *Mental Hygiene,* Volume 60, 1956, pages 535-550.

14. Curry, E. T. "Voice Breaks and Pathological Larynx Conditions," *Journal Speech Disorders,* Volume 14, 1949, pages 356-358.

15. Dalrymple, L. H. "Our Child Had a Cleft Palate," *Hygeia,* Volume 27, 1949, pages 186-187.

16. Earle, H. "The Comeback Battle of Clifton Utley," *Today's Health,* February, 1959, pages 45-46.

17. Egland, G. "An Analysis of an Exceptional Case of Retarded Speech," *Journal Speech and Hearing Disorders,* Volume 19, 1954, pages 239-243.

18. Engleberg, M. "Correction of Falsetto Voice in a Deaf Adult," *Journal Speech and Hearing Disorders*, Volume 27, 1962, pages 162-164.
19. Gardner, W. A., S. D. Hill, and H. N. Carano. "Esophageal Speech for a Ten Year Old Boy," *Journal Speech and Hearing Disorders*, Volume 27, 1962, pages 227-231.
20. Gens, G. W., and N. L. Bibey. "Congenital Aphasia: A Case Report," *Journal Speech and Hearing Disorders*, Volume 17, 1952, pages 32-38.
21. Goldstein, M. "Speech Without a Tongue," *Journal Speech Disorders*, Volume 5, 1940, pages 65-69.
22. Gustafson, C. G. "A Talisman and a Convalescence," *Quarterly Journal Speech*, Volume 30, 1944, pages 465-471.
23. Harle, M. "Dynamic Interpretation and Treatment of Acute Stuttering in a Young Child," *American Journal Orthopsychiatry*, Volume 16, 1946, pages 156-162.
24. Hauser, P. "The Talking Frog of Marion County," *Journal Speech Disorders*, Volume 12, 1947, pages 8-10.
25. Heltman, H. J. "Case Histories," *Journal Speech Disorders*, Volume 6, 1941, pages 124-125.
26. Heltman, J. J. "History of Recurrent Stuttering and Recovery," *Journal Speech Disorders*, Volume 6, 1941, pages 49-50.
27. Irwin, R. B. "Teaching a Deaf Child to Talk," *Journal Speech Disorders*, Volume 9, 194, pages 131-133.
28. Jensen, M. B. "A Case of Extreme Language Disability Concealed by Stuttering," *Journal Clinical Psychology*, Volume 4, 1948, pages 83-86.
29. Lemert, E. "Some Indians Who Stutter," *Journal Speech and Hearing Disorders*, Volume 18, 1953, pages, 168-174.
30. Louttit, C. L. *Clinical Psychology* (Read section on speech defects).
31. McKibben, S. "The Spastic Situation," *Journal Speech Disorders*, Volume 8, 1943, pages 147-153.
32. Moser, H. "Presentation of a Case," *Journal Speech Disorders*, Volume 7, 1942, pages 173-174.
33. O'Neil, James (ed.). *Foundations of Speech*, pages 449-450, 453, 465-466.
34. Platt, J. H. "Myasthenia Laryngis: a Case Report," *Journal Speech Disorders*, Volume 1, pages 187-188.
35. Pedrey, C. "Letter to the Editor," *Journal Speech and Hearing Disorders*, Volume 15, 1950, pages 266-269.
36. Pollock, M. S. "Releasing the True Intellectual Capacities of a Young Aphasic Child through the Unfettering of Emotional Bonds," *American Journal Mental Deficiency*, May, 1959, Volume 63, pages 954-956.

37. Rigby, M. "A Case of Lack of Speech Due to Negativism," *Psychological Clinic*, Volume 18, 1929, pages 156-161.
38. Rigg, M. G. "A Superior Child Who Would Not Talk," *Child Development*, Volume 9, 1938, pages 361-362.
39. Rose, R. H. "A Physician's Account of His Own Aphasia," *Journal Speech Disorders*, Volume 13, 1948, pages 294-305.
40. Shryock, H. "Speech without a Larynx," *Hygeia*, Volume 25, 1947, pages 789-792.
41. Sokolowsky, R., and E. R. Junkerman. "War Aphonia," *Journal Speech Disorders*, Volume 9, 1944, pages 29-36.
42. Strait, R. "A Child Who Was Speechless in School and Social Life," *Journal Speech and Hearing Disorders*, Volume 23, 1958, pages 253-254.
43. Tartar, G. "Report of a Case of Stuttering as a Problem in Vocational Adjustment, *Journal Abnormal and Social Psychology*, Volume 23, 1928, pages 52-56.
44. Tregaskis, Richard. *Invasion Diary*, pages 208-255; 240-241.
45. Wedberg, C. F. *The Stutterer Speaks* (read the first 50 pages).
46. Werner, L. S. "Treatment of a Child with Delayed Speech," *Journal Speech Disorders*, Volume 10, 1945, pages 329-334.
47. Whitten, I. "Therapies Used for Stuttering: a Report of the Author's Own Case," *Quarterly Journal Speech*, Volume 24, pages 227-233.
48. Will, N. "A Six-month Report on the Personality Development of a 13-year-old Stutterer," *Quarterly Journal Speech*, Volume 30, 1944, pages 88-95.
49. Wilson, D. K. "Children with Vocal Nodules," *Journal Speech and Hearing Disorders*, Volume 26, 1961, pages 19-26.
50. Young, E. H. "A Personal Experience with Speech," *Journal Speech and Hearing Disorders*, Volume 23, 1958, pages 136-142.

CHAPTER THREE

The Emotional Problems
of the Speech Handicapped

In the last chapter we described the various speech disorders in terms of their overt behavior—the peculiarities and differences in speech we can see and hear. Now we present a description of the covert or hidden behavior which often is just as important or even more significant than the visible or audible features of such problems. Speech defects are icebergs in the flowing currents of the ceaseless talk in which we live. We see them pass by but only when we come in close contact do we feel the hidden mass of abnormality that lies beneath the surface. This is the emotional fraction of a speech disorder. So long as it exists, the lopping off of the visible portion will only result in a new portion of the problem coming into view. We cannot ignore the emotional fraction of abnormal speech if we wish to understand and help those who possess it.

PFAGH

This strange word is an acronym, a coined assemblage of letters, each of which represents another word. The *p* represents penalty; the *f* frustration; the *a* anxiety, the *g* guilt, and the *h* hostility. We invent this word to help you realize and remember the major aspects of the hidden part of a speech disorder. Abnormal speech is no asset to anyone. It invites penalty from any society which prizes the ability to communicate effectively. Normal speech is the membership card which signifies that its owner belongs to the human race. Those who do not present it are penalized and rejected. Even the abnormal speaker himself often feels this rejection is justified.

Moreover, the inability to communicate, to get the rewards our society offers to those who can talk effectively, results in great frustration. To be unable to say the word when he desires to do so as in the case of the stutterer; to say "think" when he means "sink" as in lisping; to not be able to produce voice at all as in the aphonic; to seek to say something meaningful only to find that gibberish emerges from the mouth of the aphasic; all these are profoundly frustrating. The rest of the word of *Pfagh*, agh, the anxiety, the guilt, and hostility, represents the natural reactions to penalty and frustration. You too have known these three miseries transiently when you have been punished or met frustration, but many individuals with defective speech spend their lives immersed in *Pfagh*.

Penalties

Let us present some illustrative penalties culled from the autobiographies of stutterers, remembering that similar tales could be told by individuals possessing other varieties of defective speech:

> Most clerks look away when I get stuck and begin to force. It always infuriates me that they don't even have the decency to look at me. Once I even went to the manager of a store about it and he looked away too.

> My father wouldn't ever listen to me when I stuttered. He always walked off. I finally got so I'd say everything to him by having mother give him the message.

> People do not usually laugh at my other kinds of stuttering, but when I begin to go up in pitch, they always smile or laugh right out loud. I was phoning a girl today and hung up when I heard her snickering.

> My mother always hurried to say the word for me whenever company was in the house. I often asked her not to but she couldn't help herself. It used to shame me so, I'd go up in my room and cry and I never went visiting with them. Sometimes I'd eat in the kitchen when we had strangers come for dinner.

> The other boys in the school used to call me "stuttercat" and imitate me whenever I came to school. At first I always managed to be tardy and stay after school to avoid them, but my folks got after me

and then I began to fight with them. I got to be a pretty good fighter, but the bigger boys always licked me and the teacher punished me when I hit the girls. I still hate girls.

After I came to high school from the country, everybody laughed at me whenever I tried to recite. After that I pretended to be dumb and always said "I don't know" when the teacher called on me. That's why I quit school.

Every time I'd ask for a job a funny look would come over their face and some of them would say no right away even before I finished what I was going to say. Some of the others, and one of them was a stutterer too, just waited til I finally got it out and then they'd shake their heads. One storekeeper was so sympathetic I could hardly get out of there fast enough.

The worst time I ever had was when a hotel clerk saw me jumping around and called a doctor. He thought I was having a fit.

These are but a few of the many penalties and rejections which any speech defective or any other individual with an unpleasant difference is likely to experience. Imitative behavior, curiosity, nicknaming, humorous response, embarrassed withdrawal, brutal attack, impatience, quick rejection or exclusion, overprotection, pity, misin-

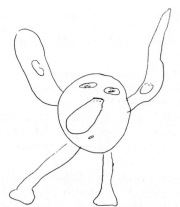

FIGURE 7. *Copy of a Crayoned Drawing of Himself by a Cleft-Palate Child.* Note size of ears, nose, and mouth. His drawings of others in his family were very normal.

terpretation, and condescension are some of the other common penalties.

The amount and kind of penalty inflicted on a speech defective are dependent on four factors: (1) the vividness or peculiarity of the speech difference; (2) the speech defective's attitude toward his own difference; (3) the sensitivities, maladjustments, or preconceived attitudes of the people who penalize him; and (4) the presence of other personality assets.

First of all, in general, the more frequent or bizarre the speech peculiarity, the more frequently and strongly it is penalized. Thus a child with only one sound substitution or one that occurs only intermittently will be penalized less than one with almost unintelligible speech, and a mild stutterer will be penalized less than a severe one. *Second,* as Bryngelson[1] has so clearly pointed out, the speech defective's own attitude toward his defect often determines what the attitude of the auditor will be. If the speech defective considers it a shameful abnormality, his listeners can hardly be expected to contradict him. Empathic response is a powerful agent in the creation of attitudes. Third, the worst penalties will come from those individuals who are sensitive about some difference of their own. Since many speech defectives have parents or siblings with similar speech differences, they are often penalized very early in life by those persons.

> You ask why I slap Jerry every time he stutters? I do it for his own good. If my mother had slapped me every time I did it I could have broken myself of this habit. It's horrible going through life stuttering every time you open your mouth and my boy isn't going to have to do it even if I have to knock his head off.

Moreover, many individuals have such preconceived notions or attitudes concerning the causes or the unpleasantness of speech handicaps that they react in a more or less stereotyped fashion to such differences, no matter how well adjusted the speech defective himself may be. Finally, as we have pointed out, the speech defective may possess other abilities or personal assets which so overshadow his speech difference that the later is penalized very little.

Why can such things happen? Why do we punish the person who is different? Why must he punish himself? Surely Americans are some of the kindest people who have ever lived on this earth. We show our concern for the unfortunate every day. No nation has ever known so many agencies, campaigns, foundations, and private chari-

---

[1] Bryng Bryngelson. "The Reëducation of Speech Failures," *Quarterly Journal of Speech,* April, 1933, pages 227-229.

ties. One drive for funds follows another. Muscular Dystrophy, the Red Cross, the United Fund, the Heart Association, Seeing Eye dogs, the coin bottle in the drugstore, the pleading on radio and television. Surely all of these activities seem to show that we help rather than punish our handicapped.

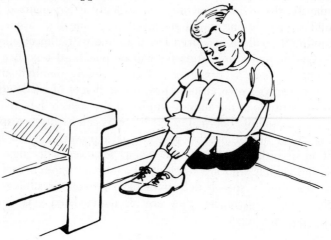

FIGURE 8. *Reaction to Penalty*

Cultural anthropologists have regarded this altruism with more than academic interest. They point out that our culture is one that features the setting up of a constant series of material goals and possessions which are highly advertised. Prestige and status seem often to be based upon winning these possessions and positions in a highly competitive struggle. We fight for security and approval, but in the process we trample underfoot the security of others. Some psychologists have felt that our need to help the handicapped is a product of the guilt feelings we possess from this trampling. Others attribute our concern for the underprivileged to fear lest someday we too will be the losers in the battle for life. They claim that we tend to say to ourselves, "There, but for the grace of God, go I," when we meet someone who has failed to find a place for himself in our world for reasons beyond his control. For this reason, we truly hunger to help those who have "never had a chance."

We Americans are also great joiners. We have innumerable clubs, societies, trade associations, recreational groups. We feel a strong need to belong. We feel uneasy when we are unable to become part of a group functioning near us. We find great security and strength from the mere fact of membership.

The person who is different—the deviant individual—is of course faced with great difficulties when he attempts to enter the normal groups, since much of their functioning depends upon communication. The speech defective cannot talk his way in; the crippled cannot join a ski club; the deafened find even the usual church services of little satisfaction; the blind find many restrictions. Such handicapped individuals usually form groups of their own. Those who have lost their larynxes form a Lost Chord Club, and speak to each other belchingly. A group of paraplegic veterans have a wheel chair basketball team. Stutterers have a Demosthenator Organization. But, at best, these are poor substitutes. Those who are different want to belong to the same groups to which normal individuals belong. And so they seek and are given the opportunities for special education and rehabilitation that may help them to rejoin the culture as a whole. We help our unfortunate now. But this was not always the case.

History of the Handicapped. No one can understand the problem of the handicapped except in terms of the penalties which their infirmity provokes. Every handicap has an emotional fraction of shame, fear, or frustration, the heritage of centuries of cruelty and neglect. Cultural history demonstrates that the stupid, the blind, the deaf, the crippled, and those who could not talk have been treated progressively as a nuisance, a disgrace, an object of mirth, a problem, and a challenge. These attitudes are still in evidence.

Rejection. Primitive society tolerated no weakness. Tribes struggled hard for survival, and those members who could not aid materially were quickly rejected. The leaders were killed by the younger men after the former had lost their teeth or their energies had abated. The inhabitants of ancient India cast their cripples into the Ganges; the Spartans hurled theirs from a precipice. The Aztecs regularly sacrificed deformed persons in times of famine or when one of their leaders died. The Melanesians had a simple solution for the problem of the handicapped: they buried them alive. Among the earlier Romans, twins were considered so abnormal that one of them was always put to death, and frequently both were killed. They left their malformed children on the highways or in the forests. If the children survived, they were often picked up by those who always prey upon the handicapped and were carried to the market place to be trained as beggars. They were not valuable enough to be slaves.

The Bible clearly reflects these early rejection attitudes. Remember Job? The prevailing belief in Old Testament times was that man's physical state was determined by his good or bad relationship with his deity. Disabilities were regarded as divine punishment for sin. A normal person could invoke similar punishment merely by associating with those who had thus incurred the wrath of God. Consequently, the blind and the crippled wailed with the lepers—outside the city wall.

During the Middle Ages the physically disabled were frequently considered to be possessed of evil spirits. They were confined to their own homes. They dared not walk to the market place lest they be stoned. Even in this century, elimination of the handicapped has been practiced. The Kaffir tribes in South Africa clubbed sickly or deformed children. The Nazis kept only the best of their civilian prisoners for slaves. The others died in the gas chamber, in the crematorium.

In this country we would hang the man who killed his crippled son. We have come far in our journey toward civilization, but perhaps not far enough. Rejection takes many other forms. Spirits, too, can be killed. This is what one handicapped person has to say:

> We think the inhabitants of old Sparta cruel for putting to death the weak, those who would be unable to compete, or to contribute much to their society; but were they after all much more inhuman than we, who nurse the weakling, keep it alive, yet as much as possible keep it from normal persons, especially the children, for fear its contact will contaminate them; then throw it out to compete with normal adults? [2]

How many of those reading this book would unhesitatingly accept an invitation to a dance if it were tendered by a hunchback?

Humor. It did not take the promoters long to discover that the handicapped provided a rewarding source of humor. One history of the subject states that before 1000 B.C. the fool or buffoon became

---

[2] R. V. McKnight. "A Self-analysis of a Case of Reading, Writing, and Speaking Disability," *Archives of Speech*, 1936, Volume 1, page 43.

a necessary part of feast making and "won the laughter of the guests by his idiocy or his deformity." In Homer's *Odyssey* comic relief from tragedy was illustrated by the vain effort of the one-eyed Polyphemus to pursue his tormentors after they had blinded him. For a thousand years thereafter every court had its crippled buffoons, its dwarf jesters, its stuttering fools. Attila the Hun held banquets at which "a Moorish and Scythian buffoon successively excited the mirth of the rude spectators by their deformed figures, ridiculous dress, antic gestures, and absurd speech." Cages along the Appian Way held various grotesque human disabilities including "Balbus Blaesus" the stutterer, who would attempt to talk when a coin was flung through the bars. In Shakespeare's *Timon of Athens* Caphis says, "Here comes the fool; let's ha' some sport with 'im." Often this sport consisted of physical abuse or exposure of the twisted limb. These handicapped fools accepted and expected ridicule. At least it provided a means of survival, a livelihood, and it represented an advance in civilized living.

Gradually, the use of the handicapped to provoke mirth became less popular in continental Europe, and the more enterprising had to migrate to less culturally advanced areas to make a living. At one time Peter the Great had so many fools that he found it necessary to classify them for different occasions. In this country today we have a much higher regard for the handicapped than Cortez found when he conquered Mexico and discovered deformed creatures of all kinds at the court of Montezuma. Now you may find them used to provoke laughter only in the circus side shows, in the movies, on the radio, and in every schoolyard.

Pity. Religion is doubtless responsible for the development of true pity as a cultural reaction to the handicapped. James Joyce says that pity is the feeling which arrests the mind in the presence of whatsoever is grave and constant in human suffering and unites it with the human sufferer. It was this spontaneous feeling that prompted religious leaders to give the handicapped shelter and protection. Before 200 B.C. Asoka, a Buddhist, created a ministry for the care of unfortunates and appointed officers to supervise charitable works. Confucius said, "With whom should I associate but with suffering men?" Jesus preached compassion for all the disabled and made all men their brothers' keepers. In the seventh century after Jesus' death the Mohammedan religion proposed a society free from cruelty and social oppression, and insisted on kindliness and consideration for all men. A few hundred years later Saint Francis of Assisi devoted his life to the care of the sick and the disabled. Following this, the "Mad Priest of Kent," John Ball, was so aroused by the plight of the crippled and needy left in the wake of the Black Death that he publicly pleaded their cause, often at the risk of his own life. With the rise of the middle class, true pity for the handicapped became much more commonplace. The oppression which the merchants and serfs had suffered left them more sympathetic to others who were ill used. The doctrine of the equality of man did much for the handicapped as well as for the economically downtrodden.

However, many crimes have been committed in the name of charity. The halt and the blind began to acquire commercial value as beggars. Legs and backs of little children were broken and twisted by their exploiters. Soon the commercialization of pity became so universal that it became a community nuisance. Alms became a conventional gesture to buy relief from the piteous whining that dominated every public place. True pity was lost in revulsion. Recognizing this unhappy trend, Hyperius of Ypres advocated that beggars be classified so that work could be provided according to their capacities. His own motives were humanitarian, but he cleverly won support for his cause by pointing out that other citizens "would be freed of clamor, of fear of outrage, of the sight of ugly bodies." His appeal was successful, and asylums and homes for the handicapped began to appear, if only to isolate the occupants so the public need not be reminded of their distress. Another motive which improved the position of the handicapped was the belief that one could purchase his way into heaven or out of hell by charity. The coin thrown to the cripple has been impelled by many motives. The longing for religious security, the heightening of one's own superiority by comparison with the unfortunate, the social prestige of philanthropy, and the desire to be freed from embarrassment have all contributed to the welfare of the handicapped. Pseudo pity has accomplished much, but true compassion would have ended the tragedy.

Present Treatment of the Speech Handicapped.   We have sketched the treatment accorded the handicapped at some length because the speech-defective person is diagnosed immediately as belonging to that unfortunate group. The moment the cleft-palate child or stutterer speaks he joins his brethren, the crippled, the deaf, the spastic, the blind, and, perhaps, the fool. He is different. He possesses an abnormality. A little child hesitates in his speech; his parents diagnose him as a stammerer; he reacts to his hesitations as though they were revoltingly unpleasant; his playmates accept his evaluation, or his parents' evaluation, and reject, laugh at, or pity him; and so he joins the unhappy tribe of the million stammerers who exist in this country today.

It may seem strange to learn that the primitive attitudes of rejection, humor, and pity, are still very common reactions to the perception of speech defects today. Listen to these:

> They got me inside a circle of them and every time I tried to break out and go home, they pushed me back. "Make a speech. Make a speech." I tried to tell them I had to get my groceries home. My mother had to have them for supper, but the men would just laugh all the harder and push me back. They told me to say different things if I wanted to get out, things like "She sells sea shells" and dirty words. I was crying and I got mad and swore at them and then they let me go but I can hear them yet.
>
> I asked the girl for a dance and had a hard time getting it out. She flushed, then blurted out, "Well, I'm not that hard up yet."
>
> I can take almost anything but that pitying glance. It's sort of as if I have a cup in my hand every time I talk and people feel they ought to put some pennies in it. I can't explain it but when they look away or down at their feet, I feel like something unclean. I can't help it that my operation tore loose, and I talk through my nose, but I can't even explain it to them.

We no longer keep our "Balbus Blaesuses" in cages, but a current radio program features a "comedian" whose main humorous appeal is based upon his substitution of *w* for *l* and *r*. The song about "K-K-K-Katy" is still being sung although "Stuttering in the Starlight" and "You-you-you tell 'em that I-I-I stutter" have been forgotten. Cartoons and comic strips do not fail to exploit the impediments of speech.

Frustrations

In our first chapter we described some of the other functions of speech besides those of its motor and acoustic patterns. We said that we use speech for communication, for social control, for thinking, for the expression of emotion, and as a means of parading the ego. All these are mighty important to all of us. Consider, then, how a person must feel if he cannot talk intelligibly. Others have difficulty in understanding the messages of the stutterer, the jargon-talking child, or the person who has lost his voice forever due to cancer. Others listen, but they do not, they cannot, understand. The aphasic tries to ask for a cigarette and says, "Come me a bummadee. A bummadee! A bummadee!" This is frustration.

Or even when the listener can understand the words, he finds himself distracted by the odd contortions of the spastic's or stutterer's face, the twitching of the cleft-palate case's nostrils, and he forgets what has been said and asks that it be repeated. This is frustration too. Communication is the life blood of a society. When it cannot flow, the pressure builds up explosively. The worst of all legal punishments short of death is solitary confinement where no one can talk to the prisoner, nor can he talk to anyone else. There are such prisoners walking about among us, sentenced by their speech and hearing disorders to lives of deprivation and frustration.

The good things of life must be asked for, must be earned by the mouth as well as by the hands. The fun of companionship, the satisfaction of earning a good living, the winning of a mate, the pride of self respect and appreciation, these things come hard to the person who cannot talk. Often he must settle for less than his potential might provide were it not for his tangled tongue. Speech is the open sesame, the magical power! When it is distorted, there is small magic in it—but much frustration.

We need safety valves for emotion. When we can express the angry evils within us, they subside; when we can verbalize our grief, it decreases. A fear coded into words and shared by a companion seems less distressing. A guilt confessed brings absolution. But what of the poor devils who find speaking hard, who find it difficult even to ask for bread? This wonderful function of speech is denied them. The evil acids cannot be emptied; they remain within, eating their container. For many of us it comes hard to verbalize our unpleasant emotions even though we know that in their expression we find relief. How much more frustrating it must be for those who feel that they have only the choice of being still—or being abnormal!

Perhaps most frustrating of all is the inability to use speech as the expression of self. One of the hardest words for the average stutterer to say is his own name. Most of us talk about ourselves most of the time. We talk so people will notice us, so we can feel important. This egocentric speech is highly important in the development of the personality. Until the normal child begins to use it, he has little concept of selfhood, according to Piaget, the famous French psychologist. If you will listen to the people about you, or to yourself, you will discover how large a portion of your talking consists of this cock-a-doodle-dooing. When we speak this way we reassure ourselves that all is well, that we are not alone, that we exist and belong. The person with a severe speech defect finds no such reassurance when he speaks. He exposes himself as little as he can. In this self-denial, too, lies much frustration.

Penalties and Frustrations as Causes of Speech Disorders. Thus far, we have been speaking of these unpleasantnesses as *reactions* to abnormal speech, but we must not forget that punishment and frustration can influence and provoke or precipitate a speech disorder.

One of our cases, an ex-soldier, came to us with a hysterical aphonia. He could not even whisper but spoke only in a silent pantomime. The disorder dated from his experience in combat when he made a mistake and gave an order that sent a large group of his comrades to an unnecessary death. Thereafter he was shunned by his fellow officers and men. No one spoke to him except when it was absolutely necessary in the course of duty. Within the month, his voice was gone.

A second-grade boy had been receiving speech therapy for over a year and had made excellent progress in mastering many of his defective sounds. In the third grade he met a teacher who was old and uncontrolled, who had had to return to teaching after her husband had died, and who hated the whole business. She used the boy as a scapegoat for her own frustrations, and, under the guise of helping him, ridiculed his errors and held him up to scorn before his fellows. Shortly after the fall term began, this boy's speech began to get worse and within a few months it had lapsed to its former unintelligible jargon.

We had been working with Ted, an eight-year-old youngster, for three years. His cleft palate had been repaired surgically but the muscles were very weak and there was scar tissue which made it a bit difficult to close off the rear opening to the nasal passages with speed. He had improved greatly, however, and only a few bits of nasal snorting or excessive nasality remained when he talked carefully. Then one day his associates on the playground, led by the inevitable bully, began to call him "Mortimer Snerd" and "Nosey-Nosey." Within one week his speech disintegrated into a honking unintelligible jargon and he refused to come to the clinic for any more therapy.

One young stutterer diagnosed his own problem for us. His speech was full of irregular and forced repetitions. He hesitated. He seldom was able to utter even a short sentence without having wide gaps in it. One day, after he had just beaten up our plastic clown punching bag he confided in us. "Y-y-y-you know . . . y-y-you know whuh-whuh-what's wrrrrong with me? I-I-I-I-I'm the lllllittlest . . . child." He was. He was the runt of the litter, the weakest, smallest, most unattractive of the eight children in that family. The others were an aggressive bunch, yelling, fighting, arguing, talking. His mouth never had an ear to hear it. When his sentences were finished, it was some brother's or sister's mouth that finished them. He was constantly interrupted or ignored. He had learned a broken English, a hesitant speech.

Neurotic Speech Disorders. In our practice we have encountered some individuals whose mutism, stuttering, lisping, baby talk, or abnormal voices seemed to be symptoms of a primary neurosis. By this we mean that the speech disorder was adopted, usually unconsciously, as a device to protect the person from the stress of an emotional conflict which he seemed to be unable to solve in any other way. The case of the soldier with aphonia is such an example. The conversion of intolerable emotional conflicts into physical symptoms is not at all uncommon. Many a headache has such an origin. When speech becomes entangled in such a neurosis, it presents some difficult problems since psychotherapy often requires the use of speech as the healing tool. But let us take a quick look at some of these problems.

Jim was eighteen, a rather shy, frail youth. He was an excellent student and had hoped to go to college and perhaps from there to the ministry, for he was unusually religious. His father, however, had other ideas. He wanted Jim to follow in his occupational footsteps and become an auctioneer. The father was a huge man, red-faced and bull-voiced. Crude, rough and gregarious, he seemed almost the very opposite of the son in every regard. Jim's life had been a series of half-rebellions and total defeats. He was completely dominated by the father at the time he came to us with a voice so weak and husky we could barely understand him. Intermittently, he lost his voice completely, and upon graduation from high school when he entered the speech clinic, he was speaking in pantomime, unable even to whisper. This pantomimic speech is almost always a sign that the disorder is hysterical in nature and so we referred him to a psychologist for psychotherapy. Since he was unable to communicate orally, the exploration of the problem necessarily was first accomplished through writing and later through hypnosis. Only after the boy was given a job so that he could support himself and work his way through college and live away from his home, did his voice begin to return.

Although the great majority of individuals with articulatory disorders seem to have problems due to a failure to learn the standard sounds of speech, we occasionally find one in which the defective speech appears to be of neurotic origin.

A. T., a girl of fifteen, suddenly began to lisp and substitute *w* for *r*. She had previously spoken without any articulatory defect for at least six years, although her first-grade teacher declared she had some kind of speech disorder when she was seven years old. Three months later the disorder disappeared as suddenly as it had appeared. The only explanation which seemed to have any evidence to support it was that the girl knew of her parents' plan to get a divorce and adopted the symptoms of an earlier age level when no family conflict was threatening to disrupt her security. At any rate, the disorder disappeared as soon as a parental reconciliation was effected.

The majority of stutterers develop their speech difficulties early in life, usually between the ages of two and four, and they begin gradually. Whenever we discover that the stuttering begins suddenly and with great severity and relatively later than the usual age of onset, we suspect neurosis. The following account comes from the autobiography of a boy who suddenly began to stutter at the age of fifteen. From the first, his stuttering was horrible, full of contorted ugliness. He retched and gagged when he stuttered. Perhaps you will understand.

My folks never knew what a rat I was, and fortunately they died before they found out. Maybe it would have been better for me if they had. It's tough when both your parents die when you're only fifteen. But I was the perfect little gentleman at home. Fine manners. You know, courteous to old ladies, run and get my Dad's slippers, help my mother, say sir to everyone, be quiet in church, read a lot at home. I sure looked good, but was I rotten inside. I learned to smoke and curse and fight and steal before I was five. I ran the gang and no one squealed if any of them who did the dirty work got caught. My folks thought I was wonderful, and I was when I was with them. When they died though it tore me apart. I lost half of myself and the other half didn't belong either. I was a good twin and a bad twin, and if one twin dies you aren't a twin any longer. I didn't know what to do. Raising hell didn't seem to be any fun any more.

When we find such problems we can be pretty sure that speech therapy alone will not suffice. These are disorders of the personality, not of speech. These are the cases we refer to the professional psychotherapist. Speech may be affected but speech, itself, is not the problem.

Some professional workers feel that all speech defects are of this variety, that they are but symptoms of a primary neurosis. There are a few psychiatrists, for example, who feel that *all* stutterers are fixated sucklings, still too deeply attached to their mothers, using

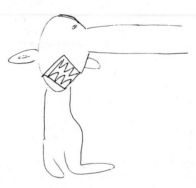

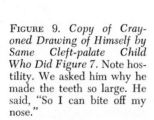

FIGURE 9. *Copy of Crayoned Drawing of Himself by Same Cleft-palate Child Who Did Figure 7.* Note hostility. We asked him why he made the teeth so large. He said, "So I can bite off my nose."

their stuttering symptoms as a kind of oral masturbation to provide a bitter pleasure. There are some psychologists who believe that *all* articulatory errors are merely symptoms of a neurotic need to remain infantile so that the responsibilities of maturity can be avoided. There are some who view every abnormal voice as indicatory of a primary emotional conflict. We feel that such a point of view is prejudiced and narrow. Perhaps these psychotherapists hold this view because those individuals who do have profound personality problems would be the very ones who would be referred to them. The speech therapist gets the ordinary, garden-variety of lisper or stutterer. The neurotics go to the psychiatrist, as well they should.

It is easy to see why such a psychiatrist would come to believe that all speech abnormalities are merely neurotic symptoms. He needs only scrutinize his patients to come to such a conclusion. But he can still be dead wrong! In our experience the large majority of speech problems have their origin in faulty learning or perceptual or organic factors. Speech is taught and it is learned; it isn't acquired instinctively. There are bound to be poor teachers and poor learners. There are people who are hard of hearing, who have cleft palates, who seem unable to identify pitches and sounds, who have cerebral palsy or brain injuries. Our own experience with thousands of cases just does not jibe with the concept that defective speech is always, or even commonly, a neurotic symptom.

Perhaps the following report from a public-school speech therapist may help to put the matter in truer perspective. We asked him, and he was not unsophisticated in the field of psychopathology, to study his 132 cases and to report to us all those who, he felt, needed professional psychotherapy.

> I am not sure, not at all certain of my findings. The more I studied and probed the children, the more emotional difficulties I discovered. In terms of obviously abnormal behavior patterns, there were only sixteen children whom I would refer to a child-guidance center for study and therapy and only two that I would refer to a psychiatrist.

> Ninety-two of the children seemed entirely within the normal range. They appeared secure with adequate self-esteem; they were spontaneous in speaking and emoting; little daydreaming, withdrawal behavior or excessive aggressiveness; they could subordinate themselves to the group activities and also accept leadership in the group; they can learn; they are flexible; they can have fun. They didn't seem too much concerned about their speech problems. Their teachers did not report any of them as problem children.

> The other twenty-two children were borderline cases. They intermittently had other problems; truancy, lying, stealing, fighting, mischief, school failures, sick-headaches, crying spells, and so on. Most of the children in this group had only one or two of the above patterns of abnormal behavior, and except for this they were just like the ninety-two normal children. They were occasionally in trouble, yet by and large they were getting along. I don't feel that I should refer them for psychotherapy, but I feel that I should be helping them a little, studying them, conferring with teachers and parents, and giving them some release therapy.

> The two that I feel should have psychiatric help are these: D. B., a thirteen year old stutterer, occasionally comes to school intoxicated; constantly curses to get speech under way; often truant; has hit several teachers; thrice expelled; parents both work; stormy scenes at home; very belligerent in speech class.

My other case is R. S., a girl with a severe articulation disorder which many people cannot understand. She just sits and looks out of the window in her fourth grade class; is becoming more and more detached daily; does not respond to questioning; seems uninterested in what the other children are doing. Keeps putting the end of her pencil under her finger-nails until they bleed. She too needs immediate psychiatric treatment.

The sixteen cases who I definitely feel need some psychotherapy (but not psychiatric help) are children usually with severe speech defects. One girl has become my silent shadow, following me everywhere, mutely begging for a kind word or glance. Another comes in regularly to speech class crying that all the other kids hate her, that she has no friends and her teacher has it in for her. A boy stutterer never speaks except in a very low voice, never looks at his listener, and constantly hangs his head. A little Latvian boy of ten is still terrified of life and trusts no one, least of all strange men. A lateral lisper of thirteen cannot stop talking, but keeps a finger always in the corner of his mouth. These, and others like them, comprise the group which I would like to work with myself, if only I had time to do some decent psychotherapy. Since I don't, I hope that the child guidance center can accept them.

Secondary Neuroses.   We have been using the term *primary neurosis* several times; now let us describe neurotic behavior as it stems from the stress produced by the speech disorder itself. We have said that neurotic behavior may be viewed as a protective measure, as a way of handling stress which has become intolerable. Abnormal speech itself produces stress. It makes communication difficult; it interferes with emotional expression; it hurts self-esteem; it frustrates social, educational, and vocational drives; it provokes rejection, mockery, and pity. We could hardly expect that such stresses would not create some need for neurotic defense. Let us cite a simple example.

Yes, I've used my stuttering in many ways to get out of things I otherwise would have to do. I don't have to go to the store to buy things for the family or run errands. I don't have to say Grace. The other day we had a flat tire and my father had to walk to the gas station two miles away to get somebody to come fix it. If I didn't stutter so bad, I know I'd have had to go. In school I never have to prepare, except for the examinations, because I know I won't be called on. There's lots of things like that and I do take advantage. I feel I might as well get some good out of my stuttering. It's no good for anything else.

Here is one a bit more complex.

> Until I was in Junior High I never minded my stuttering too much. Wasn't much mocking then. But when I had to transfer to this school the kids gave me a bad time. I could hardly stand to get on the school bus, it was that bad. If it wasn't the boys, it was the girls who gave me the works. Every day it was like that. My stuttering got much worse and that was when I began spitting and grinding my teeth when I stuttered. I never used to do that until I went to Junior High.

In this last instance we can see how the stuttering itself began to be used as a way for expressing hostility both toward others and toward himself. Stuttering in this new way was safer than slugging the tormentor; it was less painful than confronting the stuttering self. Here we see the exploitation of a speech abnormality. Stuttering had begun to yield some neurotic profit. In our experience, most of the neurotic behavior we find in our cases is of this nature. The neurosis is secondary, not primary.

Anxiety

The third letter in *Pfagh* represents anxiety. It should not be difficult to understand why people who meet rejection, pity, or mockery would experience this emotional state. When one is punished for a certain behavior, and the behavior occurs again, fear and anxiety raise their ugly heads. If penalty is the parent of fear, then we might speak of anxiety as the grandchild of penalty, for the two are not synonymous. The stutterer may fear the classmate who bedevils him or he may fear to answer the telephone since fear is the expectation of approaching evils which are known and defined. But anxiety is the dread of the unknown, of defeats and helplessness to come. In its milder form, we speak of worrying. There is a vague nagging anticipation that something dangerous is approaching. To observe a person in an acute anxiety attack is profoundly disturbing. Often he can find no reason for his anxiety but it is there just the same. At times it fades, only to have its red flare return when least expected. Few of us can hope to escape it completely in our lifetimes but there are those for whom anxiety is a way of life. It is not good to see a little child bearing such a burden.

One of the evil features of anxiety is that it is contagious. When parents of a handicapped child begin to worry about his speech, the child is almost bound to reflect and share their feelings. "Will he ever be able to go to school, to learn to read, to earn a living, to get married? Who will hurt him? Will he ever learn to talk like the fellows?" Such thoughts maybe never leave the parents' lips but somehow they are transmitted to the child, perhaps by tiny gestures or facial expressions or even the holding of the breath. Once the seeds of anxiety are planted, they sprout and grow with incredible speed.

Another of the evils of anxiety is that it usually is destructive. It does not aid learning or speech therapy. It distracts; it negates. It undermines the self-esteem. The person seeks to contain it, to explain it. Sometimes he invents a symptom or magnifies one already there. When speech becomes contaminated with anxiety the way of the speech therapist is hard. One of the first things a student speech therapist must learn is to create a permissive atmosphere in which speaking is not painful, over which no threat hangs darkly. The speech therapy room of the public school must be a gay, pleasant place, so much so that some little children hang on to their defective speech sounds so they will not have to leave. All of us need such a harbor once in a while; *these* children need a haven often, one where for once they can feel free from penalty and frustration, where defective speech is viewed as a problem instead of a curse. In the presence of an accepting, understanding therapist, they can touch the untouchable, speak the unspeakable. There they can learn. Anxiety does not help in learning or relearning.

Reactions to Anxiety.   Anxiety is invisible but it has many faces. By this we mean that it shows itself in different ways.

Edward had undergone many operations for his cleft palate but the scars on his face and the speech that came from his mouth bore testimony of his difference. Throughout his elementary and secondary school years, he had appeared a carefree, laughing, mischievous child. He was the happy clown, the gay spirit and, by this behavior, he had managed to gain much acceptance. When other people laughed at him, he laughed with them. His grades were poor although he was bright. Then suddenly, in the final semester of his senior year in high school, he underwent a marked personality change. He laughed no longer; he became apathetic, quiet, and morose. Formerly very much the extrovert, he now withdrew from contacts with others. He daydreamed. He walked alone. Our intensive study of this boy revealed that he had always lived with anxiety, that his gay behavior was adaptive but spurious. Underneath he had always ached. The compensatory pose of gaiety had brought him rewards but it had not allayed the anxiety.

When faced with the necessity for leaving school and earning a living, the anxiety flared up too strongly to be hidden and the change of personality took place. Not until we were able to provide some hope through the fitting of a prosthesis (a false palate) and some information about the possibility of plastic surgery, did the anxiety decrease sufficiently to enable us to improve his speech.

One of the common methods used to ease anxiety is the search for other pleasures. By gratifying other urges we seem to be able temporarily to diminish anxiety's nagging. Some of the people with whom we have worked are compulsive eaters of sweets; they grow fat and gross. And then they worry about their weight. Others relieve the anxiety by sexual indulgences. There are others who find a precarious and temporary peace by regressing to infantile modes of behavior, trying to return to the period of their lives when they did not need to worry about speaking. We also find a few sufferers who attach themselves to a stronger person like leeches, hoping for the security of dependency. Yes, there are many ways of reducing anxiety, but unless the spring from which it flows is stopped, it always returns. That is why people with defective speech need speech therapists.

When the anxiety clusters about speaking, one way of reducing it is to stop talking. Some persons with speech defects merely become taciturn; some lose their voices; others contract what is called *voluntary mutism* and do not make any attempt to communicate except through gestures. We knew a night watchman once who claimed that he averaged only two or three spoken sentences every twenty-four hours. "It's easier on me than stuttering." We've also known several hermits; they had either speech defects or woman trouble.

There is also a curious mechanism called "displacement" which most of us use occasionally to reduce our anxiety. We start worrying about something else besides the real problem which is causing us such distress. The shift of focus seems to bring some relief, much as a very hot water bottle on the cheek can ease a toothache. The scream of a little child in the night may reflect such a displacement, but perhaps a better example can be found in Andy.

Andy stuttered very severely when he came to us at the age of seven. He blinked his eyes, jerked and screwed up his mouth, and sometimes cried with frustration when he was unable even to begin a sentence. At times he spoke very well. But what struck us most about

Andy was his furrowed brow. Whether he stuttered or not, he seemed to be constantly worried. His face always had an anxious expression. Finally we were able to get him to tell us what he was worrying about. Surprisingly, it was not about his stuttering or his parents' very evident concern about his speech. Andy said he was worrying about the moon hitting the sun. He said that if this happened, everything would blow up. He said that on those nights when there wasn't any moon, and both sun and moon were down under there someplace, that they might crash together. Andy said he could never sleep on those nights. His mother and father had told him this couldn't happen but Andy said they had lied about Santa Claus, and how did they know anyway that it wouldn't happen. It took a lot of play therapy, speech therapy, and parent counseling before Andy was able to surrender his solar phobia and express his real anxiety, which concerned his speech.

We wish to conclude this section with a caution. Let us remember that some children with abnormal speech have no more anxiety than children who speak normally. All of us have some anxiety, probably need some. A bit of anxiety in the pot of life is like a bit of salt in a stew. It makes it tastier. But too much salt and too much anxiety ruin both. We have had to describe the anxiety fraction of a speech handicap so that you can understand it, so that you will not add to it, perhaps so that you may relieve it. Those of us who come in contact with handicapped children or adults may unwittingly make their burdens heavier if we do not understand. But there are some fortunate persons with speech disorders who are lucky in their associates and ability to resist stress, who seem to manage to get along with a minimum of anxiety. They may find themselves loved and accepted. They may possess philosophies or compensating assets which make the speech problem minor in importance. Let us just give one example.

At thirty-two, a very talented singer developed cancer of the larynx, and it was removed surgically. She reacted to the challenge with courage, mastered esophageal speech and began to specialize in the history of musical instruments, playing the lute, the Irish harp and many other of the ancient strings. She said, "I would have been only a second best vocalist and I should have spent my life in self-love, self-exhibition, and frustration. Now I have many more friends and acquaintances. I have things to give. I hardly ever think of myself. It's a good thing I lost my voice."

So let us state our caution again. If there is excessive anxiety, recognize its face where you find it no matter how it is disguised; but do not invent or imagine its presence if it is not there!

Guilt

The fourth letter in *Pfagh* represents guilt. Like anxiety, it too constitutes a part of the invisible handicap which often accompanies abnormal speech. We have long been taught that the guilty are they who are punished. Intellectually we can understand that the converse of this proposition need not be true, that those who are punished are not always those who are guilty. But let affliction beset us, and we find ourselves in the ashes with Job of the Old Testament. "What have I done to deserve this evil?" We have known many persons deeply troubled by speech disorders and other ills and most of them have asked this ancient question. Parents have asked it; little children have searched their souls for an answer. Here's an excerpt from an autobiography.

> Even when I was a little girl I remember being ashamed of my speech. And every time I opened my mouth I shamed my mother. I can't tell you how awful I felt. If I talked, I did wrong. It was that simple. I kept thinking I must be awful bad to have to talk like that. I remember praying to God and asking him to forgive me for whatever it was I must have done. I remember trying hard to remember what it was, and not being able to find it.

It seems to be the fashion now to blame parents for many of the troubles of their children, for juvenile delinquency, for emotional conflicts, for defective speech. We can blame the school if Johnny cannot read, but few parents of a child who comes to school with unintelligible speech have escaped the blame of their neighbors. The father of a cleft-palate child often feels an urge to accuse the mother, and the mother the father, for that which is the fault of neither. When guilt enters a house, a home is in danger. Children who grow up in such an atmosphere of open or hidden recrimination are prone to blame themselves. Thus the emotional fraction of a speech disorder may grow.

Reactions to Guilt Feelings. Guilt is another evil that eats its container. In its milder forms of regret or embarrassment, most people can handle it with various degrees of discomfort. However, when shame and guilt are strong, they can become almost unbearable. To protect himself, the person may react with behavior which can produce more penalty or more guilt. We have seen children deliberately soil themselves, throw temper tantrums, break things, steal things, even set fires so that they could get the punishment they felt their guilt deserved. After the punishment comes a little peace!

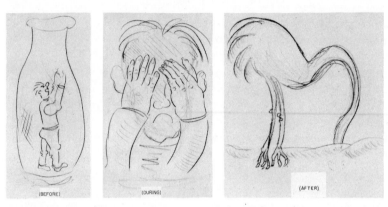

FIGURE 10. *Three Drawings by the Same Subject Illustrating the Role of Shame and Guilt.* *

Other children punish themselves. We have watched stutterers use their stuttering to hurt themselves, using it in much the same way as the flagellants of the Middle Ages flogged and tortured their bodies for their sins. We have known children with repaired harelips and cleft palates who could not bear to watch themselves in a mirror even to observe the action of the tongue or soft palate. We have heard children cry and strike themselves when they heard their speech played back from a tape recorder. We who deal with such children must always be alert to this need for punishment lest they place the whip in our hands.

Here is what one adult with cerebral palsy painfully typed for us:

> Sometimes when I lie in bed pretty relaxed I almost feel normal. In the quiet and the darkness I don't even feel myself twitching. I pretend I'm just like everybody else. But then in the morning I have to get up and face the monster in the mirror when I shave. I see what

---

* From J. G. Sheehan, P. A. Cortese, and R. G. Hadley, "Guilt, Shame and Tension in Graphic Projections of Stuttering," *Journal Speech and Hearing Disorders,* Volume 27, 1962, page 134. By permission of the authors.

other people see and I'm ashamed. I see the grey hairs on my mother's head and know I put them there. I eat but I know it isn't bread I can earn. Oh there are times when I get interested in something and forget what I am but not when I talk. When I talk to someone, he doesn't have a face. He has a mirror for a face and I see the monster again.

We who must help these people must also expect at times to find apathy and depression as reactions to the feelings of guilt. It is possible to ease the distress of guilt a little by becoming numb, by giving up, by refusing to try. Again we may find individuals who escape some of their guilt by denying the reality of their crooked mouths or tangled tongues. They resist our efforts to help them because they refuse to accept the *fact* of abnormal speech. Somehow they feel that the moment they admit the existence of abnormality, they become responsible. And with responsibility comes the guilt they cannot bear. So they resist our efforts to help them. Finally, we meet persons who absolve themselves from guilt by projection, by blaming others for their affliction, by converting their guilt into hostility or anxiety. But this brings us to the next section.

Hostility

The final letter of *Pfagh* represents hostility. Both penalty and frustration generate anger and aggression. We who are hurt, hate. We who are frustrated, rage! Here is an example to help you understand. It was written by an aphasic veteran who had been shot in the head.

The worst feature of my brain injury was the frustration. I would know exactly what I wanted to say but it would come out of my mouth differently. If I wanted to say "Please pass the cake" my mouth might say "Please part the ice" which didn't make sense to anyone else or even to my own ears. A hundred times a day this would happen. I'd find myself crying or cursing or frozen into some stiff posture or making some meaningless movements with my leg and I knew that these were just my ways of trying to handle the complete feeling of inability that characterized my life.

Reactions to Hostility. Hostility, like anxiety and guilt, ranges along a continuum all the way from momentary irritation through anger to intense hatred. Some children with severe speech problems show little hostility; yet we have known some with mild and minor disorders to show much. One child may have much anxiety or guilt but little hostility; another may reveal quite an opposite state of affairs. Some children just seem to roll with the punches and the frustrations and menace to get along with a minimum of emotional response. But often hostility and aggression are found and so we must understand them.

Aggressive or Protest Behavior as a Reaction to Penalty. Penalty and rejection by his associates may lead an individual to react aggressively by attack, protest, or some form of rebellion. He may employ the mechanism of projection and blame his parents, teachers, or playmates for his objectionable difference. He may display toward the weaknesses of those in the group the same intolerant attitude which they have manifested toward his own. In this way he not only temporarily minimizes the importance of his own handicap, but also enjoys the revenge of recognizing weaknesses in others. He may attempt to shift the blame for rejection. He will say, "They didn't keep me out because I stuttered—they just didn't think I had as nice clothes as the rest of them wore." In this way he will exaggerate the unfairness of the group evaluation and ignore the actual cause. Another attack reaction may be that of focusing all attention upon himself. He can refuse to cooperate with the group in any way, can belittle its importance openly, and can refuse to consider it in his scheme of existence. Finally, he may react by a direct outward attack. A child, or an adult with an easily provoked temper, may indulge in actual physical conflict with members of the group which has not accepted him.

The Case of the Grandmother's Nose

Ivan, whom we straightway named The Terrible, was a very agile little boy of six with completely unintelligible speech. He was a holy terror. Other mothers would sweep their children back into the house when Ivan came tricycling up the sidewalk. No baby sitter ever sat twice at his house. His mother worked days, probably in self-defense, and the boy was cared for by his grandfather and grandmother who lived upstairs. Only the grandfather could control Ivan and when he left the house to go to the store the grandmother would flee to her bedroom and lock the door, because Ivan would occasionally swarm up her and bite her, preferably on the nose. She was hard of hearing and found Ivan's garbled jargon quite impossible to comprehend. Ivan demanded that people understand him. If they did, he was well behaved and cooperative. But when they didn't, he went berserk; he scratched, bit, and attacked the object of his hatred. It took two years before Ivan was tamed and talking and our speech clinic still bears certain scars as an enduring memorial to Ivan. So does this therapist's hands.

A rejected individual may spread pointed criticism of the group in a resentful manner. In any of these methods, the object of the rejection does not retreat from reality—he reacts antagonistically and attacks those who made his reality unpleasant.

Among the speech defectives the author has examined, the behavior problems that seemed due to a protest reaction against the group's penalty include: lying, enuresis, constipation, temper tantrums, stealing, arson, suicide, use of obscene language, cruelty to pets, truancy, fighting, destruction of property, disobedience, attempted suicide, sexual promiscuity, and feeding difficulties.

Some speech defectives show few outward signs of these reactions except attitudes of sullenness or non-cooperation; in others, the protest is unmistakable. Unfortunately, these protest reactions do not solve the problem. They merely increase its unpleasantness.

The more the speech defective attacks the group, the more it penalizes him. Often such reactions interfere with treatment, for many of these speech defectives resent any proffered aid. They attack the speech correctionist and sabotage his assignments. The inevitable result of these attack reactions is to push the speech defective even further from normal speech and adequate adjustment.

Intelligent Unemotional Acceptance as a Reaction to Penalty. The reactions previously discussed ignored reality. This third type of reaction involves an admission of reality. A person may honestly state the reason for the group's rejection of him. He may even tell why his difference would be a weakness to that group. He accepts the rejection wholesomely and takes an objective attitude toward both the group's action and his handicap. The basis of his reactions is the short sentence uttered by the greatest of all mental hygienists, the cartoon character Popeye, who says, "I yam what I yam." The individual with such an attitude says, "Of course I have a difference. I stutter (or have red hair, or weigh two hundred and fifty pounds, or have a big nose), but what of it? That's just the way I am." This type of reaction destroys much of the emotionality and abnormal behavior usually built around a difference. It provides no necessity for using the tricks and subterfuges which always accompany attempts to hide or to minimize a defect. It furnishes the essential basis for subsequent remedial speech work as it brings the defect into the open and allows its possessor to study it thoroughly and to work on overcoming it. No speech defect can be eradicated when it is hidden. It must be seen as a problem to be solved before its possessor can solve it.

Relationship between Anxiety, Guilt, and Hostility

We have seen that these emotional reactions to the possession of abnormal speech may each appear in many different forms. Anxiety can show itself in behaviors ranging from nightmares to compulsive eating. Guilt and hostility too can appear in many different shapes. It is important also that we recognize that each of these emotional reactions can convert itself into another. When our fears become unbearable we may translate them into hate. A guilty child can lose some of his guilt in worry. Hate can turn into fear. The child who hates his parents for their nagging, for their insistence that he speak more clearly, may feel guilt because of that very hostility. Even in the same child, these feelings may shift back and forth, one into the other. It is important that we do not always accept at face value that which we see. That angry little hellion before us may in reality be a very frightened youngster. If we are to understand, we must look deeply.

Effects of These Emotions on Speech. Speech disorders may have their origins in emotional storms; in turn they may provoke emotion. But there is also a third important role which emotions play in the lives of those who do not speak normally. These feelings make treatment difficult. When speaking is permeated by anxiety, guilt, and hostility, it becomes difficult to confront, hard to modify. These feelings so surround speech that it becomes almost untouchable. Often the person who wishes to help finds himself in the middle of these storms. The child cannot intelligently discriminate between his lisp and the standard *s* sounds because he is torn by conflicting emotions. All he hears is the static of his own anxiety or guilt. An angry child does not learn easily.

Anxiety, guilt and hostility, the evil children of penalty and frustration, also affect all the functions of speech which we outlined in our first chapter. They spoil the laller's attempt to coordinate his tongue and, by so doing, affect the motor aspect of speech. It is possible to become voiceless or speechless with chronic anger or fear—the acoustic aspect. The aphasic who, in quieter states, can talk or write fairly well, becomes unable to do either when the frustration overwhelms him. (Thinking.) The stutterer, so full of fear and self-disgust, throws down the telephone receiver and cannot even say "Hello!" (Communication.) Overcome by shame, the cerebral palsied boy avoids the high-school parties and cannot bring himself to ask for the job he desires so much. (Social control.) Fearful to reveal herself as one who cannot talk as others do, the sixth grader with the harelip never speaks aloud. She will only whisper. This is speech as the identification of the self. The part of a speech handicap that we can hear is only a portion of the problem.

Severity of the Emotional Problems. We have repeatedly indicated that the amount of penalties, frustration, anxiety, guilt feeling, and hostility varies from individual to individual. We wish to state again that there are some fortunate possessors of speech disorders who experience not much more than a normal amount of these unpleasantnesses. They probably happened to have lived in homes that were warm and accepting. They probably were fortunate in their teachers and playmates. They may have had other personality assets which compensated for the speech disabilities.

We also suspect that the severity of the emotional problems varies directly with the severity of the speech disorder itself. A stutterer whose symptoms are visible as well as audible, whose face contorts while he struggles for utterance, is surely likely to endure more penalties and to feel more frustration than one who stutters mildly and infrequently. A child whose speech is badly garbled by articulatory errors will suffer more than one who inconsistently misarticulates only his *th* sounds. In short, the amount of emotional distress seems to vary proportionately with the amount and degree of overt speech abnormality.

Moreover, our culture tends to be more tolerant of certain types of speech abnormality than others. Deviations in voice must be rather drastic before they provoke attention and rejection. Generally speaking, we seem to react more to a stuttering problem than we do to an articulatory one. Yet even in articulation we find that a severe and salivary lateral lisp will evoke more negative attention than comparable difficulty on some other sounds.

There also seems to be more acceptance of deviate speech in the young child than in the adult, probably because we know that good speech must be learned and that the learning takes time. Many of the children with articulatory errors seen by the speech therapist in the early grades appear fairly unconcerned and unemotional about their problems. The beginning stutterer has few fears. And yet these same children some years later may show marked signs of emotional upheaval. If, in this chapter, we have seemed to magnify the importance of *pfagh* it is only because we want to prevent it. And, although the research is inconclusive with respect to the amount of emotionality in the average person with a speech disorder, we are bound to find, at all ages, certain individuals whose hidden emotional handicaps require our understanding.

SUMMARY

In this chapter we have attempted to present the main features of the emotional fraction of a speech handicap. We have described not only the penalties which our culture places upon disordered speech but also the frustrations experienced by the person who cannot talk normally. The ways in which emotional conflicts serve as the causes or results of speech disorders have been discussed. We have shown that anxiety, guilt, and hostility may arise as the result of this penalty and frustration and that these feelings may, themselves, provoke further reactions which can contribute to the total problem and interfere with its solution. Finally, we have pointed out that the extent of this emotional fraction of the speech handicap may depend upon the severity and frequency of the speech deviations, their type, the person's age, the presence of compensatory assets, and the attitudes of his associates.

PROJECTS

1. Limp *very* obviously down a crowded street or past a playground and observe the reactions of the people you meet.

2. Go into a drugstore and pretend to be deaf and dumb. Point to your lips and ears and make gestures requesting a pencil and paper. Observe the clerk's reactions.

3. Find a comic book concerning the adventures of P-Porky the P-P-Pig.

4. Stop a person on the street and ask him a direction while pretending to stutter. Observe his reaction and your own.

5. Interview some handicapped person on the penalties he has received.

6. Why did Lord Byron have such a compulsion to excel in swimming, boxing, duelling, seducing, and poetry? Did he have a happy life?

7. How did the children in Somerset Maugham's "Of Human Bondage" react to the hero's club foot?

8. Interview one of the special education teachers in your community concerning her experiences in solving the problems caused by social penalties.

9. What scenes can you recall in which a handicapped person was being penalized by society?

10. One of our cases, a spastic, with ungainly coordinations and body twitches, was walking home from school one day when a police car drove alongside, an officer jumped out and grabbed the young man, saying, "Come on, where's your home, you drunk fool?" He dragged him into the car, and searched him, finding in his wallet his address, a college dormitory. When he found out his mistake there, he turned to the spastic and said, "You've got no business out on the street anyway in your condition. Why don't they keep you at home." If you were that spastic what would you do and how would you feel?

11. Write a paper describing your own personal history of pfagh.

12. Deliberately frustrate some other person and observe his reactions.

13. Ask some psychologist to administer to you the Rosenzweig Picture Frustration Test.

14. In what ways do you characteristically respond to penalty?

15. For what behavior have you found special approvals? How do you respond to approval?

16. How do you characteristically express hostility outwardly and inwardly?

17. Keep a card in your pocket or purse all day and note each instance of anxiety and record its nature.

18. What memories of guilt feelings do you have during the period prior to your high school years?

19. Try to analyze one of your recurring dreams in terms of pfagh.

20. Visit some school for handicapped children and observe the attitudes of the teachers and children.

READINGS

21. Adams, H. M., and P. J. Glasner. "Emotional Involvements in Mutism," *Journal Speech and Hearing Disorders*, Volume 19, 1954, pages 59-69.
22. Biorn-Hansen, V. "Social and Emotional Aspects of Aphasia," *Journal Speech and Hearing Disorders*, Volume 22, 1957, pages 53-59.
23. Chapin, A. B. "A Program for a Speech Inhibited Child," *Journal Speech Disorders*, Volume 12, 1947, pages 373-376.
24. DuPont, H., T. Landsman, and M. Valentine. "The Treatment of Delayed Speech by Client-Centered Therapy," *Journal of Consulting Psychology*, Volume 17, 1953, pages 122-125.
25. Kinstler, D. B. "Covert and Overt Maternal Rejection in Stuttering," *Journal Speech and Hearing Disorders*, Volume 26, 1961, pages 145-155.
26. Matis, E. E. "Psychotherapeutic Tools for Parents," *Journal Speech and Hearing Disorders*, Volume 26, 1961, pages 165-170.
27. Murphy, A. T. "Counseling Students with Speech and Hearing Problems," *Personnel and Guidance Journal*, Volume 33, 1955, pages 260-264.
28. ———, and R. M. Fitzsimmons. *Stuttering and Personality Dynamics*, Chapter 8.
29. Perrin, E. H. "The Social Position of the Speech Defective Child," *Journal Speech and Hearing Disorders*, Volume 19, 1954, pages 250-252.
30. Stevens, E. "Psychodrama in the Speech Clinic," *Sociatry*, Volume 1, 1947, pages 56-58.

ILLUSTRATIONS

The following anecdotes and case presentations illustrate certain principles which have been presented in this chapter. Find a quotation from the chapter which each of these items illustrates.

1. A public-school speech therapist had a group of third-grade children all of whom had severe articulation problems. Feeling sure that most of them had been frequently misunderstood and frustrated in their efforts to communicate, she began the sessions with the following activity. She put on a Halloween mask and said, "I'm the big person who can't understand when you try to tell me something. Today, you can get even. Whenever this big person says 'What?' or 'What did you say?' or

'Say that again' you can stick out your tongues and yell at me. Each of you listen to what the other children say so you can help yell it so I can't help but understand." She reported later that she made more progress in that one session than she had for a period of several weeks.

2. E. G. was a cross-eyed girl of nineteen with a very severe stutter. Although of superior intelligence, she left school in the ninth grade and, from that time on, she very seldom left the confines of her home. She dominated her wealthy parents in every way and shirked every type of responsibility. When guests came for dinner, she had the servants serve her in her room. She spoke very little to anyone but read a great deal. Simulated heart attacks were used to control her parents. She refused to see any physician. Financial reverses and the death of her father forced her to do something about her speech defect after an attempt at suicide failed because of lack of courage. Enrolled in the speech clinic, she immersed herself in the literature on stuttering but failed to carry out any assignment which entailed any persistence, courage, or exhibition of her speech defect. Faced with dismissal, she pleaded that she wanted to cooperate but did not have the will power. She declared that she thought she would acquire some if she were permitted to remain. She was told that she could return if she would have an operation for her strabismus and carry out a certain set of assignments at home. The operation was very successful, and, when she returned a year later, her personality seemed to have changed entirely. She had performed not only all of the assignments given her but many more difficult ones as well. She had prepared herself for college entrance examinations, had taken dancing lessons, and had obtained and held a job in a restaurant for some time. For the first time she seemed to have some self-respect and courage to undergo temporary unpleasantness in order to achieve a future goal. Her stuttering was still present though its severity had decreased. She cooperated in every way and progressed rapidly in her speech work. Her explanation for the change was succinct: "Having my eyes fixed gave me my chance."

3. One of our most severe stutterers, a college student, used to spend three and four hours daily listening to symphonic records up in his dormitory room with the door locked. He would play each recording several times, conducting the invisible orchestra with a baton, stopping the record player every so often to scold the bassoon player or to demand another playing of the previous passage. Said he, "I know it sounds silly, but after a lot of wretched talking it's the only thing that gives me a little peace."

4. Cynthia was a frozen-faced little girl of nine. Only her eyes were alert and they were always on guard. She did what she was told but never volunteered. One day the speech therapist put on a puppet drama in which Zo-Zo the clown had a good many unpleasant things happen to him. Zo-Zo always laughed. Then when one of the other children said viciously to him, "Zo-Zo, your mother's dead," the clown stopped laugh-

ing and said sadly, "Oh why can't I cry? I want to cry. I don't want to laugh now. Please help me cry. Please!" At this point Cynthia broke into gales of tears. The class was dismissed, but Zo-Zo and the teacher had quite a long interview with the girl which, with the release, finally led to the solution of her problem and a new out-going personality.

5. A seventh-grade girl who lalled (distorted most of the tongue-tip sounds) and found it difficult to make herself understood showed no interest in her speech and refused to come to the public-school speech therapist for help. She had frequent attacks of asthma and a poor academic record despite an average IQ. Finally she was persuaded to come, and after some initial difficulty, she made rapid progress in correcting her articulation. At the end of two months her speech was almost normal, the asthmatic attacks which had kept her out of school almost once each week had disappeared, and she was making good grades.

6. "I must be pretty tough because I'm not in the bug house. The constant experience of starting to say something and never having it come out when I want it to should have driven me crazy long ago. I can't even say my own name. Once in a while I get a little streak of easy speech and then wham, I'm plugged, tripped up, helpless, making silent mouth openings like a goldfish. It's like trying to play the piano with half the keys sticking. I can't even get used to it because sometimes I can fear a word and out it pops; then again when I am expecting smooth speech and everything's going all right, boom I'm stuck. It sure's exasperating."

7. "The most wonderful thing about being able to pronounce my sounds now is that people aren't always saying 'What? What's that?' I bet I've heard that fifty thousand times. Often they'd shout at me as though I were deaf and that usually made me talk worse. Or they'd answer 'Yes' when that just didn't make sense. I still occasionally find myself getting set for these reactions and steeling myself against them and being surprised when other people just listen."

8. Another stutterer, a girl of twenty, came from the highest strata of society in the British set in Montreal, Canada. Her eye contact was perfect, her composure completely unruffled, but her face and mouth went through some of the worst contortions we had ever seen. As soon as one of these contortions had subsided and the word was said she continued as though nothing at all had happened. She too found it very difficult to modify her stuttering. She had been trained to ignore it. This is what she said. "In my set we always ignore the unpleasant, the ugly, and the uncomfortable. No one in my whole life ever raised an eyebrow or said a word about my stuttering. They always acted as though I spoke as well as they. *Noblesse oblige,* you know."

9. We once worked with an Indian from Oklahoma who stuttered. He was a very difficult case, primarily because he was completely unable to get prepared for any word on which he might stutter. It was quite apparent that he did fear certain sounds and certain words because he would

pause and hesitate for a long time before attempting them. However, during these preparatory pauses he just seemed to "blank out." He became detached from the situation and from his utterance. During these pauses he was quite relaxed and passive, but he did not seem to hear anything said to him. These were not *petit mal* epileptic seizures. Finally, we found out. "My old grandmother, a wise woman, told me when I was a little boy that if my spirit went to the mountains I would never be afraid. So when I see hard word coming I go to mountains."

10. In a hut by a wilderness in northern Michigan lives a poet with a cleft palate and harelip who is convinced that the world is not ready for his genius. He has a large folder of rejection slips. He writes constantly, and this is his masterpiece:

> Man Speaks to Man
> No?
>
> . . . .
> No!

He is quite rational and quite objective. "My parents were very fond of me, their only child. They could not bear to have my palate and lip operated on. Instead they decided to train me to be a genius. Everything I ever wrote they saved and praised. I used to hide the bad poetry but I was never quite sure what was bad. They trained me well, but only in one direction. All I can do is write poetry, advanced poetry. I'm pretty sure it's too advanced. But poets have a hard time living in this society and so do cleft-palate people. So I live by myself. Even if I could talk like other people, I wouldn't know what to say to them. Such a course would give me more problems than I could possibly cope with. This is better. Among the things I write should be a few that will be great. . . ."

CHAPTER FOUR

Speech Development

In this chapter we present the basic information about the development of normal speech and relate this information to some of the problems of disordered speech.

The Beginnings of Speech

Many of us would say that speech begins with the birth cry, although few of us would agree with Schopenhauer, the vinegar-penned old philosopher, who claimed it was a protest against having to enter this miserable world. By outrageously placing a buzzing doorbell against the mother's abdomen, researchers found they could cause an increase in the movements of the foetus, thus indicating that the unborn baby may hear. Even more incredibly, there seems to be some evidence that a few infants have vocalized while still in the uterus.[1]

All of this author's babies, fortunately, were mercifully silent during the months before birth but they more than made up for it thereafter. We heard their birth cries, however, noted that these were produced on inhalation, and wryly wondered if they would turn out to be Hottentots, whose language consists primarily of inhalatory sounds. Most of the early vocalization of all babies seems to be reflexive in nature, whether it be on inhalation or exhalation or, more commonly, both. This seems to be true for both crying and comfort sounds. They talk in and out like donkeys. We have heard such sounds in the struggling speech attempts of adult stutterers

---

[1] P. F. Ostwald. "The Sounds of Human Behavior," *Logos,* Volume 3, 1960, page 21.

and aphasics. We have heard lispers who sucked inward the air for their *s* sounds. Some of our cerebral palsied friends have never learned to speak on exhalation alone. The baby, like these cases, has a lot of untangling and learning to do in mastering speech.

The skills involved in speech begin to be acquired as soon as the child is born and are seldom perfectly mastered, even during a lifetime. Much of the speech learning during the first six months is relatively independent of the stimulation given by the child's parents. Even in the crying and wailing of infants the short, sharp inhalation and prolonged exhalation so fundamental to true speech are being practiced. Lip, jaw, and tongue movements involved in the production of all the speech sounds in all human languages are repeatedly performed. The early awareness of these movements and their accompanying sounds provides the foundation for speech readiness. Throughout the first years of life there are many ways in which parents can help or hinder the development of speech. Their knowledge or ignorance determines whether the child will learn to talk because of his parents' efforts or in spite of them. Their application of principles, so obvious that we wonder why they should ever be violated, will determine whether the child's speech will be an asset or a handicap. Time after time the speech correctionist tries to trace the cause of a stutter or an articulatory defect, only to lose it in the vague parental memories of childhood. It is vitally important for the student of speech correction to know how speech develops.

Crying versus Comfort Sounds. The first reflexive sounds are the shrill, nasal wails of a child in discomfort and struggling. As Lewis[2] writes, "At first these are the only sounds that a child makes. He cries when he is uncomfortable; otherwise he is silent." For the first month most of the child's vocalization consists of this wailing.

Even during the first month, the vocalizations vary from child to child. One infant may coo and laugh when taken from the breast; another may whimper; and still another may kick and scream. Research indicates that even at this period there are more vowels and consonants used in noncrying vocalizations than in whimpering, and more sounds used in whimpering than in ordinary crying.

Whenever we interview the mother of a child with a severe articulation disorder or a child who has not acquired any intelligible

---

[2] M. M. Lewis. *How Children Learn to Speak.* London: George G. Harrap Company, Ltd., 1957, page 15.

speech we routinely ask her if the child cried a lot more than her other babies during the first months of his life. (We never ask the father this; he is bound to say yes.) The answer may be the starting point of the trail to important information concerning the child's physical condition, family conflicts, or even maternal rejection. But we also know that a child who spends all his time in crying will not have the practice time for experimenting with other sounds, with other movements of the mouth and body.*

Many parents seek to prevent all crying, although a certain amount of it does exercise the child's vocal and respiratory coordinations as well as its parents' patience. They jounce their baby up and down, juggle it back and forth, or rock it, pat it, and whirl it until it is dizzy enough to end its crying through unconsciousness. Other parents resolutely ignore their newborn's howls because of a mistaken fear that they might spoil the child. These babies may cry away so many of their waking hours that their speech-sound repertoire will be necessarily limited. As we have seen, fewer sounds are used in crying than in noncrying speech. Again, many parents interrupt their children's automatic vocalization by embracing them or conversing with them. They should let the vocal play period complete itself. During this first period the muscular development of the tongue may be delayed and abnormally high palatal arches may be produced by bottle feeding with improper nipples. These organic conditions may delay speech development.

The noncrying sounds are composed of grunts, gurgles, and sighs, and include most of the front vowels, the consonants *k, l, g,* and the glottal catch. These particular consonants involve contacts and tongue movements similar to those used in swallowing. All of these sounds are accompanied by movements of the arms, legs, or trunk. They sometimes occur during the act of sucking or immediately after feeding. Compared to later vocalizations, the noncrying sounds produced by a healthy baby during the first month are relatively

---

* C. A. Aldrich, C. Sung, and C. Knop, in their article, "The Crying of Newly Born Infants," *Journal Pediatrics,* Volume 27, 1945, pages 89-96, state that the average crying time spent by babies less than eight days old was 117 minutes per day. Peak periods of crying occurred at 6 P.M. and at midnight. They attributed 35% of the crying to hunger, 28% to dirty or wet diapers, and the rest to unknown causes, which the present author interprets as meaning just for the hell of it. Moreover his own babies preferred the 5:30 A.M. hour to any other.

infrequent. More crying is done than whimpering, and more whimpering noises are produced than noncrying ones. Perhaps it was this fact which led one scientific father, faithfully and no doubt solemnly, to record his baby's wails, first phonographically and then in the phonetic alphabet. After a profound mathematical analysis of the records, he concluded that the wails increased in pitch. Most night-walking fathers would agree that the wails also increase in loudness and meanness.

The comfort sounds, although non-purposive, are the ancestors of true speech, and somehow most parents seem to know it. When they occur, the mother comes close and bathes the child with the sounds of love. This may be more important than one might think. There seems to be a curious phenomenon called *imprinting* at work. Scientists have found that an animal's response to certain sounds seems to be imprinted shortly after birth. For example, Hess[3] and others have performed experiments such as one where freshly hatched ducklings were given a mechanical decoy which said "gock, gock, gock" and the ducklings from that time on followed and came to the mechanical "gock" of the decoy in preference to a real goose's honking. Of course, humans are not geese, and we do not know much about human imprinting.

But we do know that orphanage babies begin to talk later and have more speech defects than babies whose parents care for them. A baby needs a mother's voice if it is to talk, and it is important that the mother's voice has love in it. Even parakeets will not talk unless they are fed and spoken to lovingly. This is why in interviewing parents we are interested in discovering whether the baby was unwanted or illegitimate, in discovering how soon the mother had to go back to work, in knowing what sort of a person took care of the infant while she was gone. We also ask about feeding problems. Some babies have a tough time getting enough milk or keeping it down. They cry more and coo less. A tired, frantic mother may forget that babies, like husbands, talk most after they've been fed. This is the time for bathing the babe in pleasant sound, partly his own and partly the mother's.

The feeding-speaking situation will always be important for many reasons. Consider the nipple on the baby's bottle. Very often,

[3] E. H. Hess. "Imprinting," *Science*, Volume 130, pages 133-141.

in taking case histories of lallers, we find the mothers mentioning that the child had great difficulty in getting enough milk, that he was a "slow feeder," and that they had to widen the opening in the nipple. To us, this is very significant, for when a baby sucks, he does not suck with the lips alone. The tongue tip is thrust forward and upward in the squeezing action. He needs to learn this coordination so basic to many speech sounds. Some babies never get a chance to learn it; it's all they can do to keep from drowning and they keep the back of the tongue high to survive. Many cleft-palate children retain this rear elevation of the tongue in speech and some authorities feel that much of the excessive nasality is due to it. There are others who feel that the design of the ordinary rubber nipple is very poor and contributes to later malcoordination of the tongue and to the habituation of the "infantile swallow." This latter term refers to a form of swallowing in which the lips are pursed and the tongue is thrust forward. In the normal swallow, these two behaviors do not occur. When a child continues to use this "infantile" form of swallowing—and he swallows on the average about twice each minute—certain tongue-thrust habits are created which have been said to produce such dental abnormalities as protruding teeth or an open bite or such speech defects as a lisp.[4] The matter is still, however, in dispute.

Private and Social Babbling.   Babbling usually begins about eight weeks after birth. It consists of odd little vowels, usually the *ee, ih, uh,* and others made in the front of the mouth, a few *m, b,* and *g* consonant sounds and assorted snorts, gurgles, and grunts, all combined with squeals and sighs and a few Bronx cheers for good measure. It is a delightful fairy language. There are times when the baby uses it when others are around, bathing him, waving huge fingers in front of his eyes, talking nonsense to him. Then it can be shared and enjoyed by all. But there are other times when the baby needs to play with his toes and his mouth, privately.

A good share of this vocal play is carried on when the child is alone and it disappears when someone attracts his attention.

One child played with her babbling each morning after awakening, usually beginning with a whispered "eenuh" and repeating it with

---

[4] S. T. Fletcher, R. L. Casteel, and D. P. Bradley. "Tongue Thrust Swallow, Speech Articulation, and Age," *Journal Speech and Hearing Disorders,* Volume 26, 1961, pages 201-208.

increasing effort until she spoke the syllable aloud, whereupon she would laugh and chortle as she said it over and over. The moment she heard a noise in the parents' bedroom this babbling would cease and crying would begin.

The parents who joyfully rush in and ruin this speech rehearsal are failing to appreciate its significance in the learning of speech. The child must simultaneously feel and hear the sound repeatedly if it is ever to emerge as an identity. Imitation is essentially a device to perpetuate a stimulus, and babbling is self-imitation of the purest

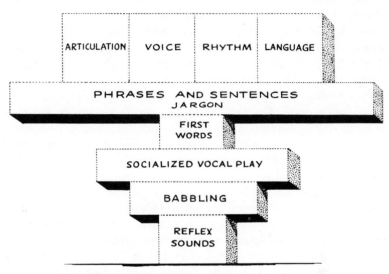

FIGURE 11. *The Development of Speech.*

variety. When the babbling period is interrupted or delayed through illness, the appearance of true speech is often similarly retarded. Deaf babies begin to babble at a normal time, but since they cannot hear the sounds they produce, they probably lose interest and hence have much less true vocal play than the hearing child. Mirrors suspended above the cribs of deaf babies have increased the babbling through visual self-stimulation.

About the fifth or sixth month, when the infant can fixate an object with his eyes, and grab a toy and maneuver it into his mouth, or hoists his hind end up to crawl, there appears a new kind of babbling which we call *vocal play.*

Vocal Play. The child begins to use his vocalization (with more vowels than consonants) for getting attention, supporting rejection, and expressing demands. Frequently he will look at an object and cry at the same time. He voices his eagerness and protest. He is using his primitive speech both to express himself and to modify the behavior of others. This stage is also marked by the appearance of syllable repetition, or the doubling of sounds, in his vocal play. He singles out a certain double syllable, such as *da-da* and frequently practices it to the exclusion of all other combinations. Sometimes a single combination will be practiced for several weeks at a time, though it is more usual to find the child changing to something new every few days and reviewing some of his former vocal achievements at odd intervals. True disyllables (*ba-da*) come relatively late in the first year, and the infant rejects them when the parent attempts to use them as stimulation.

At this time the child will often "answer back." Make a noise and he makes a noise. The two noises are usually dissimilar, but it is obvious that he is responding. In this vocal play, most of the vowels are still the ones made in the front or middle of the mouth but a few *oo* and *oh* sounds (which are back vowels) can be detected in the child's vocal play. There are also more consonants to be heard, the *d, t, n,* and *l* having appeared, but it's still hard to separate them out of the flow of unsorted utterance unless you have long, sharp ears. Some private babbling continues throughout these months, yet now the child seems to take more pleasure in public practice. He's listening to himself but also listening to you. He is talking to himself but also sometimes to you. This is *socialized vocalization*.

We must not conclude this section without pointing out some implications which babbling and vocal play have for speech therapy. Svend Smith, a Danish speech therapist, has devised a set of rhythms based on the bongo-drum chants of South African natives, and he has his patients utter strange and unfamiliar cries in unison with the rhythmic beat. We too have used his methods, and often find that children and even adults can follow our own chanting as it progresses from these strange cries into standard sounds of English. We find that they can make sounds which previously they were unable to produce. Often we use the baby's comfort sounds or the repeated syllables of vocal play in these chants. The rhythm helps to create the freedom to try new sounds. Some children become so tense when attempting a sound which they have never successfully produced, that they cannot possibly find the new coordinations. Babbling and vocal play can free them from this tension. To vary our production of sound, we must feel some of the same freedom that the baby experiences when babbling or doing vocal play. In this regard, it is interesting to note that in England and elsewhere on the continent, a speech therapy session often begins with a period of relaxation. We know of no better way to relax than by free babbling, especially when the therapist is babbling freely too. Perhaps we are returning to an earlier period when learning to speak was fun.

Inflected Vocal Play. Although some squeals and changes in pitch and loudness have previously occurred in the babbling, it is not until about the eighth month that inflections become prominent. It is then that the vocal play takes on the tonal characteristics of adult speech. We now find the baby using inflections which sound like questions, commands, surprise, ponderous statements of fact, all in a delightful gibberish that has no meaning. We not only hear the inflections and sounds of English but those of the Oriental languages as well. No baby can be sure he will end up speaking English. So he practices a bit of Hottentot now and then. We have tried hard to imitate some of these sounds and inflections and have failed. The baby can often duplicate whole strings of these strange beads of sound.

The private babbling and social vocal play continue strongly during this period from eight months to a year. The repertoire of sounds increases. There is a marked gain in back vowels and front consonants. Crying time diminishes, though few fathers would believe it. They begin to get interested in their sons and daughters about this stage, however. The infant is becoming human. He'll bang a cup; he'll smile back at the old man. He'll reach out to be picked up. He begins to understand what "No!" means. But most important of all, he begins to *sound* as though he is talking.

We have previously spoken of various stages of development, but it should be made very clear that, although most children go through these stages in the order given, the activity in any one stage does not cease as soon as the characteristics of the next stage appear. Grunts and wails, babbling, socialized vocalization, and inflection practice all begin at about the times stated, but they continue throughout the entire period of speech development.

It is during this period that the baby begins to use more of the back vowels (u, ʊ, o, ɔ) in his babbling. According to Irwin and Curry,[5] 92 per cent of all vowels uttered by babies are the front vowels as compared to the 49 per cent figure for adult speech. They say, "It is evident that a fundamental process of development in early speech consists of the mastery of the back vowels." It is interesting that when we work with adult articulation cases we prefer syllables such as *see* and *ray* and *lee* to those involving the back vowels like *soo* and *low*. Front vowels seem to be more easily mastered.

The baby, through his vocal gymnastics, gradually masters the coordinations necessary to meaningful speech. But it must be emphasized that when he is repeating *da-da* and *ma-ma* at this stage, he is not designating his parents. His arm movements have much more meaning than those of his mouth. It is during these months that the ratio of babbling to crying greatly increases. Comprehension of parental gestures shows marked growth. The child now responds to the parent's stimulation, not automatically, but with more discrimination. His imitation is more hesitant but it also seems more purposive. It begins to resemble the parent's utterance. If the father interrupts the child's chain of *papapapapapapapapa* by saying *papa*, the child is less likely than before to say *wah* or *gu* and more likely to whisper *puh* or to repeat the two syllables *puhpuh*. During this period, simple musical tones, songs, or lullabies are especially good stimulation. The parent should observe the child's inflections and rhythms and attempt to duplicate them. This is the material that should be used for stimulation at this period, not a long harangue on why mother loves her little token of heaven.

This period, too, has a message for those who wish to help the child with abnormal speech. We see that new sounds are not acquired solely in meaningful words; they appear singly, or doubly in syllables, and nonsense syllables at that. We note that they occur in the context of pleasurable contacts with others who share them. They are to be played with, not demanded. We have known many children who could make a perfectly good *r* sound in isolated words like *church*, yet who failed to say this sound when it occurred on a falling inflection as in the word *father*. Speech therapy should not

[5] O. C. Irwin, and T. Curry. "Vowel Elements in the Crying of Infants Under Ten Days of Age," *Child Development*, Volume 12, 1941, pages 99-109.

be done in monotonous drill. The baby tells us that the way to acquire new sounds is to use them expressively and socially.

The First Words

Some time between the tenth month and the eighteenth the normal child learns to say his first true words. Comprehension shows a great spurt of development at this time. The baby suddenly becomes a very human being. He learns to walk and to talk and to feed himself, three of the most fundamental of all human functions. He's quite a fellow indeed. Let us see how he masters his first words.

The Autism Theory. Experiments in teaching birds to talk led O. H. Mowrer, a famous American psychologist, to formulate what is known as the autism theory of speech acquisition.[6] He found that his birds would reproduce human words only if these words were spoken by the trainer while the birds were being fondled or fed. After this had happened often enough, the word itself could apparently produce pleasurable feelings in the bird. Since myna birds and parakeets produce a lot of variable sounds, it is almost inevitable that a few of these sounds might resemble the human word that produced such pleasant feelings. Thus when the bird hears itself making these similar sounds it feels again the pleasantness of fondling and being fed. So it repeats them and the closer the bird's chirp-word comes to resemble the human word, the more pleasant the bird feels. By properly rewarding these progressive approximations, we can facilitate the process. However, finally the bird will find that "Polly-wants-a-cracker" or "To-hell-with-Iowa" * is pleasant enough to be self-rewarding. The word "autism" refers to the self-rewarding aspect of the process. At any rate, these phrases seem to sound almost as good to the bird as a piece of suet tastes.

When this theory is applied to the child's learning of his first words, it seems to make a lot of sense. Certainly, the mother says

[6] O. H. Mowrer. "On the Psychology of 'Talking Birds'—A Contribution to Language and Personality Theory," in *Learning Theory and Personality Dynamics*. New York: The Ronald Press Company, 1950.

* One of the author's graduate students taught a parakeet to say this most reprehensible phrase, knowing well that the author had received his doctorate at that excellent institution. The author is presently engaged in teaching the bird to stutter when it says it, having found it impossible to extinguish the phrase, or, for that matter, the bird.

"Mama" or "baby" a thousand times while feeding, bathing, or fondling the child. Also it is certain that the baby will find *mamamama* or *bubbababeeba* sometime in his babbling and vocal play. If these utterances flood him with pleasant feelings, he will repeat them more often than syllables such as "gugg" which have no special pleasant memories attached to them. It is also true that the closer the child comes to the standard words, the more reward he will get from the mother. There still remains the problem of giving meaning to utterance and this is explained in terms of the context. "Mama" is used when the mama is present; "baby" is used when he sees himself in a mirror or plays with his body. This theory raises some objections, but it seems to be the best explanation we have yet been able to formulate.

The Imitation Theory. This theory has been formulated in several ways, some of which are circular and nonexplanatory. Certainly there seems to be no primary instinct of imitation at work. If by imitation we mean that the baby suddenly begins to reproduce exactly what he sees or hears, the facts do not support the theory. Nevertheless, during the last months of the first year, most children seem to make some attempts to reproduce movements which they witness, but rarely are these movements exact. Imitation, as used in the larger sense to denote attempted reproduction, seems to be motivated by the desire to perpetuate the stimuli which intrigue one's interest. It is the child's way of maintaining his interest. The child's memory span is very weak and short, and to compensate for this deficiency he seeks to perpetuate the stimulus by repeating it. This accounts for the doubling and repetition of syllables in the vocal play and for the persistence with which he pounds the rattle on the table.

When the process of speech imitation is studied, we discover that it begins when the parent starts to imitate the child. This may sound paradoxical, but its truth will be apparent when the situation is defined. During vocal play the child happens to be repeating the syllable *ma*. The hearing of the sound interests him, and so he repeats it again. Suddenly the sight of his mother interrupts his response to his own stimulation, and he lapses into silence. But the mother, unaware of the perfection of her technique, says to him, "Mama? Did you want mama?" and immediately the interesting stimulus is there again. Wishing it to continue, he makes the same vocal coordinations he made when alone, and again the same interesting sounds are heard, *mamaamaama*. Whereupon the mother rushes to the phone to tell her husband that the child has spoken his first word.

Only when the child uses the word as a definite tool of communication with such a meaning as "Mother, come here," or "Mother, lift me up!" can we say with certainty that he has acquired his first word. Nevertheless, the process of word acquisition has been described. The first step in teaching a child to talk should be the imitation of the sounds being made by the child during his vocal play. This should be preceded, if possible, by the parental imitation of other movements, such as pounding the table. If the child can be stimulated to return to his own former pounding by watching the parent pound, half the battle is won, for the first requisite is gained: the perpetuation of a stimulus given by another person. In imitating the speech of the child, the parent should seek to interrupt the child's activity before it is completed. For example, if the child is saying *da-da-da* over and over, it is wise to interject the parental *da-da* as soon as the child's first *da* has been produced. This will produce the most favorable conditions for getting the child to return to his own former activity, and usually he will maintain it much longer and much more loudly than he usually does. At first only a few sounds should be used in this way, preferably those that later can be used to represent the people doing the training. Thus the child will acquire *mama* in a situation which always represents her presence, and it is wise for her to say the word whenever she picks the child up. Thus the child will come to associate the interesting sound with the person, and it will thereby come to have meaning.

The child should be given such training until he responds consistently with eager repetition whenever the parent has interrupted vocal play by imitating his vocalizations. After that it is wise for the parent to utilize the silence periods which occur during the babbling as intervals of strong stimulation with the sounds previously used by the child. For example, the child has been babbling and suddenly becomes silent. The parent then attracts his attention and repeats *mamama* (or any other syllable which the child has been practicing). If the child will respond to this stimulation by attempted repetition, a second step in word acquisition has been taken. After considerable training involving the practices of both steps, the parent having been careful to pick the appropriate times, the child will suddenly surprise everyone by using the word very meaningfully, perhaps accompanying it with the gesture of reaching. In similar fashion, other early words may be taught.

In one sense, it may be said that the first words are acquired through stabilization. Out of all the vocal tangle of sounds produced by the baby, certain monosyllables or repeated syllables appear as familiar entities. They already have meaning for the child since they have expressed his needs or bodily conditions. He has played with them on so many pleasant occasions that they are old friends. He knows them well. Now, these same syllables become associated with certain conventional gestures (*bye-bye*) or consistent objects (*mama*) which appear repeatedly in his daily life. The first words have been his for a long time. They merely get a stabilized adult meaning.

> One parent, whom we studied with some interest, tried by every device of conditioning known to educated idiots to have his boy say the word "Ralph" (the father's name) as his first meaningful word. He worked with the boy for hours. When the first word did arrive (fourteen months late) it was "teetee" and referred to a cat.

Even as certain gestures such as reaching become stabilized from the wild undifferentiated arm-swinging of the infant, so, too, do the first words from their early matrix of vocal play.

Gesture is very important in stabilizing the first words. Sometimes it is almost too powerful.

> We observed one child who had the following history. At nine months the mother stretched out her arms to the child whenever the latter asked through gestures to be taken up. At nine months, eight days, the child would imitate the mother by reaching out bimanually whenever the mother did so. The mother then began to say "mama" whenever she used the gesture. At 9:14, the child would say it with the mother as they stretched out their arms. At 9:16, the child said "mamama" as she responded to the mother's silent gesture of reaching. On the same day she also said "mama" as she reached for her cup. At 9:19 she said "mama" to the father when he reached out to take her. Long after she could say "Daddy" imitatively and spontaneously, the gesture of reaching was always accompanied by "mama."

Fortunately, the effect of the accompanying gesture is seldom so persevering. Phonetic and intonation patterns of adult vocalization usually accompany the gesture and are perceived by the child as a whole. He responds not merely to the warning shake of the parent's head but to his own imitative head wagging and to the peremptory tone of the phrase "No. No!" and, if these fail, to the swat on his bottom as well. Even the mother's turning of her head or body as she recognizes and says "Daddy" is a meaningful gesture. Comprehension of speech for the baby consists of his interpretation of gesture, intonation of patterns, and the presence of syllables which he has previously practiced. Those gestures spontaneously used by the child are much better than any that parents could think up. If you interrupt his hand-waving by your own similar gesture, and say "bye-bye" and then take him outdoors, the word will be learned fairly easily. But if you try to teach him to kiss his father's picture and say "Daddy" at the same time, the work will be long and hard and perhaps useless.

These first words of the child may sound very much like those of adult speech, but they differ greatly in meaning. Some of them are no doubt "abracadabra" words. The child says "mama" and magically she appears. Other early words are mere signs of recognition or acquaintanceship. "Ba" may mean, "I know you. You're a ball. You're that round smooth thing I throw and bounce." He utters it with the same smug self-satisfaction that our friends manifest when, hearing a familiar musical phrase, they pat their egos and murmur, "Brahms, of course!"

Again we find some important clues which can be used in helping the child who does not talk or who talks defectively. Speech is not acquired through demand or command. A recent study[7] shows that most parents use demands and commands for speech as their preferred method in helping their children who have difficulties in mastering normal speech. "Say this . . . Say that . . ." are the common phrases heard by such children. "Say it again . . . Say it right!" These are the phrases which ring in a little child's ears. Few speech therapists use such primitive methods. They know that good speech will come if they can create the proper conditions, and the proper conditions are much like those used by parents in teaching the baby to say his first real words.

---

[7] R. L. Shelton, W. B. Arndt, and J. Miller. "Learning Principles and Teching of Speech and Language," *Journal Speech and Hearing Disorders*, Volume 26, 1961, pages 368-376.

Speech Development in the Last Half of the Second Year

At eighteen months, the child is toddling about the room pushing chairs and toys from one position to another. He climbs without discrimination. He spills with a spoon but manages to feed himself after a fashion. His handedness is pretty well established. Extremely active, he seldom plays with any one object or activity very long. As fond of music as before, he now prefers marches to lullabies except before bedtime. When angry, he screams, kicks, or holds his breath, but this mass activity is not focused or directed against any particular person. He initiates games such as "Peekaboo" and seems to take great pleasure in "making" adults cooperate. A large empty box is his dearest toy. He usually plays beside other children rather than with them, and he plays better alone. He relies on adults for assistance and attention but shies away from strangers. He should never be asked to speak to them at this age.

At eighteen months the child's speech activity consists of a *few meaningful words,* a little solitary *vocal play,* some *echolalia,* and a great deal of what we shall call *jargon.* Again, let us repeat that we are discussing the mythical average child. The average child has acquired from ten to twenty meaningful words with which to manipulate his elders and express his needs. He not only has names for members of his family but for many other things. Some typical examples are: (mo) for *snow;* (ɔgɔn) for *all gone;* (baɪbaɪ) for *bye-bye;* (aɪt̪) for *light;* (kækə) for *cracker;* (pɑp) for *pot.* Many of these are used as one-word sentences and they are very general in their reference. (kækə) can refer to *cracker* or *bread* or even to the fact that the dog is chewing a bone. Many parents lose a great deal of pleasure by not trying to solve these little crossword puzzles of infancy.

> Parents of our acquaintance put the problem to us in these words: "Why does our eighteen-month-old daughter refer to both the cat and a champagne bottle by the same word *dih* (dɪ)?" At the time we could not answer, but during the child's third year the word *dih* changed to *ding* (dɪŋ), then to *dink* (dɪŋk), and finally to *drink.* The child had been fascinated by the sight of the cat drinking its milk.

Occasionally the use of one word will spread to include a great many unrelated objects. The child feels little of his parents' confusion when he uses the word *behbuh* (bɛbə) to mean first "baby," then "bib," then "bread and butter." In this instance, the referential spread was no doubt due to the phonetic similarity of all these words. Had the parents taught them at different times or with different intonation or stress, the spread would not have been so great. Soldiers and others who suffer damage to the brain show these same symptoms.

Many early words are generalizations because they are so few and must serve a child so often. When a child who learns the word *puppy* as the designation for his varying perceptions of dogdom is suddenly confronted by a pony, he must needs make *puppy* do for both until he gets a new term. One child used the sound *fffff* as a generalized word for flowers. We also use a similar generic term. But he used *fffff* for perfume, for cigarette smoke, and for the figures on the wall paper. As the child comes to discriminate between objects, he needs terms to fix the contrasts involved. As long as ponies and dogs are merely big creatures with four legs on the corners and a hairy coat, they require but one word, and *puppy* is adequate. But when he realizes that ponies neigh, and he can ride on them, and they are bigger and eat carrots and never sleep by the fireplace—then a new word is needed, and it is acquired.

How, then, do children acquire these new words? The answer seems to be that at the moment when the child is undergoing some new experience in perception, or has an urgent desire to manipulate some new object in order to know it better, the adult intervenes, supplying a new word. If the child perceives this vocalization as part of the total experience, and at the same time produces the word through imitation, he finds he has a more efficient tool than the old generalized word. As the process repeats itself, the child comes to realize the greater expressiveness of conventional language forms. The whole process is, of course, also influenced by other factors: by the child's growing discrimination, by the strength and constancy of adult intervention at the crucial moments, and even by the natural responsiveness of the child.

These first words are used by the child even in his play. He yells "bell-bell-bell" (or a reasonable facsimile thereof) to himself as he rings it. He repeatedly labels the eyes, nose, and ears, not only of the mother who taught him but of his dog or doll, and he pokes them in the labeling. The early words are still accompanied by gesture or pertinent activity. He needs the parents' gestures in order to comprehend their utterances, and so he gestures and speaks in his turn. Only about one fourth of his speech attempts on these words can be understood by strangers. Each family seems to elect one of its members as interpreter. Nevertheless these first ten or twenty words of the eighteen-month-old child are a wonderful achievement. His manner shows that he knows it even if you do not. One child beat his chest and war-whooped whenever he used a new word successfully.

Jargon. The largest share of the average eighteen-month-old child's speech is *jargon*. This unintelligible jabber is probably more important for speech development than people realize. It is the lineal descendant of vocal play, but it differs from the earlier babbling in its rich variety and its seeming purposiveness. The child seems to be talking to other people or to his toys, rather than playing with the sounds themselves. He seldom repeats the same syllable.

> One boy, aged nineteen months, was observed banging a teddy bear with a hammer and between wallops addressing his victim as follows: "Gubba! Dadda bo-bo!" (Another hammering.) "Show gubba mahda." (Hammers again.) "Ashlee? Baá!" (Throws teddy bear over his shoulder.) In phonetics, the discourse was transcribed: gʌbə dædə bobo . . . ʃo gʌbə madɑ . . . æʃli . . . ba . . .
>
> Often this conversational jargon includes words he has mastered. Reaching out his dish for more ice cream he said, "ɛ:ɛ adə <u>mamə</u> i ɪ <u>nænə</u> <u>aɪ kim</u> ʃlæ?" The words which we have underlined are certainly understandable, and perhaps (nænə) refers to "banana," a favorite food, but the other syllables are difficult to interpret. And most of the child's jargon is even less intelligible.

As Gesell [8] phrases it, "At eighteen months her jargon was beguiling. She would talk confidentially for minutes at a single stretch, uttering not a single enunciated word but conveying much emotional content." As this quotation hints, jargon is probably the child's practice of fluency. Most young children swim in a river of fast-flowing meaningless adult jargon. Why should they not imitate their elders in fluency even as they copy their speech sounds and inflections? Certainly the gap between the few halting words of the child and the ceaseless ebb and flow of adult speech is very wide. Jargon

[8] A. Gesell. *The Psychology of Early Growth Including Norms for Infant Behavior and a Method of Genetic Analysis.* New York: The Macmillan Company, 1938.

is the bridge. It reaches its peak at eighteen months, dropping out rapidly, and it is usually gone by two years. A few children never use any jargon. When words fail they gesture or cry or remain silent. Most babies are like adults. They must talk whether what they say makes sense or not.

Vocal Play and Echolalia. The babbling play of infancy still appears, usually when the child is in bed or alone. He plays with repeated syllables or prolonged sibilant sounds. His new teeth enable him to produce new whistling sounds and so he must practice them. Often you can hear him whispering to himself and working up to the crescendo of vocalization. Prolonging sounds with his finger in mouth, or fumbling rhythmically with lips, he discovers again (and not for the last time) how fascinating he is. Jargon is his vocal response to a vocal world. Vocal play is his private rehearsal.

Echolalia appears very markedly in some children during this period, and it probably occurs in all children occasionally. By this term we mean the parrotlike echoing of words he hears. Occasionally whole phrases and sentences will be repeated so faithfully that the parent fairly jumps. In one instance a year-and-a-half-old girl almost wrecked a church service by saying, "and ever and ever amen!" fourteen times in the middle of the preacher's sermon. She had only spoken a few words prior to this event and she never uttered the phrase again for years. Parents frequently use echolalia to teach their children nursery rhymes, most of which are first learned backward. The parent says, "The cow jumped over the moon." "Moo," says the child automatically. Soon the parent begins to hesitate before the last word, and the child fills in.

Echolalia occurs almost instantly and unconsciously as if in a dream. The child's attention is elsewhere. Feeble-minded adults show a great deal of echolalia, as do aphasics and some psychotics. Any fairly normal person who has ever held a conversation with one of these echolalics will never forget the experience:

Are you ten years old?
Ten years old?
Yes.
Yes.
I mean . . .
I mean . . .

When is your birthday?
Birthday?
Yes.—Oh let it go!
Let it go.

There madness lies. But in little children echolalia is a normal stage of development and, sensibly, they pass through it in a hurry. It is seldom observed in the normal child after two and a half years.

Speech at Two Years. By the time the child reaches his second birthday he should be talking. Speech has become a tool as well as a safety valve or warning siren. He is saying things like: "Where Kitty?" "Ball all gone." "Want cookie." "Kiss baby." "Go bye-bye car." "Shut door." "Big horsie cry." "Put 'bacco in pipe."

Simple and compound sentences are often heard. The jargon is almost gone. His articulation is faulty; his speech rhythms are broken; his voice control ranges from loud to louder, but he has learned to talk. He may still turn out to have any of the speech defects, but he isn't mute. Not by a good many decibels, he isn't.

In summary, we may say again that children *learn* to talk. Their parents do the teaching, and it is usually very poor. Because of the widespread ignorance concerning speech development and the teaching of talking, many children: (1) fail to practice their speech sounds in vocal play; (2) do not learn how to imitate sounds; (3) do not learn that sounds can be meaningful and useful tools; (4) do not practice or profit from their jargon; (5) resort to gesture and other substitute behavior rather than develop a growing vocabulary, and therefore they (6) lay the foundation for defective speech.

Later Speech Development

The third and fourth years of life are especially important in the development of speech for it is during these years that most of the speech disorders might be said to begin. Certainly it is then that articulatory errors become fixed, stuttering starts, and voices begin to assume characteristics which may last throughout the person's life.

The young child has much to learn in the months that surround his third birthday. Prohibitions become important in his life and he becomes negative in turn. Bursting with energy, he meets frustrations at every turn. He must learn to become a social being, whether he wants to or not. The world of words becomes vastly important to the three-year-old. Through speech he finds expression for his emotion. By means of talking, he manipulates his associates and satisfies his needs. He has great need for fluency and precision of utterance.

The few infantile words that he learned during his first two years cannot possibly serve his growing needs. He now needs to express relationships and qualifications. He needs plurals and gender. He becomes conscious of the past and the future, and these demand new verb forms. The whole problem of English syntax presents itself as a challenge to the three-year-old. At the same time, his needs for a larger vocabulary are increasing. "What's that? What's that?" is a game which every parent learns to play, on the answering end. The three-year-old is into everything strange. He tests and tries everything, including the patience of his associates. These explorations yield him many moments of confusion when something never before seen has no name to identify its impact. Thus one three-year-old, who had shown precocious speech development with few if any breaks in fluency, suddenly observed a parachute descent and cried out "ε-ε-ʌ-ʌ-ε -bʌ (gesture of pointing and excited breathing), -bʌd-bʌd- goʊ-bum." At the time, her normal speech was being recorded, and therefore the transcript was accurate. Her usual speech was rhythmic and fluent. It is interesting also that she showed a return to earlier phraseology: "go boom" for the "fall down" which she had been using for over a year. Under the pressure of haste, the unfamiliarity of the experience, the confusion of *airplane* (ε˞) and *bird* (bʌd), both of which were probably felt to be inadequate, the child's fluency broke down and she showed hesitant speech similar to that of primary stuttering.

Besides learning the conventional forms of syntax and acquiring a new vocabulary, the young child must also perfect his pronunciation and articulation. He has many errors to eliminate: the reduplications like "goggy" for "doggy"; the use of the labial *w* for the tongue-tip *l* and *r* sounds; the use of the *t* and *d* for the *k* and *g* plosives; the omissions of many of his final sounds. He also has many new coordinations and sound combinations to master: the precise grooving of the tongue for the sibilants; the transitional timing of the vocalization and movement on the affricatives (tʃ) and (dʒ) and the glide (j); the preparatory positioning of the tongue for the second sound in such blends as *sl, fr,* and *pl.* If these seem like a lot for a three-year-old to master, it must be said that we have only mentioned a few of them. All these and many other articulation skills must be mastered and perfected until they can be used at fast speeds and under conditions of excitement.

Parents often wish to know how well their child is doing in mastering the speech sounds. All we can offer are averages and these often are unfair. Girls acquire the difficult consonants earlier than boys. Children from homes in the higher socio-economic bracket speak more clearly than those from the economically poorer homes. There are many factors which may influence a specific child's progress and so we hesitate to provide any norms. We do so only with the caution that you use these averages as averages and not as yardsticks.

Generally speaking, we can say that the research indicates that children of three years should have mastered most of the vowels and diphthongs, and the *p, b, m, w, t, d, n,* and *h* consonants, should be speaking in short sentences, and should have a vocabulary of about nine hundred words. Many of the other consonants may be heard at times but their use is not consistent and errors of omission, substitution, and distortion occur. However, over 90 per cent of the three-year-old's speech should be readily understood. By five years of age all of his speech should be understandable and the *k, g, f,* and *v* sounds should be used with fair consistency except in the blends (gr, cl, st, etc.). Then during the sixth year the *l* sound, the *s* and *z,* the *sh* and *ch,* and occasionally the *r* which seems often to be very difficult, begin to show themselves regularly. Most of the research indicates that the average child should be speaking standard English by the time he enters first grade or about the time of his seventh birthday. Let us say again that these are averages, that there are always some children developing faster and others more slowly than these norms who must be considered normal.

But there are also children who vary so far from the norm that they need help. Indeed, we feel that every child should be helped by his parents to learn to talk. If the mother would stimulate the child with isolated and nonsense sounds in verbal play, the child would find it easier to master those sounds. Many children have to master their alphabet of sound the hard way, by catching the sounds on the wing. They need easier models. They need to hear what these sounds are like. In our next chapter we will describe ways of teaching the alphabet of sound, and tell you how to help a child recognize that words have heads and tails, and show you how a parent should set models for self-correction. If parents had this information, we feel, many articulatory disorders could be prevented.

Attaining Fluency. If we may return for a moment to the crucial third and fourth years, we will find the child learning to be fluent, learning to keep the utterance flowing. The basic need here is to provide good models for the child, models which are within his reach. Many children go through a temporary period of hesitant speech at this time which, we feel, presents a danger that might be avoided if parents knew what to do.

Just as he imitates his father's pipe-smoking or his mother's sweeping with extreme fidelity, so, too, will he imitate their inflections and voice quality *and* attempt to imitate their fluency. It is in this last item that much of our trouble with stuttering begins. Children of this age do not have the vocabulary to keep their fluency up to adult standards. The adults about them speak to one another and to the children themselves in compound-complex sentences, in paragraphs that flow one after the other in endless series. If they pause, it is for so short an instant that the child cannot get his speech under way. Grownups often penalize interrupting children, but they will interrupt the child's speech with impunity. They finish the child's sentences before he has been able to get them half said. They interrupt to correct a plural or a pronoun or a past participle, and often seize the opportunity to rush on with their own flow of verbalization. When a child tries to adopt an adult fluency pattern of which he is not capable, or if he is bombarded by many of these parental interruptions, he will have hesitant speech. Anyone who has tried to speak a half-learned foreign language with a fluent native will understand what little children undergo. The average parent does not realize what has happened until the child's speech fails to develop normally.

If this childish urge to speak as fluently as his parents when he has neither the vocabulary nor the other necessary skills can precipitate stuttering, we should try to decrease its intensity. Whenever frustration is produced by having an aspiration level far above the person's performance level, we should try to reduce the former. In the case of the child learning to talk, the problem can be solved fairly simply. If the parents will speak to the child, using short phrases and sentences, using simple words whose meaning he can comprehend, using the simplest of syntax, the child will never need to feel speech frustration. He can achieve these fluency patterns without too much difficulty. We have been able, clinically, to free many children from primary stuttering by merely getting their parents to speak more simply. As an example let us quote from a parent's report:

> Each evening, as you suggested, we have been holding a family conference and confessing to each other our errors in handling Ruth. Among other things, we found ourselves constantly talking over her head. Today, for instance, I said to her, "Ruth, do you suppose you could go to the bath room and bring down some of the dirty towels and washcloths? Mama's going to wash." She looked at me intently, then went upstairs and came down with some soap, and said, "Woothy wa-wa-wa-wash bath bath. . . ." and she stuttered pretty badly. So I thanked her for the soap and said, "Ruthy go upstairs. Bring Mama washcloth, please." Her face lit up, and she ran upstairs and down again in a hurry, bringing me the washcloth and a towel too. Then she said, "Woothy bwing wash coth. Nice girl." I begin to see what you mean by speaking more simply.

One need not talk baby talk in order to speak more simply. We must merely give our children fluency models within their performance ability.

If we are to prevent speech defects, we must prevail upon parents to change their present policy of sporadic correction and *laissez faire*. They must learn how to help the child master the difficult skills with which he is confronted in adult speech. They must learn how to keep from making speech-learning difficult. They must not do all the wrong things so blithely.

Acquiring Language and Vocabulary. You will remember that speech consists of a set of symbols. The aphasic's set of symbols has been disordered and perhaps some of the pieces have been lost. This is why he has trouble talking or listening or reading or writing. Let us now see how children acquire these symbols in the first place.

Most parents are eager enough to help the child to get his first twenty or thirty new words. Some parents are even too ambitious at first; they try to teach such words as "Dorothy" or "Semantha." But their teaching urge soon subsides. The child seems to be picking up a few words as he needs them. Why not let him continue to grow

at his own pace? Our answer does not deny the function of maturation in vocabulary growth. We merely say that parents should give
a little common-sense help at moments when a child needs a new
word, a label for a new experience. When parents notice a child
hesitating or correcting himself when faced with a new experience,
they should become verbal dictionaries, providing *not only the
needed new word, but a definition in terms of the child's own vocabulary*. For example:

> John was pointing to something on the shelf he wanted. "Johnny
> want . . . um . . . Johnny want pretty pretty ball . . . Johnny
> wanta pretty . . . um . . ." The object was a round glass vase with
> a square opening on top. I immediately took it down and said, "No
> ball, Johnny. Vase! Vase!" I put my finger into the opening and let him
> imitate me. Then we got a flower and he put it in the opening after
> I had filled it partially with water. I said, "Vase is a flower cup.
> Flower cup, vase! See pretty vase! (I prolonged the *v* sound slightly.)
> Flower drink water in vase, in pretty vase. Johnny, say 'Vase!'"
> (He obeyed without hesitation or error.) Each day that week, I asked
> him to put a new flower in the vase, and by the end of that time he
> was using the word with assurance. I've found one thing though; you
> must speak rather slowly when teaching a new word. Use plenty of
> pauses and patience.

Besides this type of spontaneous vocabulary teaching, it is possible to play little games at home in which the child imitates an older
child or parent as they "touch and say" different objects. Children
invent these games for themselves.

> "March and Say" was a favorite game of twins whom we observed.
> One would pick up a toy telephone, run to the door of the playroom
> and ask his mother, "What dat?" "Telephone," she would answer,
> and then both twins would hold the object and march around the
> room chanting "tɛpoʊn tɛpoʊn" until it ended in a fight for pos-
> session. Then the dominant twin would pick up another object, ask
> its name, and march and chant its name over and over.

In all of these naming games, the child should always point to,
feel, or sense the object referred to as vividly as possible. The mere
sight or sound of the object is not enough for early vocabulary acquisition. It is also wise to avoid cognate terms. One of our children
for years called the cap on a bottle a "hat" because of early confusion.

Scrapbooks are better than the ordinary run of children's books for vocabulary teaching because pictures of objects closer to the child's experience may be pasted in. The ordinary "Alphabet Book" is a monstrosity so far as the teaching of talking is concerned. Nursery rhymes are almost as bad. Let the child listen to "Goosey Goosey Gander, whither dost thou wander" if he enjoys the rhymes, but do not encourage him to say the rhymes. The teaching of talking should be confined to meaningful speech, not gibberish. The three-year-old child has load enough without trying to make sense of nonsense. When using the pictures in the scrapbooks, it is wise to do more than ask the child to name them. When pointing to a ball, the parents should say, "What's that?" "Ball." "Johnny throw ball. Bounce, bounce, bounce" (gestures). Build up associations in terms of the functions of the objects. Teach phrases as well as single words. "Cookie" can always be taught as "eat cookie." This policy may also help the child to remember to keep it out of his hair.

Review of Speech Development in the Child

It would seem appropriate here to summarize the acquisition of speech in all of its aspects. First let us consider its motor characteristics. Beginning with a fairly stable set of reflex behaviors which allow the child to inhale and exhale, to close and open the vocal folds and to move the jaws, lips, tongue, and palate, the child through crying, grunting, sucking, and swallowing becomes able to produce variations in his vocalization. At first, when he makes his noises, large bodily movements accompany this activity. Gradually he becomes able to differentiate the finer from the larger movements. At first, tongue movements are accompanied by jaw and lip activity; later the tongue can move alone. In the laller who finds it difficult to produce a good *r* or *l* sound we often find the lips and jaw still working. That may be why he says "wabbit" for "rabbit" or "witto" for "little." The first speech sounds to be mastered seem to be those which involve relatively easier or less complex coordinations than those which come later. When articulatory errors are present, they usually represent more simple coordinations than those required for the standard sound. The ability to control the breath and voice also shows a progression of mastery.

When we consider speech from its acoustic aspect, we find at first only a limited number of sounds in the baby's repertoire. Irwin (20) tells us that in babies under ten days of age, 92 per cent of all vocalization consists of the front vowels only. Gradually, he begins to use more back vowels and by about three years of age all the vowels should be mastered. The first consonants are those produced by the lips (*p, b, m,* and *w*), the tongue tip (*t, d,* and *n*), or the back of the tongue (*k, g, ng*). The last sounds to be acquired are the *s, l, r, th,* and the blends. We also find growth in fluency and in voice.

When we view speech as a form of symbolic language (speech as thinking), we note a progression beginning in meaningful gestures and tones, proceeding through a period in which the child acquires the first words, then gains vocabulary and finally learns how to use it in the complex formulation of sentences involving commentary, prediction, and recall. In this sequence, comprehension always seems to precede expression. The young child in his preschool years does much of his thinking aloud.

We have seen how speech as communication and social control has its beginnings in the last half of the first year of life. The baby learns to send the important messages to the mother both by wailing and by speech and gesture. The cry sends the message that he is wet or hungry; the nasal grunt and the aversion of the head tells her that he's had enough. In turn, he learns that a horizontal shaking of the mother's head or a curious little sound means "No." Later, he learns that he can manipulate big people by using sounds, can get what he wants by using words. With proper models and rewards, he rapidly learns the magical utility of speech as communication and social control. He finds that although talking is a rather complicated business, it's well worth learning. Some children never discover this.

Finally, we again come to speech as the expression of the self. Beginning with the cry for attention, the banging of the cup on the high chair, the baby learns that he exists and that he can force others to recognize that important fact. As Walt Whitman put it, he learns "to celebrate myself and sing myself." When the baby begins to explore his toes and mouth (occasionally at the same time) the concept of self is vague but eventually he learns who he is. At first the baby almost seems to regard himself as another object in a world full of interesting things. He uses his first name to designate himself or says "me go bye-bye." Piaget, the famous French psychologist, long ago pointed out that when a child first begins to use the perpendicular pronoun "I," a huge step has been taken. This generally occurs in the third and fourth years. Much egocentric speech occurs during this latter period and many of the child's insatiable questions and demands are used more for calling attention to himself than for communication. Again in this use of speech as an expression of the self, we find learning, growth, and development.

PROJECTS

1. Visit a nursery school and report on the ways the speech of these children differs from that of adults. Note voice, rhythm, and language as well as articulation.
2. Spend an hour with an awakened baby less than one year old and report your observations of his communicative behavior.
3. Interview the mother of a child about a year and a half old to discover her methods for teaching the child to talk.
4. Go to a pet store and locate the owner of a talking bird. Visit the owner and interview her to determine how the bird was taught to talk. Also report the bird's repertoire and the conditions under which it talks best.
5. Tape-record some infant vocalizations.
6. Write an answer to a mother who has asked you how to teach her child to talk.
7. Visit a school for mentally retarded children and evaluate their speech development.
8. How did Helen Keller, blind and deaf from birth, learn to talk?
9. Prepare a paper on subhuman communication.
10. Dolphins seem to be able to communicate with each other very well. One research center sought a speech therapist to try to teach them to talk to humans. Conduct a library search on this topic and report what you find and whether or not you think the project would be feasible.
11. How did speech develop in the human race? Read Chapter 1 in Travis' *Handbook of Speech Pathology* (28) and report.
12. Interview parents of young children to compile a vocabulary list of infant words which differ from the adult forms of these words.
13. We have a recording of a dog saying or rather growling "Hamburger!" How can you explain the methods used for teaching him to do this?
14. Prepare a chart illustrating speech development.
15. Describe the language of bees. Read *Bees, Their Vision, Chemical*

Senses and Language by K. von Frisch. Ithaca: Cornell University Press, 1950.

READINGS AND REFERENCES

16. Battin, R. R. "Two Methods for Presenting Information on Speech and Language Development," *Journal Speech and Hearing Disorders,* Volume 27, 1962, pages 17-22.
17. Berry, M. F., and Eisenson, J. *Speech Disorders.* New York: Appleton-Century-Crofts, 1956, Chapter 3.
18. Goda, S. "Vocal Utterances of Young Moderately and Severely Retarded Non-Speaking Children," *American Journal Mental Deficiency,* Volume 65, 1960, pages 269-273.
19. Greene, M. C. *Learning to Talk.* New York: Harper & Row, Publishers, 1960, pages 1-76.
20. Hawk, S. S. "Can a Child Be Taught to Talk?" *Journal Speech Disorders,* Volume 4, 1939, pages 173-179.
21. Irwin, O. C. "Speech Development in the Young Child: II. Some Factors Related to the Speech Development of the Infant and Young Child," *Journal Speech and Hearing Disorders,* Volume 17, 1952, pages 269-279.
22. Lewis, M. M. *Infant Speech.* New York: Harcourt, Brace & World, Inc., 1936.
23. Metraux, R. W. "Speech Profiles of the Pre-school Child 18 to 54 Months," *Journal Speech and Hearing Disorders,* Volume 15, pages 37-53.
24. Morley, M. M. *The Development and Disorders of Speech in Childhood.* Baltimore: The Williams & Wilkins Co., 1957, pages 1-55.
25. Mowrer, O. H. "Hearing and Speaking: An Analysis of Language Learning," *Journal Speech and Hearing Disorders,* Volume 23, 1958, pages 143-152.
26. Myklebust, H. R. "Babbling and Echolalia," *Journal Speech and Hearing Disorders,* Volume 22, 1956, pages 356-360.
27. Poole, I. "Genetic Development of Articulation of Consonant Sounds in Speech," *Elementary English Review,* Volume 11, 1934, pages 159-161.
28. Travis, L. E. (ed.). *Handbook of Speech Pathology.* New York: Appleton-Century-Crofts, 1957.
29. Van Riper, C. *Teaching Your Child to Talk.* New York: Harper & Row, Publishers, 1950, pages 1-96.

CHAPTER FIVE

Delayed Speech: Its Nature and Causes

The Problem

When most children reach the age of seven or eight, they have learned the basic motor skills needed to produce speech which is acoustically satisfactory, which sounds normal. They are then using inner speech as well as overt speech for thinking—for commentary, prediction, and recall. They certainly have learned to employ speech to control others and to satisfy some of their wants. They have learned to use it in sending and receiving messages. Most of them, with more or less efficiency, have found how useful speech can be in expressing their happy and unpleasant feelings. And they have also discovered the joy of employing speech for the display of the self. They will make gains in all of these aspects of speech, but the essential first learning has taken place. The process has been a gradual one but a normal one.

This chapter concerns those other children who show marked retardation in speech development. Some of them were slow to say their first words. Some of them were still unable to speak in sentences when they came to us for help. There are children who speak only through gestures or grunts; others who speak copiously but in a jargon not even their parents can understand. Some have difficulty in receiving messages; they do not hear or comprehend the spoken word. For a few, the problem seems to be focused in emotion— they do not want to talk or dare to talk. We have worked with children who used, not speech, but the lack of speech, mutism, to control others, to get the special consideration they could achieve in no other way. There are mentally retarded children who do not talk because they have nothing to say. We have known twins who invented their own language and preferred it.

To find some term which could cover such a hodgepodge of children, speech therapists have come to use the phrase *delayed speech*. Although Myklebust[1] and others have disliked the term and feel that it contributes to sloppy diagnosis, yet it still describes the essential feature of the complaint. These children have failed to acquire normal speech as a usable tool. They have been slow in speech mastery. They cannot use speech as other children do to serve the various needs which speech can serve. Some of them are not only delayed but seem to be fixated, unable to progress. The parent who brings us such a child, brings him because he seems to be markedly retarded in acquiring usable speech. We wish to emphasize this concept of usable or *tool speech*. By tool speech we mean the use of speech to fulfill the person's communicative needs. We can consider speech as a tool, or speech as an ornament. Without belaboring the point, we would say that *when a child's articulation, vocabulary, sentence structure, and speech output are so deviant from normal standards that listeners often cannot understand him,* he can be said to possess delayed speech. Such a child has not yet acquired the ability to communicate, to control others (or himself), or to express his feelings in speech so others can understand them. A child who lisps is not so denied. A laller's speech may not be ornamental but it is useful. The child who has delayed speech is a deprived child; he doesn't just have a blemish. He lacks the tools and the skill to use them. Our task with the lisper is to remove the flaws in a tool he already can use. When we work with a child who has delayed speech, we often have to help him build a tool and teach him how to use it.

Case Presentations

At this point it might be wise to provide some glimpses of the actual pictures presented by these children with delayed speech.

Dick is a post-encephalitic child with no motor or hearing defect. He was first seen at 4.8 years of age. An occasional grunt, used indis-

[1] Myklebust, H. R., "Aphasia in Children." Chapter 16 in Travis, E. E., *Handbook of Speech Pathology.* New York: Appleton-Century-Crofts, 1957, page 515.

criminately comprised his total verbal output. No imitative oral responses could be elicited. Communicative contact was pointedly evaded and he was extremely hyperactive. Gestures were infrequently used to indicate what he wanted. The prognosis made by physicians was that he would never develop the use of speech. At 6.8 years he was imitating sounds and producing word approximations. Spontaneous speech was limited to one-word sentences, but symbol meaning was clear only when the subject was known to the listener. Responsiveness and contact were improving. At 8.2 years he was able to imitate most of the consonant sounds; spontaneous speech was frequently understandable although still limited in output. Phrases and sentences such as "open the door," "your green car," "boy drink milk," objects and picture naming, and ready responses to greetings were indicative of a much improved communication adjustment.[2]

Here is the description of a wedding as narrated by a ten-year-old British girl:

I went to Reading. See, see bus. Long time. Went swimming. Mummy. Me. And the black man by. Mummy job. Down a stream. Quiet. Married. Long way. Very long way. Church. When I went there, fell I did. And I went soon, soon. Know her, she bride. Went to Reading, bus. Went to seaside. Not. Only next. Next. See the bridge. Way to holidays.[3]

Some children with delayed speech use only grunts and gestures. Here is such a child:

Don was five years old, physically normal, and his parents were completely convinced of his intelligence. His hearing was good and so were his coordinations. He seemed to comprehend speech very well and could follow directions with ease. Possibly because of an early isolation on a farm with few playmates, he had few friends and preferred to play alone. He was well behaved and his lack of speech and of interest in socialization seemed to be his only real difference. His parents had become quite anxious about his delay in learning to talk but seemed to love him. He was an only child. With this brief introduction, let us give you the observer's report. The observer watched the child and his parents through a one-way mirror and heard him over a hidden intercommunication system.

---

[2] Schlanger, B. B. "A Longitudinal Study of Speech and Language Development of Brain Damaged Retarded Children," *Journal Speech and Hearing Disorders*, Volume 24, 1959, pages 358-359.

[3] Renfrew, C. E. "Speech Problems of Backward Children," *Speech Pathology and Therapy*, Volume 2, 1959, page 35.

Father told Don to take off his hat and coat and to hang them on the rack. Boy did this without hesitation, then returned to play table and looked at toys. Father told him to help himself. He worked the little pump and when the little ball came out of the spout he smiled, looked at the father and said, "uhn, uhn, uhn" and pointed to the ball. Father told Don to put ball back into upper hole of pump. Don did, then pumped handle but ball was stuck. Looked at father who was not paying attention. Took pump to father and said, "oo." Father shook pump and ball came out. Don put ball back and shook pump. Ball did not come out so he put it down and put his thumb in his mouth. Father withdrew it without comment. Don said, "no," and put thumb back in mouth. Father said, "Cut it out, you hear me?" Don obeyed but held thumb in other hand. Father opened picture book and said, "See cow? Say cow." Don looked but did not respond. Father said, "Say cow. Try it anyway." Don said, "uhn."

This was typical of the entire half-hour of observation. The only recognizable word was "No." Boy used monosyllables to call attention and then conveyed his meaning with gestures. If he could not make himself understood, he just gave up, waited quietly, or turned to something else.

This case is not typical. In fact, one of the major characteristics of delayed speech problems is its variability. But the child's reliance upon gesture, grunting, and attention-getting phonation is commonly found. Some of these children have so little interest in speech that they not only will not make any effort to talk but also they show no interest in listening. Some of them have in consequence been sent to feeble-minded institutions or to schools for the deaf or treated as aphasics. Children who cannot send messages by mouth have little incentive to receive them by ear. In examining them we must be careful to explore thoroughly for instances in which they did respond or attempt to communicate. The general picture may lead to a false diagnosis.

Another fairly common pattern of delayed speech is the child who vocalizes constantly but speaks a gibberish which cannot be understood:

One of the children we examined vocalized every minute of her stay with us. She was a restless, wandering child whose attention constantly shifted. As she picked up one toy, threw it down, ran to the window, tapped at the pane, shook her skirt, sucked her thumb, laughed at her reflection in the mirror, and performed a hundred other consecutive activities, she accompanied each with a constant flow of unintelligible jabber. By using a hidden microphone, we were able to record some samples of her speech. The speech sample together with the object of her attention ran like this:

"Yugga boo booda . . . iganna min . . ." (jʌgɔ bu budɔ igæ nɔ min.) Picked up the toy automobile and threw it down. "Annakuh innuhpohee . . . tseeguh . . . tseekuh . . ." (ænakɔ inɔpohi ʈsigʌ ʈsikɔ.) Looked out window and tapped at pane.

In this case we were unable to recognize any mutilations of familiar words, though in most cases of delayed speech careful analysis will isolate a few words, consistently used, which bear some resemblance to their conventional cognates. Both of these general types of delayed speech can result from fixation at an infantile level of speech development. They can also occur regressively as the result of a sudden accident, illness, or emotional shock, even when the previous speech development has been excellent. Both mutism and unintelligibility are relative terms, since noises are made by all mutes, and even in the worst jargon faint resemblances to meaningful words are occasionally found. The problem of delayed speech, however, is more than that of a severe articulation defect. These children are also handicapped linguistically and semantically. They often do not comprehend the language of others, nor are they particularly interested in vocal symbols even when they can understand them. The longer they go without receiving help in attaining a normal method of communication, the more they tend to ignore the speech of others. Jerry and Larry were fraternal twins with normal speech development in their first year. They had begun to speak in one-word sentences when Larry became ill and was hospitalized for six months, during which Jerry learned to speak in sentences, but Larry regressed to grunts and babbling. Speech therapy was begun at once, and the parents cooperated fully, but Larry stayed behind Jerry's speech level until they were in the third grade. Neither emotional factors nor residual effects of the illness seemed to have caused the delay. Instead, it seemed that Larry had by-passed the critical period of speech readiness.

Incidence

There are few studies which report the frequency of occurrence of delayed speech, perhaps because many of these children do not go to school and hence are omitted in the usual surveys. Perhaps some idea of the incidence may be gained by the fact that in two years, 454 cases of delayed speech were examined by the hospital services of the University of Iowa.[3] Although most of the very severely handicapped delayed-speech cases never enter school, all speech therapists meet some children with delayed speech and so do most early elementary school teachers. Perhaps the best normative study to date is that of Morley,[4] in England, who reports, in her long-term study of 114 children, that at the time of school entrance (four years, nine months) 4 per cent were still unintelligible, and at the age of six and a half years only one child had speech which still could not be understood. We may perhaps conclude that fewer than 1 per cent of our children have delayed speech. If this seems like an insignificant fraction, let us say immediately that for the parents of such a child or for the child himself, the inability to communicate is far from insignificant. Homes have been wrecked, lives have been distorted, all because a little child never learned to talk. We have saved some of these children from a life of custodial care in a state institution for the feeble-minded. We have seen some of them end in an institution for the insane. We have known many others who eked out a miserable existence in school and in life, unable to read or write or speak well enough to take their place in the human family. These children need proper diagnosis and special care. Many of them can be taught to communicate effectively if given early treatment.

Onset

Since delayed speech might be considered a developmental failure, it is difficult to state at what time it begins. However, in their review of the age at which the first words are acquired by babies, Darley and Winitz[5] conclude that when a child has not acquired his first

---

[3] Goodwin, F. B. "A Consideration of Etiologies in 454 Cases of Speech Retardation," *Journal Speech and Hearing Disorders,* Volume 20, 1955, pages 300-303.

[4] Morley, M. E. *The Development and Disorders of Speech in Childhood.* London: E. and S. Livingstone, 1957.

[5] Darley, F. L., and Winitz, H. "Age of First Word: Review of Research," *Journal Speech and Hearing Disorders,* Volume 26, 1961, pages 272-290.

words by 18-24 months, there is indication of "severe retardation or disability." Our own review of the research on the onset of speaking in phrases and sentences leads us to conclude that any child who is not using at least a few understandable two-word phrases or sentences by the age of thirty months should be referred to a physician or speech therapist immediately. According to Stinchfield and Young[6] there seems to be a restricted period, which these

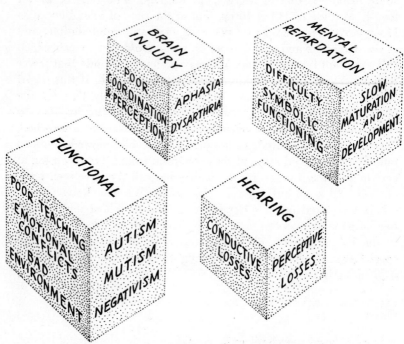

FIGURE 12. *Causes of Delayed Speech*

authors call the "speech readiness period," which encompasses the time between the ninth and twenty-fourth months, during which the child seems especially ripe for speech learning. He may be taught to talk much later, but it is during this period that he will learn his speech skills most quickly and thoroughly. We are here speaking of

---

[6] Stinchfield, S. M., and Young, E. H. *Children with Delayed or Defective Speech*, Stanford University Press, 1938.

the normal child, not of the child with mental retardation, brain injury, or deafness. In later sections we shall discuss their problems.

The causes of speech retardation fall into four main categories: (1) mental retardation; (2) functional causes; (3) brain injuries; (4) hearing loss. Of these, the first—mental retardation—accounts for a substantial number of our cases. The admittedly vague classification of functional causes includes not only those of emotional conflicts but also the environmental influences which make it difficult for a child to learn to talk. Brain injuries such as those resulting from accidents, disease, or birth traumata are represented in the speech delay we find in cerebral palsy, postencephalitis, aphasia, and similar organic problems. Hearing loss includes the congenitally deaf, the deafened, and those who are hard of hearing.

The relative importance of these factors in producing delayed speech is revealed in studies by Wood,[7] Goodwin,[8] and Morley.[9] Wood found that one third of her delayed-speech cases seemed to be due to brain injury and showed aphasic language disturbances; one fifth of them seemed to be due to mental retardation; and the rest were listed as falling under the headings of hearing loss, immaturity, and unintelligible articulation. In about 5 per cent the cause could not be diagnosed. Goodwin's cases came from children referred to the hospital services of the University of Iowa and 35 per cent were mentally retarded; 26 per cent showed brain-damage origins; 11 per cent were due to functional causes; 11 per cent to hearing loss; and in 21 per cent the cause could not be determined. Morley's figures show a higher incidence of delayed speech due to hearing loss.

[7] Wood, N. E. "Communication Problems and their Effect on the Learning Potential of the Mentally Retarded Child." Cleveland: Western Reserve University; U.S. Office of Education, Department of Health, Education and Welfare Cooperative Research Project Number 184 (6539), 1960.

[8] Goodwin, F. B. "A Consideration of Etiologies in 454 Cases of Speech Retardation," *Journal Speech and Hearing Disorders,* Volume 20, 1955, pages 300-303.

[9] Morley, M. *The Development and Disorders of Speech in Childhood.* London: E. S. Livingstone, 1957, page 63.

Mental Retardation

It is interesting that the research corroborates what every parent of a delayed-speech child tends to fear (and what the neighbors are certain is the problem)—that low intelligence may possibly be the cause of the delay. In our discussion of the many aspects of speech, we have tried to show its complex function. Learning to talk is a complicated business. It is not easy. Since the mentally retarded child finds it difficult to learn even simple skills, we should not be surprised to find them slow to talk. Various researches show that the mentally retarded are significantly delayed in uttering their first words, first phrases or sentences. Those who are very deficient operate on a vegetable-like level of existence and never learn to talk at all. However, those who are educable can certainly be taught to speak well enough to find a place in our society. Unfortunately few of them are given the professional help they need daily. As a result, their speech age is usually much lower than their mental age, to say nothing of their chronological age. They are truly delayed in speech.

But let us make very clear that mental retardation is not always, or even generally, the cause of delayed speech. There are other reasons. Moreover, we must distinguish between mental deficiency and mental retardation. In the former, we usually have a constitutional problem. There is a basic impairment in intellectual functioning which is incurable and which allows us little hope for social or vocational adequacy. A famous American psychologist once defined, in jest, the zero level of intelligence as one which could be determined by the following test: "When ordered to bite off one's own toes, will do so." We have known children with very low IQ's but when they show profound mental deficiency such as that of the so-called low grade idiot, they would not even understand such a direction even if they could carry it out. We worked with one of these children daily for six months using every ounce of intelligence and effort at our disposal and finally got him to say "Ugg" occasionally when we entered the room. It may have been disgust.

We have been more fortunate with the mentally retarded. "It isn't that they don't have their buttons. They do have some but they don't seem to know how to use them," was a comment of one of our student therapists. We have found that patient, daily training can be successful if we use rewards, and try to get one-word commentary or commands, first through parallel talk (which will be described later in this chapter), then through simple phrases and short sentences. We emphasize tool speech, not display speech. We try to create the same conditions of interaction which produce speech in the normal infant: love and mutual sharing of activity and imitation. Many of these children seem to think in gestures and postural symbols rather than in words. They code their perceptions in a "body English" rather than in language. They have trouble in remembering or in predicting because it is difficult to remember or to predict with gestures or postures. They have trouble in perceiving because they have no labels. We provide the simple words they used for these functions, and finally they begin to use them. Our mouths must at first be their brains. We have attained some surprisingly satisfactory results.

Indeed we suspect that more intensive language training will eventually be the key feature of special education for the mentally retarded. Many of these children, once they learn to talk, show remarkable growth in functioning. Socially they become more adequate. Their tested IQ's go up somewhat. In part these increases in IQ are due to a more improved ability to comprehend the examiner's directions. Children who cannot send messages are not particularly interested in or adept at receiving them. We are not speaking here of the results of verbal intelligence tests such as the Stanford-Binet which are not at all appropriate for the child with delayed speech, but of such performance tests as the performance section of the Wechsler[10] or the Arthur Adaptation of the Leiter Scale[11] or such picture-pointing tests as the Ammons.[12] Even on these "non-verbal" tests, children do much better once they have learned to speak a bit. It is quite possible that many children appear, or even become, mentally retarded because they never learn to speak. Thinking, perceiving, remembering, predicting—all of these require the use of symbols. When the human race invented

---

[10] Wechsler, D. *Wechsler Intelligence Scale for Children.* New York: Psychological Corporation, 1949.

[11] Arthur, G. *The Arthur Adaptation of the Leiter International Performance Scale.* Washington, D.C.: Psychological Service Center Press, 1952.

[12] Ammons, R. B., and Ammons, H. S. *The Full-Range Picture Vocabulary Test.* New Orleans: R. B. Ammons, 1948.

speech, it devised a set of symbols which enabled it to conquer the earth. Some little children, for want of special teaching early enough, never share that heritage. It is true that mental deficiency can cause delayed speech; it is also true that delayed speech can contribute to mental retardation.

Functional Causes

Under this admittedly vague heading we should like to place two sets of problems: (1) those in which emotional disturbance seemed to be the basic reason for the speech delay and (2) those in which environmental conditions or poor methods of teaching made the learning of speaking very difficult. In the individual case, it is often difficult to separate the two, since both may be involved. But there are children who are bright who do not talk, who have no brain injury or hearing loss.

Emotional Disturbance. The range of problems encountered in this category is wide. In it we find children who are psychotic or autistic at one extreme, and children who are emotionally immature or negative at the other. They do not learn to talk because, perhaps, they fear the communicative relationships which speaking demands or because their flood of inner emotional static prevents them from hearing the models they need. Some of these children live in a world of their own. Others find their *lack* of speech a powerful tool for controlling others. There are children who find the awaiting world of adult life too unpleasant a prospect after they hear their parents screaming at each other, and so they prefer to remain infants all their days. What better way than to refuse to talk? Why should a child wish to put something into his mouth if it is unpleasant or painful? Why should a child speak if that speaking puts him in contact with someone he fears or hates? Speaking is revealing; there are children who cannot bear the exposure. We cannot possibly sketch all the ways in which emotional problems can produce speech delay, but we will touch on some of them.

Voluntary Mutism. This term is not an exact one. Often the refusal to attempt to speak is not voluntary but compulsive. In the histories of some of our cases of delayed speech we find that at one time they had begun to talk, not only in single words but also in sentences. Then something happened—a shock, an accident, a severe illness, a frightening experience, a stay at a hospital. The parents can often tell you only that the child suddenly stopped talking.

Austra was a Latvian girl of seven who had experienced many of the terrors of displacement and bombing raids. She came to us two years after her father had finally managed to get to the safety of the United States. Her mother and brother and two sisters had been killed. Austra seemed to comprehend everything we said to her and her performance on the Wechsler Intelligence test was superior but she talked only in grunts and gestures. The father told us that she had spoken very well until the age of three. She seemed to be a very happy child. Her father put the matter succinctly: "Austra has forgotten, but her mouth remembers." It took a lot of doing, but Austra learned to talk and is now in college.

Very often we find some indication that the onset of the disorder seems to lie in a situation where the child was in the act of talking when the traumatic experience occurred.

As an illustration, the treatment of the child who lost the power of speech after being knocked down by a dog may be described:

The speech correctionist to whom the child was referred spent a week of fifteen-minute daily periods in gaining the child's confidence. In these periods games were played in which the child's dominance over toys, teddy bears, and so on, was stressed. The clinician never spoke to the child but used sign language entirely. Gradually, games were introduced in which activity was accompanied by vocalization. There was a spiral maze in which a little train traveled the grooves when pushed by the humming clinician. If the child pushed the train without humming, the clinician shook his head and took the toy away from him. Pictures of dogs were hidden about the room and the child learned to say "dah-dah-dah" until he found them. A stuffed toy dog was provided and the child was encouraged to roll a large ball in the attempt to knock it over. The clinician then held the toy dog and made it prance and dodge the ball. All activity by this time was accompanied by some kind of vocalization, and the clinician occasionally used one or two words such as *dog, train,* and *here.* A puppy which had previously been trained to play the ball game was brought in, and when the child appeared for his conference the clinician was playing ball with it. The child was given the ball, and, rolling it at the puppy, knocked it over. "Look, look, I did it," he said spontaneously, and from that time on, speech returned swiftly. The child seemed very cruel to the puppy for a while, but gradually this attitude changed. Later, the clinician taught the game of "Knock-down," in which alternately the child and the clinician and the puppy pretended to attack and to be knocked over. The child was very amused by this game and kept a running conversation going all the time in imitation of the clinician.

Negativism. Our culture demands much of its young. At the very time that the child is learning to talk, a hundred other demands are put upon him. He must learn how to eat at the table, how to control his bowels, how to be quiet, how to pick up his toys, how to behave himself. And this is the age at which we find out that we are *selves*, not objects, that we are important in our own right. This is the "bull-headed" obstinate age, when the child learns how to say that favorite word of his parents: "No!" There are children who fiercely resist the constant pressure to conform, who fight a gallant but losing battle against incredible odds. And there are a few children who actually win, by discovering the one way they can refuse and get away with it. They refuse to talk.

You can't make a horse drink. You can't make a child talk. The tenacity with which some children resist their parents' efforts to eliminate thumb sucking is minor compared to that shown by some children who triumph by not speaking. It's a tough problem to handle, once it has existed for a few years. At times the negativism is widespread; often it seems to be focused on speech alone. First, we must convince the parents and associates of the child to stop making the usual demands that he say this and say that, and inhibit their complaining expressions of anxiety. We must remove the rewards which negativism brings. Here is one brief account of a child who had but one word in his vocabulary.

> The teacher said to the child in a rather peremptory tone, "Johnny, you go down to the drugstore this very minute and get yourself an ice-cream cone!" The child answered "No" and the teacher asked another child, who accepted and returned to eat the ice-cream cone under Johnny's regretful nose. Such a program soon brought a discriminatory answer to requests and commands, and when reward for positive response was added, together with humorous attitudes toward the negativism, the child's whole attitude changed, and his speech soon became normal.

Many of these children profit from a change in environment— placement in a nursery school—where they can learn from other children that speaking can be more pleasant than refusing to speak.

Autism. The autistic child is a strange child, sometimes very intelligent. It almost seems as though he is too hypersensitive to be able to bear the barrage of stimulation in which our children must live. Alexander Pope once wrote of the sensitive soul who "dies of a rose in aromatic pain." Autistic children are threatened by too much noise (and even a little noise is too much), too much color, too much movement, too many people—and sometimes even one parent is too much. They build walls around themselves, barriers to stimulation. Some of them do not seem to hear because they refuse to listen. Some of them sing the same little nameless tune over and over again to mask out the sounds and speech that can overwhelm them. Certain autistic youngsters concentrate on puzzles or mathematic manipulations to keep the world's fingers out of their lives. They may rock back and forth interminably to keep everything the same. Some of them do not talk at all or talk to themselves in a strange tongue. Other autistic children will talk a little, and even answer questions, but always in a detached and perfunctory fashion with a minimum of meaning and little feeling. They are strange children, not of this world. We have worked successfully with a few of them and have failed with more than a few. They require time and devotion which few of us can afford.

Improper Teaching Methods. In the previous chapter we described the facilitating environmental conditions and parental practices which resulted in the baby's learning to talk. Some children do not have the sort of conditions or teachers they need. Few parents understand enough about the principles of speech development to provide the special help some children require. They make too generous an assortment of mistakes. They may overstimulate or understimulate the child. They demand the wrong kind of speech at the wrong times. They may not create the kind of an interacting loving relationship out of which speech evolves. There are many other reasons.

An authority on child care once said that children learn to speak not because of parental teaching, but in spite of it. The average child certainly does seem to exhibit a remarkable ability to acquire speech when the teaching is so poor that it hardly merits the name. All that most young parents know of the teaching of talking is that they should hold out an object and repeat its name over and over. Meanwhile, they hope that the miracle will happen, and it usually does. But some children need more skillful teaching and do not acquire speech until such teaching is forthcoming. Some of the common errors made by parents in the teaching of talking are: stimulation at the wrong time, too much or too little stimulation, the wrong kind of stimulation, disregard of the need for motivation, and improper use of association to provide meanings.

Some parents begin to try to get the child to imitate them as early as the third and fourth months, whereas no attempts should be made until about the seventh month, and imitation of motor behavior should always precede imitation of speech. Stimulation at a time when the child has not reached the proper level of maturation is not only useless but also actually harmful, since it merely reduces the child's interest in the stimulation. Other parents will wake the child out of a deep slumber or will interrupt such prepotent activities as feeding to ask him to say "bye-bye." The first teaching of talking should be confined to the child's vocal play periods.

Even intelligent parents frequently overstimulate or understimulate the child and use improper types of stimulation. Children who are neglected, even in the interests of modern child education, will be delayed in their speech. Then, too, children who are bombarded from every side by crowing parents, by masses of endearing or admiring verbiage, can hardly be expected to respond selectively. Parents who have heard of the evils of using baby talk (which certainly is an evil at a later stage of speech development) confine their stimulation to such words as *bicycle, mother,* and *nurse,* and they occasionally rebuke their unlucky offspring for such achievements as *ba* for *ball.* As we have seen, the first stimulation should be the imitation of the child's own vocal play; and the next should be monosyllables or double syllables which the child has practiced previously. Later, after the child has learned to enjoy and to use speech and shows eagerness for new names, the true disyllables (such as *water*) can be used.

Many parents, made unintelligent by the presence of a new object for their self-love, seek to anticipate their child's every wish. They rush to give the ball to the child if he so much as looks at it. Were they wise, they would move it a little closer and provoke some speech attempt, thus using the situation for the teaching of talking. Probably the most frequent functional cause of delayed speech is this parental overeagerness. Children won't talk unless they profit from the attempt. Speech is a tool, and if it is not needed, it will not be used. Parents should be very careful to prevent the formation of such a condition, for only by careful and systematic retraining can it be broken down.

Finally, parents make the mistake of tearing down associations as fast as they are built. Instead of concentrating their teaching on a few simple words and their associated objects, they overwhelm the child with synonyms and adjectives and terms of endearment, a hodgepodge of stimulation which would make a nonspeaking adult with an IQ of 150 give up in despair. The use of a little applied intelligence, and some consideration of the child's outlook, will solve this problem.

Poor Speech Standards. Another cause of delayed speech is the prevalence of poor speech standards in the home. This condition is closely related to a lack of motivation, although the latter usually refers more to the substitution of a gesture language than to the presence of a primitive vocal language which results from the parental acceptance of distorted speech. Many a child of four and five is brought to the speech correctionist with speech so unintelligible that no one save the mother can understand what the child is trying to say. Twins and children of similar ages often develop a serviceable speech of this sort. One pair of twins used much vocalization when communicating with each other but used only gestures when speaking to adults. In their primitive vocabulary, the following words seemed to be used consistently: "we-we" (meaning either "I" or "you"); "eee" (any adult); "bam" (ball); "bam-aa" (apple). There were other similar distortions and substitutions. In general, this type of speech consists of the more primitive lip, nasal, and tongue-tip sounds used with the neutral or front vowels. Most of the words are approximations of those used by adults, with the distortions produced by substituting easier sounds for more difficult ones. Since the parents or associates of these children accept this counterfeit speech, the child has no incentive to improve it.

These poor speech standards are occasionally due to parental baby talk, but more often they are the result of illness or handicap which has made the parent reluctant to put any extra pressure on the child. After the illness, the parents resolve to insist upon good speech, and so they nag and correct and scold the child for a period of days. This procedure seldom produces any great change, because a strong penalty or pressure placed upon any activity as unconscious as speech tends to stamp in the error and to make it more permanent. Moreover, the mere command, "Don't say 'eee,' say 'mama' !" does not show the child how he can make the new coordinations. And again, constant nagging about the child's poor speech will surely arouse an emotional conflict, for not even an adult can watch his speech continually. Therefore, the parents usually give up the attempt and hope the child will outgrow his poor speech habits.

Better methods than those suggested in the last paragraph will be discussed in some detail later in this chapter. But it can be emphasized that good speech standards must be built gradually and that the child must be shown how to make the desired words. The parents should concentrate their efforts on not more than five words, and these words should be composed of the easier speech sounds. The child must be taught to make the sounds which comprise these words and should be able to make them at will. This teaching of sounds should be confined to a few situations or speech periods which are part of the child's daily routine. Only good-natured and humorously vivid penalties should be used, and rewards should be stressed. When the child is first able to make the desired word, corrections should still be confined to these nucleus speech periods. But as these words and nucleus situations become completely mastered, the requirements may be extended until all words and all situations must conform to the adequate speech standards.

Unfavorable Environmental Conditions.   Some children are born into homes where conditions are unfavorable to speech development. There are silent homes where the parents rarely talk to each other. There are homes so confused with the noise and distraction of ten other children that the harried mother has no time to create the relationship out of which speech comes. Sick children are slow to talk and there are sick homes too. Some children hear little but angry speech. One of our cases who had lived with his grandmother, stopped talking when he was returned to his real parents who were deaf-mutes. Often we have seen speech decay and disappear when an orphan child was shuffled from one foster home to another. When two languages are spoken in a home, one by the older children and the other by the parents, some children get too confused to talk.

If a child is to talk there must be some identification with the parent. We knew one little girl whose mother was a sodden drunken bum with whom no child could identify as she staggered around the house, dirty, cursing, and in half collapse. We have worked with children too hungry, too weak, or tired to talk and had to take care of these basic needs before they had a chance to learn. The county sheriff once brought us three almost-wild children from a hut in a swamp only a few miles from Kalamazoo. The father was a feeble-minded junk scavenger who fed them when he could. The mother had abandoned them. The tale is too incredible to put in a text book, but those three nonspeaking children in the observation room were animal children. Yes, there are environmental conditions which prevent speech development.

Brain Damage. Some children get off to a bad start on the road of life by having birth injuries. Others start well but fall victim to severe illnesses or accidents along the way. When the brain is damaged by any of these traumata, there is always the possibility of speech delay. If the central nervous system is damaged, we may find a general mental deficiency causing delay in most functions, but, in other instances, we may find instead the awkward coordinations of cerebral palsy or the inability to use meaningful symbols as in aphasia. In other injuries, a central hearing loss may be the result. There are also some less conspicuous aftermaths of brain damage—hyperactivity, irritability, inability to tolerate stress, perceptual difficulties—all of which may make it difficult for the child to learn to talk. To learn to speak, we must hear; we must be able to coordinate our muscles; we must be able to handle symbols; we must have good auditory perception. Brain injury can affect any or all of these items.

Dysarthria. This term refers to distorted speech caused by injuries of the central nervous system which make the coordinations needed for speech very difficult. Tongues may be clumsy; the lips may flutter tremulously, the jaw may fail to move on time or move sidewise; the larynx may be wrenched out of place; the chest may be expanding as in inhalation at the very time the child is trying to talk. The degree of involvement may be either widespread or almost hidden to all but the expert eye. We have worked with individuals whose only dysarthria was in the utterance of the tongue-tip sounds. Some cerebral palsied individuals find the task of coordination so difficult they never learn to speak. Many of them can be taught to do so, even though arms and legs quiver and jerk, and the face contorts with the effort. We also find *apraxias* associated with the dysarthrias in some of our cases, and in others, the apraxia occurs alone. By apraxia we mean the inability to make a movement voluntarily which can otherwise be produced involuntarily. Some children, for example, can curl up the end of their tongues to lick a tantalizing bit of peanut butter from an upper lip but cannot, no matter how they try, do the same thing voluntarily. Such a child might be able to pick up a toothbrush and move it around but could not brush his teeth. It almost seems as though the failure is in the ability to command these muscles.

Aphasia. The term aphasia refers to the loss of speech and so it may seem inappropriate to use it in children who have never developed speech. Some speech therapists prefer to use the term "developmental aphasia" instead. As we have seen in Chapter II, aphasia refers to disorders of symbolization, to disorders of language rather than speech. It may include disabilities in reading, writing, gesturing, calculating, drawing, as well as in speaking. The basic problem revolves about the use of symbols. So far as speech is concerned, these children find difficulty in formulating their thoughts in words, in expressing them verbally, or in comprehending what others are saying. It's hard for them to send messages or, less frequently, to receive them. Formulating, expressing, comprehending, these are the functions which trouble the person who is aphasic. Some aphasic children have more difficulty with visual symbols; others, more trouble with symbols involving sounds. Some who cannot read (alexia) can write or copy the symbols they see on the printed page. Others can read but cannot write (agraphia). There are many varied disabilities lumped under the name of aphasia, but we hope that we have made our point—that aphasia refers to the difficulty in using symbols meaningfully; it is a disorder due to brain damage.

There is no doubt that aphasia can occur in children who have had speech and then lost it as a result of brain injury. We have worked with many such children. Here is one.

Walter had been speaking very well, indeed much better than most children his age, when the automobile accident occurred on his fifth birthday. Thrown from the wrecked car, his head had struck a concrete abutment and he was unconscious for over a week. When he was able to leave the hospital, he was almost mute although occasionally a snatch of jargon would pass his lips. He had difficulty recognizing his parents and sister but a gleam of recognition came when the family dog nuzzled him once they were home. His first word was "Tiber" which he used for the dog's name (which was Tiger). Even his gestures were confused at first. He shook his head sideways for yes and vertically for no. He had forgotten how to cut with the scissors or to hold a crayon. Emotionally, he now appeared very unstable. He cried a lot and had uncontrollable outbursts of temper. It was difficult for him to follow directions or to remember. Occasionally he would come out with swear words his parents had never heard him speak. Gradually the speech returned, aided by our patient tutoring and the parent counseling which was so necessary. At the present time, four years later, he is speaking very well but has a marked reading, writing, and spelling disability.

There exists some argument among certain speech pathologists concerning the concept of congenital or developmental aphasia. These terms refer to disabilities in the *learning* of symbols or language as contrasted with the *loss* of ability previously learned which is what we find in true aphasia. Our own position, based upon our clinical experience, is that such congenital or developmental aphasias do exist. These aphasic children present different problems than those whose delay in speech is functional or due to mental retardation or hearing loss, although they may not become apparent until after some speaking has been learned. They may have gaps in their comprehension; intermittently appearing almost deaf, they may show inabilities in finding or uttering words which they have often used before. They confuse opposites, saying *hot* for *cold;* they use associated words instead of the ones they should use. One of our cases who could always name a chair when he saw its picture, could not say anything but "sit" when he desired to talk about it.

> You want to sit down in that little chair?
> Yes . . . No-no-no! Me want baby sit. . . .
> You want the little chair?
> No, no, no, no. Me no, no. Want baby bear, no, big man sit, sit down.

We gave him the big chair that he wanted and noted the repeated perseverations, the confusions of opposites, the use of the rhyming word *bear* for *chair* and, once more, the use of the action verb *sit* for the noun *chair*. We do not find this sort of thing when we teach the non-brain-damaged child to talk.

The aphasic child also often shows difficulties in perception, not only of sounds but also visual forms. They may make a cross when trying to draw the square in front of them. They show inversals or reversals of letters and words: *d* for *b* or *p*; *tac* for *cat*. Sometimes they get them badly scrambled not only in writing but in speaking. One of our aphasic children kept saying his own name, Tommy, as "Ommty," and he called his father "Addad." The auditory memory span—the ability to retain sequences of sounds—is often very short. We must speak to such a child in short sentences and give him enough lag to let the meaning filter in. Some of these children get the necessary delay for comprehension by using echolalia, repeating exactly and automatically what others say to them until they can scan the meaning and respond appropriately. We also see them try out words silently, in pantomime, before speaking them, to make sure they are correct. They obviously hunt for words, and produce some which have a few odd articulation errors in them: *nap* for *cap* or *chig* for *pig*. At times in the middle of very clear speech will appear a single jargon word: "I plush my eraser in school." (He meant "lost.") The aphasic child often shows a telegrammic form of speech, omitting all the little words. "Tuck (truck) go fall hill down boom." Prepositions such as *under* or *in* or *of* seem to be very difficult, no doubt because they are abstractions involving relationships. By now you are probably feeling a bit confused, trying to sort some kind of sense out of this barrage of language symbols. If so, you are probably feeling much like the aphasic child.

Perhaps it is because of the many frustrations experienced by an intelligent brain-damaged child trying to live meaningfully in a world full of words that he often seems hyperactive and excessively irritable. In working with these children you often almost seem to have to do speech therapy on the wing. They are squirrelly, on the move constantly. It's hard for them to sit still, to concentrate, to be patient. Their frustration tolerance may seem abnormally low, but we suspect it is only that they are overloaded with frustration. Occasionally they may go berserk, and show what in the adult aphasic is termed the "catastrophic response." One such boy, who had been working at his table quietly, suddenly began to scream, ran around wildly, tearing his clothes and shuddering. It was not a seizure. We held him firmly but soothingly for a while until he calmed; then he went back to his work. If these children find it harder to inhibit emotional displays than the normal child, it is probably due to the brain damage. We must understand and help.

Can they be taught to talk? Or read or write, or understand speech? We feel that the answer is yes although we have had enough failures with some children to say the word hesitantly. It's so hard to get through to a child who cannot talk, who sometimes cannot understand. Somehow it's harder for a therapist to remember his successes than his failures. Perhaps the best way to put it is to say that many of the children can be taught to talk and do all the other things if given the *proper* help.

The aphasic child, as we have indicated, needs special help. We must first of all determine which type of sensory stimulation he seems to respond to most easily. If he seems especially interested in noisy things, in sounds, we use this approach. In teaching such a child the first words we might perhaps use animal noises and associate the *miaow* with the word *cat,* or the sound of water rushing from a faucet with the word *water.* If he seems to prefer drawing, we would begin with that activity, using self-talk and parallel talk (in one-word sentences) to describe what is being drawn by the therapist or child. If the tactile sense seems especially interesting, we have him feel objects without seeing them and provide the appropriate words for the objects and what we do with them. We might have him feel in a bag and find the *big ball* or the *little ball,* or to locate the *pencil* we tell him we have hidden therein. If he is especially interested in visual stimulation we may even teach him to talk by teaching him to lip-read the names of the pictures or objects we show him. There are many roads to Rome. We use the one which seems easiest to the child.

When working with the aphasic child we are careful to decrease or to desensitize the child to outside stimulation. We help him concentrate by removing distractions. We work slowly, very slowly. We give him extra time to understand, to start talking. We use familiar materials and concrete things whenever it is possible. We use an egg first, then the picture of an egg. We repeat our activities and stimulation until they are no longer strange or confusing. We provide release from frustration. These children can be taught to talk.

Hearing Loss. It is obvious that speech development can be retarded as a result of impaired hearing. Even adults who have learned speech early and have used it adequately all their lives begin to find a decay in the precision and intelligibility of their utterance when they become deafened. Consonants become fuzzy, the vowels distorted. We need a monitoring ear to speak a language without abnormality. One can readily see how difficult it must be for the child who does not hear well. The sounds of speech may be faint or missing or unintelligible. It would be like learning to speak Chinese with your fingers in your ears. You might give up; you might even manage to learn a little, but it wouldn't be very good Chinese. Children who are born deaf seldom, if ever, acquire a normal voice or natural speech sounds despite the best of teaching. Some of them can master enough intelligible speech to get along.

However, not all children who have impaired hearing are deaf; some may merely have hearing losses. By hearing loss we mean that some usable hearing still exists. The person can hear certain sounds at a certain loudness level. He may hear some of what you say. He may be able to hear sounds which are low in pitch yet fail to hear the high-frequency sounds. He may be able to hear pretty well by bone conduction although when sounds come through the air they seem muffled and distorted.

There are two major kinds of hearing losses: conductive and perceptive. By the first, the conductive, we mean that the loss is caused by some defect in the outer or middle ear. There may be wax in the ear canal; there may be fixation of one of the tiny bone transmitters in the middle ear behind the ear drum. There are many possible reasons for conductive loss but the important thing to remember is that the lower and middle frequency tones are usually heard as being more muffled or fainter than they should be. Children with conductive loss usually learn to speak, though a little retardation may occur. They often, however, show many severe articulation errors of substitution and omission.

The other type of hearing loss is perceptive. It may be due to an injured or malfunctioning cochlea in the inner ear, or to a damaged acoustic nerve, or to injury to the brain itself. Of the two types of hearing loss, this is usually the more serious for speech learning or maintenance, because it introduces distortion as well as muffling of sound. The reason for this is that the hearing loss is not equal for different frequencies of sound. Most children with perceptive loss have a harder time hearing the high-pitched sounds than they do those lower in pitch. Sounds such as *s, th, f, ch,* and *t* are some of the high frequency sounds. If you had a perceptive loss, these would be faint or unheard at the same time that the vowels and the *m, n,* and a few other consonants would be quite loud enough. If you could not hear the announcer on the television because you had such a perceptive loss, turning up the volume wouldn't help you much because the low sounds would seem to be blasted out so much louder proportionally. The tiny high-pitched overtones would still be lost. A person with a high frequency loss can never hear normal speech as it really is. What he is able to hear will be a distorted facsimile. Engineers have invented filters to cut out all the high frequency sounds of speech. When we listen to recordings played through such filters, we are lucky to understand barely forty per cent of what we hear, and even then we have to guess.

By now you can readily understand why children with perceptive hearing loss usually have delayed speech. The models they attempt to match are always distorted. They do not even hear themselves accurately. They get confused and frustrated and lose interest in trying to speak. There is little reward from talking when others do not understand. These children need special professional help in auditory training, in lip reading, in identifying sounds by their postures and movements, in phonetic recognition. We will not touch on these matters here except in brief outline. When we find such a child, he should be referred to a hearing therapist.

DIFFERENTIAL DIAGNOSIS

It is one thing to describe these various causes of delayed speech in a text book and quite a different business when a nonspeaking child sits beside you, jabbering or grunting or gesturing. How can we find out what's wrong? Is there any way to recognize the aphasic child and be sure that he isn't deaf or autistic or mentally retarded? These are tough questions when you must observe an actual child and try to diagnose his problem. Perhaps the only way is to observe enough of them long enough, to work with them, test them, play with them, teach them to talk. We have read most of the research

on delayed speech and know what others have said about how to
tell one problem from another, but often we find that only trial therapy can give us the answer.

Nevertheless, there are a few major guidelines. Some of the clues
come from the interview with parents, some from examination. If a
child is slow to walk, feed himself, or to say his first words (and has
no basic coordination problems as in cerebral palsy) we suspect
mental retardation. If a child has much trouble sleeping, cries often,
has nightmares, is highly negative or destructive, shows marked conflicts with his siblings, finds it hard to relate to others, remains detached or shows autistic behavior, we tentatively conclude that his
speech delay is likely to have been caused by emotional conflicts.
If a child gestures very well, fails to respond to ordinary sounds or
requests, watches your face, does pretty well on form boards, fears
strange situations, we suspect hearing loss. If there is a history of
severe brain damage, intermittent difficulty in comprehension, interest in sounds but not in speech, marked delay in onset of first
words and a long lag before phrases appear; if the child uses inappropriate words or peculiar sound errors, has poor coordinations,
shows signs of perseveration, has difficulty in perceiving designs or
colors, and shows hyperactivity under stimulation, we would feel
the child has been brain-damaged. If the child has walked and
said his first words fairly early, demonstrates a lot of jargon with
some recognizable words within it, comprehends everything said to
him but refuses to try to talk upon request, we suspect poor teaching methods or interfering environmental conditions. This is about
the best we can do for you, except to warn you that some children
show not one, but a mixture of causes.

Examining the Delayed-speech Child

In order to understand the problem with which we are confronted
we must first find out the extent of the disability. To do this we
must place the child in a situation where the need to communicate
is very strong, and yet one in which the child's security is not so
threatened. If the therapist can see the child in his normal home
situation, the examination is more likely to be adequate. But we can
observe the child and his parents, or the child with his playmates
in school, or the child in the schoolroom and begin to understand

the problem. At times it is possible to establish a pretty good rapport with the child immediately and personally and to create the communicative conditions necessary for the diagnosis. However, we must always remember the difference between leading a horse to water and making him drink. Most of these children refuse speech when it is demanded of them. They have heard too often: "Say this!" and "Say that!" But when the conditions are appropriate and they do not feel under threat, most of them will interact enough to help us understand the problem.

The first task, once the child is responding, is to estimate the amount of communciative ability possessed by the child. The following summary of the examination of another delayed-speech case will make this clear, and also demonstrate the exploration into the causes of the disorder which is always required.

Examination for Delayed Speech

Case: James B. *Age:* 5:2 *Observer:* Kay B. *Interviewer:* Ruth F. *Informant:* Mother

A. Symptom Summary:

Observed situation: (Describe in detail.)

Father and child were playing with the airplane that comes apart. Child was helping to take it apart and put it together. They appeared at ease and unaware of the fact that I was watching and listening through the one-way mirror.

1. *List recognizable words and phrases actually heard:*

Da . . . (Dad?); uh-uh (no?); no, puh da (put down? Gesture of lowering); meemee (uttered questioningly while looking at door, perhaps referring to mother. Father said, "Mama will be back pretty soon."); bye; ow (ouch.)

2. *List words reported by parents to have been spoken meaningfully* (not repetitively, but spontaneously). Give informant:

Mother: bye-bye, milk, no, go car, all wet, down, cookie, no, mama, daddy, baby, night-night, potty (and others she could not remember).

3. *Frequency of above word usage: and conditions under which words occur:*

Direct observation: Never spoke these words except when father failed to understand pantomime and gesture. Most of the time played silently.

Mother's testimony: Seldom tries to talk. "Usually speaks his few words when frustrated or distracted." Silent most of the time.

4. *Jargon and babbling:* (Give frequency and conditions for occurrence.)

Jim only grunted twice and this was when he was making a strong effort to take the tail off the airplane. Said, "uhng-uhng" once when spinning the propeller.

Father says the boy occasionally talks to himself when in the workshop alone, but that "He doesn't make sense and stops as soon as he knows someone is listening." Cries loudly enough and laughs normally. Scolded puppy once "for quite a while" but father couldn't understand him.

Mother claims child babbled very little during first year of life. "He was sick too much of the time." "Has babbled little since." "What he says, he says clear, but he doesn't say enough."

5. *Comprehension:* Boy understands everything, according to both parents. Was unable to follow directions given by examiner verbally. It was occasionally hard to hold his attention, but when examiner had it, the boy could cooperate. Seemed normal for his age.

6. *Response to verbal stimulation:* Refused to attempt any sound or word given by examiner or parents. No anger, just refusal. Would not automatically finish unfinished sentences. No mouth formations of words presented by examiner.

7. *Gesture and pantomime:* Unusually good, parents could always understand. So could examiner.

8. *Reaction to listener's failure to comprehend utterance or gesture:* Child was quite passive. Just gave up trying to communicate.

9. *Interest in speech:*

Always listened when we were talking about him. Ignored other conversation.

10. *Interest in sounds:*

Quite normal. Reached for bell rung behind his back. Played with whistle and varied tone duplicately. Listened to record and laughed when recording laughed. Refused to respond to recorded appeal.

11. *Imitative ability:* Very good, but only motor activities—not speech.

B. Possible Causes: (Cite appropriate case history, interview or test data.)

1. *Low Intelligence:* Parents feel child is bright. Gesell Developmental Schedule shows boy up to age norms except in speech. Terman-Mc-Call-Lorge Non-Language Multi-Mental Test indicated child was superior. Can follow directions intelligently. This cause very doubtful.

2. *Hearing loss:* Unable to give audiometric examination. Parents are sure child hears normally. Heard watch tick when watch was unseen. Child seems normal in this area.

3. *Poor coordination:* No evidence. Generally well coordinated. Ties shoes, cuts with scissors, draws well. No athetosis or evident spasticity. Walked crack well. Moved tongue independently of jaw and rapidly in lifting to hard palate when imitating.

4. *Illness:* Parents claim "Child was ill during most of first and second

years." Cried a lot. General intestinal upsets, colic, pneumonia, frequent colds and chickenpox. No high fevers or coma.

5. *Lack of motivation for speech:* A probable cause. Parents anticipate desires and understand gestures. Child has been out of contact with other children most of his life. Parents baby him "because he was so sickly."

6. *Poor teaching methods:* A probable cause. Parents have not been consistent. Much speech demand at inappropriate times and for difficult material. Labeling, and demand for imitation, only techniques used. Much fast adult talk.

7. *Bilingual conflicts:* None.

8. *Shift of handedness:* None. Seems thoroughly right handed.

9. *Emotional conflicts, trauma, etc.:* Parental anxiety over child's speech retardation. No shocks or accidents. Some trouble over family finances. Parent relationships seem pretty good.

10. *Aphasia:* No evidence except lack of speech.

Another child with delayed speech might present a totally different picture, but the need for sizing up the problem in the terms of the above items will be equally necessary. Before we can cope with a disability we must know what that disability is. But this information is far from complete. We must also know something of the causes for the child's speech retardation.

PROJECTS

1. Make a list of all the taboos and pressures to conform which confront the child at the time he is learning to talk like an adult.

2. Procure and explain contrasting audiograms illustrating perceptive and conductive hearing losses.

3. Make a list of parental errors in the teaching of talking.

4. A mother phones you saying that her son is four years old and still no one can understand him. What questions would you ask her before giving an appointment?

5. Outline the main areas you would explore when she does come for an interview.

6. How would you examine such a child? Prepare an imagined play-by-play account of what you did in examining such a child.

7. List the similarities and differences in behavior characteristic of the brain-injured and the deaf child.

8. List the similarities and differences in behavior characteristic of the autistic child and the child whose speech retardation is due to poor environment or methods of teaching him to talk.

9. Find out about encephalography, then visit a hospital or clinic to observe how an electro-encephalogram is made. Find out how an e.e.g. could be used in diagnosis of delayed speech.

10. Make a glossary, with definitions and explanations, of the new technical terms found in this chapter.

PERIODICAL REFERENCES

11. Bangs, T. "Evaluating Children with Language Delay," *Journal Speech and Hearing Disorders,* Volume 26, 1961, pages 6-18.

12. Beckey, R. E. "A Study of Certain Factors Related to Retardation of Speech," *Journal Speech Disorders,* Volume 7, 1942, pages 223-249.

13. Bennett, D. N. "Home Teaching of Young Deaf Children," *Journal Speech and Hearing Disorders,* Volume 22, 1957, pages 68-74.

14. Carrell, J. A., and Bangs, J. L. "Disorders of Speech Comprehension Associated with Idiopathic Language Retardation," *Nervous Child,* Volume 9, 1951, pages 64-76.

15. Gens, G. W., and Bibey, M. L. "Congenital Aphasia: A Case Report," *Journal Speech and Hearing Disorders,* Volume 17, 1952, pages 32-38.

16. Hannigan, H. "Rh Child: Deaf or 'Aphasic'? 3. Language and Behavioral Problems of the Rh 'Aphasic' Child," *Journal Speech and Hearing Disorders,* Volume 21, 1956, pages 413-417.

17. Lewis, S., and Van Ferney, S. "Early Recognition of Infantile Autism," *Journal of Pediatrics,* Volume 56, 1960, pages 510-512.

18. Lubic, L. C. "A Neurologist Discusses the Evaluation of a Non-verbal Child," *Monographs in Social Research in Child Development,* Volume 25, 1960, pages 35-38.

19. McCarthy, D. "Language Disorders and Parent-Child Relationships," *Journal Speech and Hearing Disorders,* Volume 19, 1954, pages 514-523.

20. Myklebust, H. "The Differential Diagnosis of Deafness in Young Children," *Journal of Exceptional Children,* Volume 17, 1951, pages 97-128.

21. Nance, L. "Differential Diagnosis of Aphasia in Children," *Journal Speech Disorders,* Volume 11, 1946, pages 219-223.

22. Peacher, W. G. "Neurological Factors in the Etiology of Delayed Speech," *Journal Speech and Hearing Disorders,* Volume 14, 1949, pages 147-161.

23. ———. "The Etiology and Differential Diagnosis of Dysarthria," *Journal Speech and Hearing Disorders,* Volume 15, 1950, pages 252-265.

24. Rigby, M. "A Case of Lack of Speech Due to Negativism," *Psychological Clinic*, Volume 18, 1929, pages 156-162.
25. Schlanger, B. B. "A Longitudinal Study of Speech and Language Development of Brain Damaged Retarded Children," *Journal Speech and Hearing Disorders*, Volume 24, 1959, pages 354-360.
26. Weiss, D. A. "Speech in Retarded Children," *Nervous Child*, Volume 9, 1951, pages 21-30.

BOOK REFERENCES

27. Gesell, A., Amatruda, C. S., Castner, B. M., and Thompson, H. *Biographies of Child Development*. New York: Paul Hoeber, 1939, pages 129-146.
28. Johnson, W. (ed.). *Speech Problems of Children*. New York: Grune and Stratton, 1950, Chapter 5.
29. Levin, N. M. (ed.3. *Voice and Speech Disorders: Medical Aspects*. Springfield, Ill.: Charles C. Thomas, Publisher, 1962. Chapter 14 and 15.
30. Travis, L. E. (ed.). *Handbook of Speech Pathology.* New York: Appleton-Century-Crofts, 1957. Chapters 15 and 17.

CHAPTER SIX

❋ Delayed Speech: Treatment

In the previous chapter we provided the basic information concerning the nature and causes of delayed speech. In this chapter, we wish to outline the methods for teaching these deprived children to speak. The task is often a difficult one, demanding much of the speech therapist or parent. We must discipline ourselves not to become impatient, not to try too hard, nor to try too much too soon. Progress will be uneven. Often it is difficult to get started. But when a non-speaking child first discovers the magical power of intelligible speech, angels sing. We have helped persons with many different kinds of speech disorders to speak normally but there seems to be a special sort of glory in sharing a little child's achievement in mastering this most essential of all the human skills. We help them to join the clan, the human race. We know no pleasures of status, bed, or belly half so sweet. We hope you may share the experience too someday.

As we have stressed earlier, there is always a need to determine the cause or causes of the speech delay. Where they still are operative, it is necessary to eliminate them or to compensate for them. The aphasic child needs special training in handling symbols, in sending, formulating, or receiving messages. The autistic child needs to lose his fears and to accept a relationship with others. We have already outlined the special treatment which these children require. Now we wish to describe the general principles underlying the treatment of all these children.

Motivation. Many of these delayed-speech children have learned to exist without intelligible speech. They manage to get along without it, using gestures to supplement their grunts or garbled utterance. We might say that they have taught their parents or older siblings to understand their own primitive language. We have seen mothers aching and struggling to understand, trying desperately to translate the sounds and movements of such a child. Too often they succeed, thereby rewarding and reinforcing the garbled jargon or sign language.

Again, most of these parents have done much drilling, made many demands for display speech, asked for names, commanded utterance. "Say this and say that!" Their children, having a long history of failure in trying to please, give up. Attempting to speak has become unpleasant. There have been too many such sessions ending in tears or reproach or frustration. Attempting to speak has become punishing.

Creating a Need to Communciate Verbally. Some of our delayed-speech children already have accomplished this aim. They cannot refrain from jabbering. But there are many others who have not realized how important and how satisfying a tool speech can be for manipulating their elders and satisfying their desires. They simply don't think that learning to talk is worth the trouble. They find it possible to get along without verbal communcation. Pantomime and gesture are sufficient for a child in a home where everyone else tries to learn *his* language instead of the reverse. Parrots and myna birds have little incentive to talk either until their trainers pay some attention to motivation.

Silent gestures must therefore remain unrewarded. The best policy to follow is to withdraw the parents' granting of the pantomimic requests in a gradual fashion. The first day, collect two instances in which they pretend not to understand the gesture requests, guessing incorrectly until the child is pretty frustrated by their stupidity. The next day they do it four times, scattering the misunderstandings at random. Gradually most of the child's gesturing is being unrewarded. The guessing part of this technique should always be in single words:

> Today I was carrying out your suggestions. Bobby wanted me to hand him down the ball from the shelf. He kept pointing and reaching and saying "a . . . a . . . a." I looked at him in a puzzled sort of fashion, saying, "Dish? Dish? Bobby want dish." Then I tried "cap" and "cup" and "box," reaching up and taking down each, and pre-

tending to be trying hard to understand. It certainly seemed cruel, but I did it. He finally got mad and began to suck his thumb. Is this what you want me to do?

It was, but it should not be used alone. All spontaneous utterance should be rewarded by providing attention, sharing through imitation, and a little extra loving. With a severe case, even grunts and babbling should receive rewards. If the child makes any attempt at all to say the right word, or indeed for some children who do not talk at all, if any utterance accompanies the gesture it should be reinforced by pleasantness.

Another technique which creates a need to talk is to have the parent or therapist do a lot of self-talk, commenting on what they see or do. A sample of this running commentary is as follows:

> Mummy do dishes now. Wash cup . . . put cup here . . . Where glass? Oh, here glass . . . Glass dirty . . . Now glass soapy . . . Wash . . . Jerry wipe . . . Towel . . . Rub, rub . . . Glass clean . . . Glass on shelf . . .

If some of this simplified self-talk is done several times each day, the child who watches will begin to participate, first silently with inner speech and later aloud.

It is important in the speech therapy sessions that the therapist talk in this abbreviated way. Often in the first meetings it is wise to do as little talking as possible. Try to get down on the child's own level of non-verbal, gestural communication, then accompany gestures with single words, and then go to these brief phrases and sentences. The consonant flow of adult speech is so fluent and complicated that most delayed-speech children feel it is too difficult to achieve. Once it is simplified it seems easier and within his reach. For the same purpose we should cut down on the amount of reading to the child that parents do. Its fluency provides an almost unobtainable goal. We have had several cases in which the elimination of oral reading by itself created the climate productive of spontaneous speech attempts.

In counseling these parents, and in our own attempts to help these children, we must use a different approach. We must first make speaking fun. This means that all direct demands for naming, for repeating after us, for commanding utterance, must be stopped. We are not interested in display speech, in teaching birds to talk.

Instead, there must be a return to speech play, even to babbling a bit. Here is a portion of a letter from a mother:

> I did what you told us several times today and even though it made me feel silly to be making animal noises and nonsense sounds, I could see that Timmy was enjoying it. I'd say "Bubba-bubba," give him a quick hug and then run off into the kitchen. Sure surprised him the first few times. Then I'd waggle my tongue up and down in the bathroom mirror while he was watching and say "lalalalalala." Also, when I heard him making sounds when he was playing on the floor, I'd go over there and make them too. Once when he was pounding with a spoon on the frying pan, I made some other sounds first and then said "Bang-bang" and he imitated me, I think. Finally we got to making faces at each other with sounds attached to the faces. There was a kind of back and forth talking in it although he didn't say any real words. I've had to hold myself back to keep from asking him to say what I say though.

However, we must do more than this. Speech must be made pleasant, it is true, but we must not forget that the child's jargon and gestural communication must be freed from its reinforcement. We knew one silly mother who had starved her boy for two days by insisting that he say the name of any food he wanted. And that he say it right! She came to us in tears and we told her instead to pretend to misunderstand some of the boy's jargon when she really knew what he wanted, then aloud to try to guess what he was trying to say, and finally to say something like this: "Oh, you mean 'ball,' O.K. ball, here ball!" We asked her to put this delay and fumbling attempts at translation between his utterance and her fulfillment of his desire several times a day and gradually to increase the dosage. Children want what they want when they want it. The use of judicious delay, coupled with gradual translation into standard but simple English, will soon produce a real hunger to speak better.

Teaching the Child to Imitate. As in teaching the normal baby to talk, it is important that parents and therapists encourage all types of imitative behavior. We must identify with the child before he can identify with us. Accordingly, much of the early training of a child with delayed speech consists of sessions in which the parent or therapist shares the child's activities. If he scribbles, we scribble. If he explores the bottom drawer, we join him. If he hides under the table, under it we go. If he grunts, we grunt too.

Sooner or later he will engage in repetitive activities such as banging a pan on the floor, clapping hands, bouncing up and down. By interrupting these activities by our own performance of them, he will usually return to the same behavior with renewed zest. This means that he is actually duplicating our behavior as well as his own. It is the beginning of imitation. Soon we can be playing follow-the-leader in many ways, and he may occasionally enjoy being the follower. If such teaching of imitation in physical behavior is made very pleasant, it will soon generalize to speech behavior, and the child will enjoy imitating our speech. Most children respond to such play very swiftly.

The Alphabet of Sound.   Many unintelligible children try to talk without enough sounds to talk with. They need more arrows in their quiver, more keys on their verbal typewriters. Any of us would have a hard time making sense if we had but seven or eight, or even fifteen sounds. They need to learn something about the characteristics of the individual speech sounds. They need to master the sound alphabet. This should be done in play sessions. Here is a picture of some of this therapy:

1. Blindfold the child. Make the sound from several different places in the room. Ask the child to point to where the sound came from or to find you.
2. Pretend that each of you is a certain animal or machine that makes the sound. Have him run around the room with you as you produce the sound.
3. Procure a calendar mailing tube or similar device. Hold one end to the child's ear as he winds a string upon a spool. The moment the teacher stops making the sound, he must stop winding.
4. Certain objects are set aside as demanding the hearing of the correct sound before they can be touched. Such rituals appeal to children and compel attention.
5. Prolong or repeat the sound rhythmically. Ask him to clap his hands or put his fingers in the ear whenever you make it very loudly.
6. Tell the child a story or rhyme and prolong the selected sound whenever it occurs in a word. The important thing is to accent the particular sound you are working on.
7. Tie a rope on the child and tell him to walk back and forth as you pronounce the sound. Whenever you cease making the sound, jerk the rope.

Indirect Methods for Combining Sounds and Movements.   (Do these first in unison, making the sound a part of the activity.)

1. Snap off the light—say *ow*.
2. Shoot a toy gun—*bang, ba, boom,* or *pow*.
3. Turn an egg beater—any vowel on which you rhythmically change pitch.
4. Saw a board—*ee-ee*, or *ay-ay*, or *zzz-zzz*.
5. Hit piano or xylophone and sing any vowel.
6. Wind a toy—*mmmm-mmmmm*.
7. Pull the cork out of a bottle—*puh* or *buh*.
8. Pull or push any toy animal and say its sound: Cow—*moo*, dog —*bow-wow*, and so on.
9. Move a zipper: *zzz* or *sss*.
10. Rock in a chair or bounce—any vowel or consonant.

Direct Methods for Combining Sounds and Movements.

1. For *m*: Have child flip or stroke your lips as you make the *m* sound. Then you stroke his lips as he makes it.
2. For *puh*: Have child hold his whole hand flat over your closed mouth with cheeks full of air. Ask him suddenly to pull it away as you explode the *puh* sound. Reverse the process.
3. For *buh*: Hold or have child hold a feather or strip of tissue over your mouth. Then explode the *buh* sound so that the feather or strip moves or falls. Reverse positions.
4. For *tik*: Cup hands around your mouth and ask the child to look inside and hear the clock. Say *tik-tik-tik*. Then have him be the clock.
5. For *dee*: By folding a cardboard provide yourself with a series of ten holes each large enough to insert a finger in. Have child hold it in front of himself and as you insert your finger in each hole say *dee*. Then you hold it, refusing to let him hit the hole until he says *dee*.
6. For *nnnnnn*: Have child place finger on side of your nose as you open your mouth and say *nnnnnn*. Ask him if he feels the little noise. Then ask him to open his mouth so you can feel his little noise (and nose).
7. For *oo(w)*: Have child watch your rounded lips as you blow into a tube of paper or into a bag or horn. Then have him do it. Then blow the *oo* sound "out loud." Always call this the "blowing sound."
8. For *guh*: Call this the "squeezing sound" or the "choking or collar sound." Ask the child to choke you with both hands as you laugh and say *guh-guh-guh*. Reverse, but be gentle.
9. For *kuh*: Call it the "coughing sound" and play some sort of a coughing game. For example, put a feather into the mouth and cough it out with *kuh-kuh-kuh-kuh-kuh*.
10. For *f*: Call this the "blow on the finger" sound. Hold your finger laterally across the child's lower lip, pushing it inward. Then ask him to blow on your finger to cool it off. Then set his own finger in position and repeat.

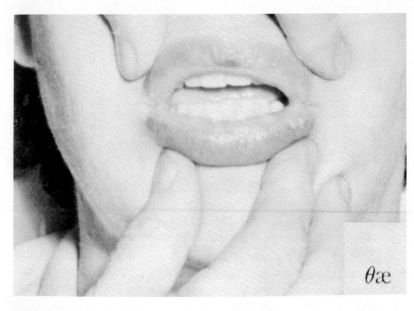

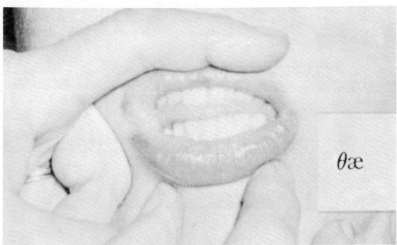

FIGURE 13. *The Motokinesthetic Method* *

* From Edna Hill Young and Sara Stinchfield Hawk, *Moto-Kinesthetic Speech Training.* Stanford, Calif.: Stanford University Press, 1955. By permission of the publishers.

11. For *v*: Ask him to watch you in the mirror as you "bite your mouth (or lip) and blow out loud." Then ask him to do it.

The Motokinesthetic Method. Some modifications of the motokinesthetic method can also be used to teach the isolated speech sounds, but this method itself is focused on the teaching of the syllable and word as units. As originated by Edna Hill Young, it consists essentially in the manipulation, touching, and stroking or pressing of the child's face and body. The therapist by these procedures helps the child to locate the muscles needed to produce the sound, indicates the direction of the desired movement, provides the proper timing of the movements, and gives some clues as to the amount of air pressure required. At the same time, the therapist stimulates the child with the proper sequences of sounds composing the syllable or word so that he hears it as he feels his mouth movements. Appropriate rewards are provided also. For a more extensive treatment of the subject we refer you to Reference 30 at the end of this chapter and to Figure 13.

Vocal Phonics. Children during their third and fourth years are fascinated by rhymes and word play of every kind. They chant such sequences as these even when alone:

> High chair, high tair, high bear, kigh kare, care care, bear tear, tear bear all up.
> Sally, mally, silly sally, sabby, babby, sally babby.
> I got a letter in the mail, in the pail, in the tail.
> I like soup, sook, soos; do you like soot?

When their playmates seem puzzled by this punning, they laugh uproariously. If word play is the lowest form of wit, it may also be the earliest. But its major significance in the development of speech lies in its phonic training. Many children persist in their articulation errors because they never learn that words are composed of a series of consecutive sounds. They hear words as wholes—as chunks of sound. The word *fish* to these children is not a series of three sounds, *f*, *ɪ*, and *ʃ*, but a single sound. Thus the pronunciation of *fish* and *pish* if spoken quickly enough are much more alike than they are different, and the child fails to perceive any error. Very often, he may echo the word after his parent without error, and yet in the very next sentence he may use the *pish* again. Many parents consider their children obstinate because they do not use these words consistently with correct sounds. Yet, parrotlike repetition has little to do with mastery of true speech. The Mongolian idiot can often echo very long words and yet be speechless in the true sense of the word. The child must be able to perceive his own errors and to create his own standards of pronunciation before he can be expected to speak correctly.

The child must learn that words have beginnings and endings—heads, middles, and tails. He must learn that the word *fish* must start with the "lip-biting, breathy, finger-cooling sound" (or some similar identification) and with no other. He must learn that *cup* must end with a lip-popping puff of air. (kʌ) is not enough. There must be one more sound.

Most children learn these elementary facts of vocal phonics unconsciously through vocal play and listening. Many articulation cases never learn that words are made up parts, and that if one part is wrong, the whole word is incorrect. These observations may seem absurdly simple to the student of this text, but he will appreciate their truth once he starts to teach some lisper an *s* sound.

> Say *sssssssssssss*.
> S*ssssssssssssss*.
> Fine! Now say *soup*.
> *Thoup.*
> Oh, oh. You said *thoup*.
> No, I didn't. I thaid it right: *ssssthoup*.

The best way of teaching vocal phonics to young children is through guessing games, rhyming, indexing, and rhythmic vocal play. Here are three typical vocal phonics games which we have used successfully with children of three to five years:

1. Make circles on the floor with chalk and give each circle a "sound name" (*ssss* or *mmmm*). The child must make that sound whenever he is in the circle. Thus, as he jumps from circle to circle, he could produce the word (s) (æ) (m) or *Sam*.

2. *Guessing game*. "Show me your *n-o-se* (nouz)." Separate the sounds at first, but gradually shorten the intervals until the child realizes that (n-ouz) is a slow way of saying *nose*. Then use other words such as (ʃ u), (f-eɪ s), (mauə), and so on.

3. *Collection game*. Give the child some gaily covered boxes and have him collect toys or objects whose names begin with an *s* sound and put them into the *m* box, and other objects whose names begin with an *s* sound and put them into the other box. Demonstrate first, and be sure

to sound out the words so that he hears the *m* or *s* sound of the objects collected. Also demonstrate rejection thus: "Let's see. Here's a phone. Does this belong in the boxes? Let's see: *f-f-f-o ne*. No, that begins with a *fff* sound, not a *mmmm* or *ssss*. We don't say *mone* or *sone* do we? Let's just get things that begin with the *mmmm* or *sssss*. You bring them to me and I'll sound them out."

One reason why so many children develop a jargon or gibberish is that they fail to realize that a word is made up of a series of sounds blended together. They hear the word as a whole and pronounce some sound which bears a certain likeness to it. Some children can be taught some real words immediately by these sound-sequence games. The majority, however, need much practice in "vocal phonics," in combining and blending sounds without regard to meaning, before true words are taught. Most successful teachers of delayed-speech cases first teach blending sounds as an interesting game and skill; then they teach sound combinations which they call nonsense names; then, finally, real and familiar words.

1. Let the teacher perform two of the previously practiced movement-sound combinations, then ask the child to imitate her. If this is too difficult, alternate before combining.
2. Let the child perform the activities while the teacher makes the sound, then reverse.
3. Trace a circle to form syllables. Have top arc of circle represent one sound, bottom part another. Trace slowly first, faster gradually for advancement, and divide circle into more parts and sides and sounds.
4. Have squares on floor for certain sounds. Say these sounds while stepping in squares. Form words or syllables.
5. Use different notes on the piano for different sounds.
6. Mount two or more cardboard bells on a piece of tag board so that they can be moved when strings are pulled. Color differently and let each represent a sound. Have child pull the strings as you make the sounds. Then exchange places.
7. Cut shapes of paper for various sounds. Arrange two or three in a row on the table for child to sound out after he learns the sounds for them.
8. Roll a ball across the room, having child say the sounds as the ball moves in the various spaces.

Exercises for Sound Sequences

1. Select short one-syllable words, which begin with the continuant sounds: *m, n, w, y,* or *v,* or any vowel. (*Examples: nose, yell, neck, man, way, egg.*) Prolong the first sound, pause, then say the rest of the word,

asking child to point to object, or indicate by pantomime, what was spoken. Then prolong the pause for several seconds and try the same procedure except for this variation. Next, separate the vowel from the final sound also and repeat exercise. Then increase number of sounds in the words used, allowing child to guess the word. If difficulty is experienced, repeat sounds more swiftly and with shorter pauses between sounds.

2. Show the child some pictures which include a number of objects. Sound out one of them.

3. Select some simple word, sound it out, ask child to help, and then sound it in unison. Ask for identification of word sounded out.

4. With chalk, divide the floor into sections, a sound for each. As child walks across the room saying each sound, ask what word is formed.

5. Sound out words and have child listen to see if he can count the sounds.

6. Tell child to say some nonsense syllables such as *an* just after teacher has pronounced another sound. (*Example.* Teacher says *mmmmm*, child says *an*. Teacher asks child what word they have spoken together. Child should guess *man*.) Then use other combinations, *puh-an pan, can,* and so on.

7. Sound out, in the fashion indicated, direction which the child must carry out. (*Example:* "Sh-uh-t th-uh doh-r.")

8. Give each finger the name of a sound. Child says each sound as he lifts (or teacher lifts) the appropriate finger.

Self-correction.   In addition to using these methods, the parent should occasionally talk gibberish herself, or use grunts and gestures, trying earnestly to get the child to understand. When he is thoroughly puzzled, she should catch herself and say, "Oh, I didn't say it right. What I mean is 'Bring me the shoe. Sh. . . .oo. Shoe!" She does not ask the child to say it. She is merely creating a model for him to follow. She is showing him that even big people make mistakes and find it hard to make themselves understood if they don't talk right. She is showing him that it doesn't hurt to correct oneself. Later on, this can also be done on single words.

Providing Proper Speech Models.   Our last suggestion illustrates the importance of presenting the proper speech models. We have to begin where the child is. If he is only grunting and gesturing, then we must share some of his own mode of communciation. If he is speaking in an unintelligible gibberish, we must share this but also contrast it with the correct forms. In other words, we are suggesting that the parent or speech therapist provide simple models which are within the child's reach. Many children fail to learn to talk simply because the language of big people flows so unceasingly and appears so complex. They can't match it. They give up and grunt or they try and talk a jargon unintelligibly. We must learn to talk simply, to return to the one-word sentences of the baby, or to the phrases and simple sentences of the very young child. These models may be within his reach.

Building a Basic Vocabulary. For the delayed-speech case it is as necessary to teach a basic vocabulary of tool words as it is for the normal infant. Some of our delayed-speech cases already have a good many words when they come to us but they are hidden and buried in the jargon. It is necessary to separate them out, get the child to use them meaningfully, and then reward them. Many of these children show great spurts of progress as soon as they come to realize that they can speak many words correctly. They also show surprise, since over-correction, rejection, or other penalties may have convinced them that they cannot talk correctly and they have accepted this judgment and made no further attempt to improve.

With the child who has little or no speech, it is necessary to teach the first words. The first project should not contain more than five or ten words, and they should begin with the easier sounds, *m, b, p,* or *w.* If possible, they should be monosyllabic or should consist of repeated syllables, such as *mamma.* They should be names of things or activities which the child enjoys. If the child has some distorted speech sounds which he habitually employs for naming favorite objects, it is wise to select new toys or new activities which he has not previously named. When this principle is followed, no unlearning is necessary. Nonsense names can be used if the true names are too difficult or begin with the wrong sounds, since the object of this first training is to teach the child to use speech as a tool and to set up proper speech standards. Later on, the child can be given the more difficult task of unlearning old incorrect names and substituting correct ones for them. The parents and teacher alike must use the nonsense name, however, when referring to the object in the presence of the child. We usually include about two true names among each set of five words used in building the primary vocabulary. Thus, one child was taught the following names in the order given:

1. "Moop" (the name given to an oddly shaped mass of modeling clay which was used in a hiding game). 2. "Wap" the sound made by the child and teacher in unison as a signal for a Jack-in-the-box to pop out).

3. "Boom" (the name of a toy cannon). 4. "Papa" (the name he used for himself when he pretended to be his father, a physician, engaged in treating the teacher, who pretended to be sick. The boy was given an old medical satchel and tongue depressor and left the room to knock at the door. Whereupon, the teacher asked "Who's there?" and refused to open the door until she knew who was knocking). 5. "Ba" (the name for "ball," or the sound used as the boy bounced it).

After the child has been taught to make the sounds that are included in the five or ten words previously selected, the teacher's next task is to teach him to combine those sounds to form words. There are two major ways of accomplishing this: by teaching whole words and by teaching sound sequences. Both methods should be used for almost all cases of delayed speech, and, for both, ear training should precede actual performance. Generally speaking, the whole-word method should be used for simple monosyllabic words, whereas the sound-sequence method should be used for those of more than one syllable.

In one case, the word *mop* was among the first five words to be taught. After the child had been given ear training in saying the *m* and *p* sounds by themselves, the teacher began the ear training necessary to the production of the whole word. She left the room in a very mysterious manner, returning with a bottle of colored water and a mop. As soon as she entered the room, she went solemnly to each corner and said "mop, mop, mop." Then she made another circuit of the room with the child, and in each corner she said the word *mop* into the ear of child. On her third circuit, she spilled a little water in each corner, uttering the same word three times, prolonging the *m* slightly and emphasizing the *p*. On the fourth circuit, she took the mop itself and wiped up the water with it, saying the word rhythmically as she worked. She motioned to the child to help her, and as he took hold of the handle he began to say the word in unison with her, somewhat to her surprise. In this case, the vivid stimulation and identification with an activity were sufficient to produce the spontaneous response.

When the sound-sequence method is used, the word should not be broken into all of its component sounds, for the vowel should always be spoken in connection with the consonants that precede or follow it in the syllable. Thus the word *wipe* should be sounded as *wi-p*, and the word *cookie* as *kooh-kee*, never as *w-i-p* or *k-oo-*

k-ee. The reason for this is that consonants vary in their formation according to the sounds that follow or precede them, and the child must not be asked to break up words into any finer elements than necessity demands.

Useful Words for a Basic Vocabulary. The following words employ the easiest sounds and are most frequently used in children's speech. However, if a child prefers others or seems interested in learning others, always follow his desire.

The words that are the easiest to say are: *baby, bacon, bee* or *be, bib, big, bite, boat, book, bow, boy, buggy, cake, can, coat, comb, come, cookies, cow, cup, dig, eat, egg, eye, go, got, gum, gun, hat, home, hot, ink, keep, keys, kitty, man, me, meat, neck, pig, pin, no, talk, tie, top, two, wagon, walk, window,* and *wood.*

Those not quite so easy to say are: *bag, bone, can, cap, come, daddy, deep, do, door, egg, fat, game, gate, hand, he, make, mamma, milk, money, moon, night, open, point, pound, put, talk, top, wait, walk, want, we,* and *you.*

Those that are the least easy to say are: *bad, ball, banana, big, book, car, cold, corn, dinner, dog, farm, fight, goat, good, hide, monkey, nose, O.K., paint, paper, pen, potato, take, tongue, water, wind, wing,* and *yes.*

Other suggestions:

1. Keep a list or notebook dictionary of all words correctly spoken without help. Make the child feel that each new word is a wonderful accomplishment.

2. Reward the child for each new word acquired.

3. Tell a story but omit the new word whenever it occurs. The child must say it. Also use the word to end a rhyme.

4. Hide objects or pictures representing the new words, then cover your eyes. The child must hunt and tell what he finds.

5. Make a phone call and ask the child to say a word for you. (Use this method in ordering groceries.)

6. Send the child home, or to a friend's house, with the picture and word to "show off" how well he can talk.

7. Whenever the child masters a new word, his mother must write it in one of the squares of a large calendar. He should "read" these every day.

8. Pin a picture to the door of a room or to a favorite chair. Child must say its name whenever he sees it.

As soon as the child has mastered a few words, have him use them in as many meaningful ways as you can invent. Review frequently. Draw pictures of them. Send them home or to the regular teacher to practice. Have the child play games with them, perhaps combining them with activities. Make the child realize that the words are useful in these games and give him great praise for their acquisition.

As soon as the child has had some experience in making words, you should begin the building of a group of words which can serve as a foundation for good acceptable speech. Scrapbooks of pictures clipped from magazines and catalogues, and certain comic strips or cartoons, carefully selected so as to produce certain words, are useful devices to review and "set" this basic vocabulary. Try to get the child to speak these words as spontaneously as possible. Work them into his contacts with other children and adults, into his errands as well as his play. Drill is much less important than use in real life situations. Provide them.

Self-talk and Parallel Talk. The speech models should have more than simplicity; they must also have utility. No child will ever learn to talk unless he sees that it is a useful tool. The way we teach him this lesson is through *self-talk* and parallel talk. By self-talk we mean that we talk aloud to ourselves, verbalizing what we are seeing, hearing, doing, or feeling. Here are some samples of a mother's self-talk and parallel talk.

> Where cup? Oh, I see cup. Cup on table. Here cup. . . . Milk in cup. . . . Mummy drink milk. . . . Johnny want cup? . . . O.K. . . . Johnny drink. . . . Milk all gone. . . . Give Mummy cup. . . . Mummy wash cup. . . . Here water. . . . Here soap. . . . Give cup bath. . . . All clean. . . . Where towel? . . . Here towel. . . . Wipe, wipe. . . . Give Johnny cup. . . . Put on table. . . . Johnny good boy.

This child was only making a few vowels, grunts, and gestures at the time but he was alert and interested. Note the mother's simple speech, within reach of the child's ability. Note the commentary accompanying what she did or saw. Note the recall and prediction. Here there is no demand for display speech. Here is self-talk used as verbalized thinking. It wasn't long before the boy was talking to himself too. Mothers and speech therapists must learn to talk this way for the time being, to build the bridge between where the child is and where he should be in language usage. He cannot jump the chasm. As he begins to talk, they can gradually increase the complexity of their models. With some children who are speaking only in grunts or gestures, we would begin therapy by doing our own self-talk in a similar fashion, then progress to single-word utterances, then to short phrases, and finally to sentences which gradually increase in complexity and completeness. We have to begin where the child is. We must join him before we can lead him.

A surprising bit of behavior comes when we get to the early sentence stage. If we occasionally fumble a bit, leave a self-talk sentence hanging uncompleted in mid-air, omit a key word, the child will often say it for us. When this occurs it is unwise to make much of an issue of the achievement. Just feel good and use the technique more often. If we put words in his ears he will find them in his mouth. This is especially effective when we are doing parallel talking.

In *parallel talking*, the mother verbalizes not her own thoughts but those of the child. She tells him what he is doing, what he is feeling. If he appears to be predicting that Jack will jump out of his box, she might say, "Jack pop out, pretty soon." If he is about to turn off the light, she says, "Light go away now." If he is remembering where she hid the cookie, she says, "Cookie in bag." As he bounces, she tells him what he is doing. When he tumbles from the chair, she says, "Johnny fall down. Ow, ow. Hurt foot. Ow!" Emotions can be expressed in self-talk and parallel talk too.

This parallel talking is fascinating stuff. Ideally, we should say the necessary word or phrase or sentence at the very instant that the child should be needing it. Practically, we seldom get the timing so precise. It is a skill which develops with use. We have known mothers become wonderfully adept after a little practice. It requires careful study of the child and a lot of guessing, imagination, and the ability to identify with the youngster. Every speech therapist should learn the art, for it is very useful in treating the adult aphasic as well as the child who cannot talk. Training in empathy is vitally important in speech therapy.

We have spoken earlier of the importance of speech as a magical tool for controlling others. Nowhere do we see this so clearly as in delayed speech. As soon as we possibly can, we teach this function. We have used puppets, dolls, even ourselves as our victims. We command these beings. We tell them to fall down, to cry, to clap hands, and they must obey! The child watches us and sees the power of speech. Soon he is commanding too. Our knees still creak from a session with a little boy who insisted that we get "Unduh taybo!" thirty-seven times by actual count. This spontaneously achieved command had been preceded by much self-talk on our part, commanding first a puppet and then ourself to follow orders.*

We also use self-talk to set models for egocentric speech, for the expression of the self. Yesterday, with the same little boy, we crouched on the floor and said, "I'm little. . . . I baby. . . ." Then we got up on all fours, and said, "I kitty . . . meow!" Then we stood up and said proudly, "I big man . . . big as a house." The boy liked the display and gestured that he wanted us to do it again. We looked puzzled, paused a bit, then said, "More? . . . You want more?" He grunted. So we did it again and again, and soon he was imitating first our postures and our animal noises, and finally a little of our speech. He climbed aboard the table, stuck out his chest and arms and crowed, "Man . . . bih MAN!" This was the beginning of speech as the display of the self.

We teach speech as communication a little later. Often it begins to come in by itself, once speech as thought and speech as social control are activated. Usually, we combine it with command at first. "Mummy blow bubble. . . . Big Bubble . . . Oh, oh . . . No more bubble. . . . All gone. . . . Go ask sister for soap. . . . Ssssss-soap. . . ." If he's interested enough he might just possibly do it.

Terminal Therapy: Its Problems. Children differ in their response to treatment. Those whose delayed speech seems due to poor teaching methods and bad environmental conditions make the swiftest progress if these can be changed for the better. Those with emotional conflicts (with the exception of the autistic child) also progress very swiftly when the conflicts are resolved. They also speak very clearly. We have known many instances of children, whose voluntary mutism or infantile jargon made them non-talkers, who suddenly began to talk very well. The aphasic child, children with cerebral palsy, will make slow progress and need help for a longer time. So will the mentally retarded.

Among the problems which may be viewed as the residue or aftermath of delayed speech are severe articulation disorders: cluttering, stuttering, odd voices, and a pattern of behavior which has been termed "specific language disability." The latter is often designated

---

* A psychological rationale for commentary and command in self-talk in terms of "tacts" and "mands" may be found in the book *Verbal Behavior* by B. F. Skinner, New York: Appleton-Century-Crofts, 1957.

by its initial letters *SLD*. Many of these unfortunate remnants of delayed speech can be prevented with proper understanding and treatment.

Dyslalia. This term, we wish to remind you, refers to the presence of errors of articulation due to functional causes. In the elementary grades of the public schools we often encounter children whose speech is barely intelligible. The use of language is adequate but there are so many errors of omission, distortion, and substitution that only the other children seem to understand them. In scrutinizing their histories we commonly find a history of delayed speech. Children who begin to speak at four or five years have a long way to go, a lot of sounds to master before they begin to read and write. They are usually children who have not had professional help. They come to us confused by too many targets in their mouths. Again, our task is to help them untangle the problem by helping them to recognize the different speech sounds, to analyze the sound sequences within words, and to build a basic nucleus of good speech.

Cluttering. When a child has discovered the pleasures of intelligible speech, he sometimes takes off like a skyrocket. He wants to talk all the time, to say everything at once. He grabs every ear in sight and fills it constantly. Communicatively, he has been starved and so he fills his mouth with too many words too fast. If, as often occurs in cluttering, there is a family predisposition and some evidence of minor brain damage, his speech will become almost incoherent the moment he speaks swiftly, although he can speak very well when he is careful. He falters, repeats, changes words, slurs his speech sounds, transposes syllables, and generally makes a hurried mess of his communication. This is cluttering. To some degree it may be prevented by decreasing the urgency of communication, by removing the need for haste, by providing speech models which are themselves unhurried. The tempo of the home, the tempo of the mother's speech, should be slowed. Parents should respond by saying that they do not understand the torrent of tangled syllables, by showing the child how he has spoken, and by providing a willing ear which has plenty of time to listen.

Stuttering. There are times when a child seems to travel a crooked path down which first delayed speech, then cluttering, then stuttering appear sequentially. In other children, the stuttering emerges directly from the delayed speech. Too much pressure for speech output by the happy parents who finally see their child beginning to talk may cause a need to talk without having anything to say. Such children will falter. We don't want them to learn a broken English so we must counsel parents to wait rather than to urge. There are also many moments in learning to talk when words must be hunted, changed, revised in articulation, sorted out in sentences. This places a heavy burden upon fluency. Some children almost seem to face a choice between stuttering and defective articulation when they emerge from delayed speech. If there is such a choice, we would counsel parents to accept the defective sounds. Learning to talk takes time.

Voice Problems. These are not common residues of delayed speech but they do occasionally occur. One of our six-year-olds who began to say his first sentences at five had two voices, his own and one that his mother called his "frog voice," because it was pitched so low and possessed a croaking sort of quality. David spoke an almost unintelligible jargon in his natural child's voice but his frog voice spoke very good English. The problem was one of identification. He had been a very isolated child, living on a farm. Dave's mother worked in a drugstore during the day and his father worked at night in a local factory but managed to care for him during part of the daylight hours. Dave had received help in the speech clinic and also at home under our guidance for several months when suddenly he began to speak very clearly but in the deep bass croak of the frog voice. It became apparent that he was identifying intelligible speech with his father's speech and felt that he had to match it in pitch as well as in clarity and form. We got the child placed in a nursery school and soon he was speaking well in his own voice. Other children finally learn to conform to adult speech standards but keep an infantile voice as a last defense against the pressures of a too-demanding environment. These are often the active ones. Autistic children who begin to talk also may show odd voices.

S.L.D. When there has been a history of brain damage or symptoms thereof are present the child may show long-lasting effects in other functions besides speech. The term *specific language disability**[*]* has been used to designate this pattern of difficulties. These children have difficulty in school because of reading, writing, and spell-

---

[*] De Hirsch, K. "Specific Dyslexia or Strephosymbolia," *Folia Phoniatrica*, Volume 4, 1952, p. 231.

ing problems. Deficiencies and abnormalities in visual perception, in visual-auditory associations, in symbol manipulation are frequent. Coordinations are poor. There is often hyperirritability and excessive restlessness. In many respects the picture is one of residual aphasia. Such children need special teaching and long term treatment.

Summary

In treating the child with delayed speech, we must attempt to remove or reduce the impact of the various factors which have caused the retardation in speech development. We must create the necessary motivation, convince the child that it is possible and rewarding to use intelligible speech. The child must come to know the characteristics of the individual speech sounds and the ways in which they occur in words. We must provide simple speech models within his ability to duplicate. Through self-talk and parallel talk we must provide the language symbols needed for thinking, communication, social control, emotional expression, and the development of a self-concept. After a child has begun to speak intelligibly, we must take the necessary measures to prevent the appearance of articulatory disorders, cluttering, stuttering, and voice problems, and we must continue to help the brain-damaged child so that he can be successful in the other language activities.

PROJECTS

1. Summarize the treatment of a child with delayed speech as gleaned from his clinic case folder.
2. Do a follow-up study of three cases who were treated in your training center more than four years ago for their delayed speech.
3. Draw a series of faces showing the positions and directions of the therapist's hand movements in teaching the *b*, the *f*, the *s*, and *l* sounds using the motokinesthetic method.
4. Turn down the sound on the television and do some parallel talking in a running commentary on what you see on the screen. Tape-record, if possible.
5. Observe some child at play and empathically assume his postures and movements as they occur. Report what you did.
6. Think aloud for five minutes. Be able to demonstrate before the class.

7. Say five nursery rhymes, using only the vowels of the words. Practice until you can do them fluently before the class.

8. Communicate to your roommate only through gestures for an entire evening. Report your experience.

9. A child says to you, "Ah wah oo tay me to duh baawoo na." What do you say and what do you do?

10. Outline the home treatment for a child with delayed speech in terms of five main principles. Tell the mother what to do and how to do it. Do not use any "Don'ts" but keep your suggestions positive.

11. Invent three activities which could be used to teach a four-year-old delayed-speech child the concept of sound sequences.

12. Explain to a hypothetical mother how to teach the alphabet of sound. Invent a dialogue in which you and the mother participate in this situation.

13. Tape-record a conversation with a friend in which you speak very simply but naturally. Use a very simple vocabulary and only simple sentences, no compound or complex ones.

14. A four-year-old child, formerly without speech, has now gained it due to your efforts and is talking all the time. His parents are delighted. What should you tell them to prevent other difficulties from arising?

15. A three-and-a-half-year-old child, subjected to too much demand for adult forms of speech, has become mute. What concrete suggestions could you offer his parents?

PERIODICAL REFERENCES

16. Egland, G. O. "An Analysis of an Exceptional Case of Retarded Speech," *Journal Speech and Hearing Disorders,* Volume 19, 1954, pages 239-243.

17. Greene, M. C. "Diagnosis and Treatment of Late Speech and Language Development in Children," *Folia Phoniatrica,* Volume 12, 1960, pages 101-107.

18. Mowrer, O. H. "Hearing and Speaking: An Analysis of Language Learning," *Journal Speech and Hearing Disorders,* Volume 23, 1958, pages 143-152.

19. Plotkin, W. H. "Situational Speech Therapy for Retarded Cerebral Palsied Children," *Journal Speech and Hearing Disorders,* Volume 24, 1959, pages 16-20.

20. Rigg, M. G. "A Superior Child Who Would Not Talk," *Child Development,* Volume 9, 1938, pages 361-362.

21. Werner, L. S. "Treatment of a Child with Delayed Speech," *Journal Speech Disorders,* Volume 10, 1945, pages 329-334.
22. Westlake, H. "A System for Developing Speech with Cerebral Palsied Children," *Crippled Child,* Volume 29, 1951, pages 10-11.

BOOK REFERENCES

23. Beasley, J. *Slow to Talk.* New York: Teachers College Bureau of Publications, Columbia University, 1956. Read all of this little book.
24. Johnson, W., Brown, S. F., Curtis, J. F., Edney, C. W., and Keaster, J. *Speech Handicapped School Children.* New York: Harper and Row, Publishers (revised edition), 1956. Chapter 6.
25. Levin, N. M. (ed.). *Voice and Speech Disorders: Medical Aspects.* Springfield, Ill.: Charles C. Thomas, Publisher, 1962. Chapter 15.
26. Myklebust, H. *Auditory Disorders in Children.* New York: Grune & Stratton, Inc., 1954.
27. Stinchfield, S. M., and Young, E. H. *Children with Delayed or Defective Speech.* Palo Alto: Stanford University Press, 1938. Read all of this book.
28. Travis, L. E. *Handbook of Speech Pathology.* New York: Appleton-Century-Crofts, 1957. Chapter 16.
29. Van Riper, C. *Your Child's Speech Problems.* New York: Harper and Row, Publishers, 1961. Read all of this book.
30. Young, E. H., and Hawk, S. S. *Moto-kinesthetic Speech Training.* Palo Alto: Stanford University Press, 1955. Read all of this book.

CHAPTER SEVEN

Voice Disorders

The Problem

Disorders of voice represent only a small fraction of the case loads of most speech therapists as compared to the disorders of articulation. A few professional workers, who like to call themselves "phoniatrists," specialize in this part of the field of speech pathology, and in speech clinics, hospitals, or private practice concentrate their efforts to help singers, teachers, or politicians who are losing their voices, persons whose vocal cords have been paralyzed or removed through surgery, or those with other major abnormalities of voice.

However, all speech therapists are certain to have persons with voice problems referred to them. Many of them we ourselves can help; others we should refer to the specialists in our own field or to our medical colleagues. No speech therapist can afford to be ignorant of the basic information in this area. One severely abnormal voice in a public school situation will call so much attention to itself that the speech therapist's competency may well be judged on the progress made thereon, no matter how much speech improvement has occurred in the articulation of fifty other children. This is patently unfair, but this is not the best of all possible worlds. The voice case or the stutterer who does not improve stands out like a third thumb. Moreover, in order to refer a given case to a specialist, one needs to present that case in a professional manner. Again, often we must work with voice problems referred to us by the physician and again our professional competence will be evaluated in terms of our understanding and skill. Even for those who do not intend to become professional speech therapists, some basic information concerning the voice and its disorders has real importance. We all have voices; many of us abuse those voices; and some of us are using voices which are far from being assets in a vocal world.

Variability of Voice

Chaliapin, the famous basso, once said that going to a party was like going to a symphony played by instruments all of which were out of tune. "All around me are voices blowing discords, squeaks, rasps, whines, grunts, and growls. I can hardly bear it." Fortunately for most of us, our ears are not so sensitive. His observation, however, is more accurate than our calloused ears would be likely to admit. All about us are voices which could be improved, made more pleasant and efficient. And there are some so markedly unpleasant or peculiar that they are referred to the speech therapist. The singing teacher gets some of these, the speech teacher gets another group, the physician sees the pathological ones, and the speech therapist is usually called upon last.

The human voice is a tremendously variable thing, ranging all the way from the soaring splendor of a Metropolitan Opera soprano to voices which should be used only for cooling soup. What is more, each of us possesses not one voice but many, a fact which is probably the most important one to be found in this chapter, for it provides us with that most valuable possession of all—hope. Voices can be changed, or, perhaps, we should say, discovered since the potential for producing them has always been present. It is the speech therapist's job to help the voice case explore his bag of many voices and to find one that fits his needs for both normal communication and self expression. It is certainly true that each of us finally settles on a characteristic way of phonating which is almost as individual as our fingerprints. We need say only a few words on the telephone and we are recognized—unless we disguise our voices. Some of this identification comes from the articulation and tempo of our utterance, but much more from the voice. Although we are easily recognized by others, oddly enough when we hear our own recorded voices, they sound strange and sometimes unpleasant. We are not sure why it is so hard to hear ourselves objectively, but we know that this difficulty is always encountered in voice therapy. Perhaps it is because we must use our ears to hear our thoughts and those of others. Perhaps it is because the sound field is different, our ears being behind our mouths but in front of the ears of others. Perhaps, as has been suggested, we monitor our voices by bone conducted sound. Perhaps, if we heard them more objectively, we'd revise them, and choose better ones.

The Determinants of Voice

What then were the forces which led us to choose the voices we use? We know that they have changed since we were children as a result of the changing larynx at puberty. We know that they vary with different circumstances, as in public speaking, praying, or making love in the moonlight. Anger can make a pleasant voice harsh; depression can leave it weak and monotonous. The voice of authority is not the voice of the helpless. To put these various observations together, we may say that our voices are determined by age, sex, physical structure, by emotion, and by the roles we play in living. Our voices are the result of selective learning. Hitler's harsh and strident voice was only one of many available to him, but this was the social-controlling one which brought him his rewards. The hypernasality of the whining infantile housewife has been rewarded too often by its service in emotional expression. Relief is a powerful reinforcer. In contrast, we have known people with beautiful voices who seemed entirely unaware of them, and yet we suspect that these voices too were habituated by the favorable responses of many listeners.

Again, some of us acquire our voices by what is said to be imitation but what probably is identification. We assume the voices of the models we admire and, if they are not incompatible with our other needs, we find security therein. Perhaps, by identifying through the adoption of our mother's voice, we feel we get all her other virtues. At any rate, we feel better when we hear such an admired voice coming from our lips and we use it until it becomes a part of us. It is much the same sort of reinforcement which enables us to teach parrots to talk. These then are some of the factors which determine the choice of voice. We shall meet them again when we investigate the reasons why some individuals have voice disorders.

As we have described earlier in this book, there are many terms used in designating voices as abnormal. The general category is *dysphonia* and it embraces many individual disorders. We will spare you such jaw-breakers as *phonasthenia, myasthenia laryngis,* and *rhinophonia* and refuse to use such layman's adjectives as *thin, metallic, or hollow.* Instead we will describe those disorders of pitch, intensity, and quality which are likely to come to the speech therapist for referral or help. Let us begin by giving some brief pictures of some cases as described by some of our public-school colleagues:

I have an eight-year-old boy with a very deep, low-pitched voice which is also harsh. The voice quality has a buzz in it and this, I think, accounts for the impression of harshness. The boy is not at all tense, either generally or in the laryngeal area. He has quite a range, going way up into the treble, and his singing voice is quite normal for his age so far as pitch is concerned. The singing voice is, however, somewhat breathy. The speaking voice is pitched almost at the very bottom of his range. When he is heard for the first time, the effect is quite startling, and he has received a lot of teasing about it, to which he reacts good naturedly. The other children have nicknamed him "Bullfrog."

My most frequent voice cases are those of excessive nasality. Phoebe is typical. She whines when she talks, although she is not at all a chronic complainer. Instead she is rather shy and noncommunicative. Most of the nasality is of the assimilation type. Every word containing an *m* or *n* sound is completely nasalized and so also is the vowel *ae* and *ai*. For example, she can say the sentence, "If we are to go we'd better hurry," without a trace of this excessive nasality. But if she says, "Many men make money," it's one long whine. The effect on the listener is odd. Even I find myself wondering why all of a sudden she seems to be complaining, wondering what's wrong with her now. The palate seems to be entirely functional and there's no emission of air from the nose on the isolated vowels mentioned above. Maybe the velum is too short or sluggish. It's hard to tell. I have had a hard time with these cases and they haven't shown much progress. Would appreciate a few suggestions.

My worst voice case is a senior in high school this year and he's the son of the superintendent of schools. He's big for his age. A good athlete. No ear for music nor interest in voice improvement. What's wrong is that his voice keeps breaking, just like a boy's voice sometimes does when he reaches puberty. It will shoot up an octave from his usual baritone. It (the break) occurs most often when he gets excited or emotional. Very noticeable to others but boy comes to speech class under protest. His father insists or I'd get rid of him. He's been shaving since he was fourteen. He's eighteen now. Help, help!

The ones that trouble me the most are the children with soft voices, who just can't talk loudly enough to recite in class without having the teacher demand over and over again that they make themselves heard. Most of them are terribly shy, afraid of their classmates and, I think, of themselves. They just can't let go in anything. I've had my only success with these, and not too much at that if I'm to be honest about it, by working with them individually, building up their faith in me, giving them a chance to talk about their troubles and having them help me. One little girl though, Alice, isn't a bit shy; actually, she's quite aggressive but her voice is as soft as a baby chick's peeping, even when she tries to yell on the playground. She just doesn't seem to have any breath support for her tone, though she's full of energy.

I have trouble with the foreign kids, especially those who come to this country when adolescent. Their articulation clears up pretty good, but the foreign melody pattern of inflections stays with them, and they sound just as foreign as ever. The Latvians seem to be the hardest of them all. I can't seem to get them to stop going up in pitch before every pause. They're worse than the Swedes.

From our own current practice come these brief summaries of other types of voice cases:

Mary M. is a forty-year-old teacher of mentally retarded children. Her husband is very hard of hearing and so is her only daughter. She began to show a very hoarse and husky voice shortly after a prolonged bout of laryngitis during which she continued to teach. When intermittent aphonia began to occur, she went to her physician who in turn referred her to a laryngologist. The latter diagnosed the problem as vocal nodules, tiny growths on the vocal folds, which he then proceeded to remove through surgery. He prescribed voice rest but she continued to teach and to handle her duties at home as soon as her voice returned. Soon the nodules returned and the laryngologist recommended voice therapy under our direction. We are now engaged in teaching her a new voice and altering her speech environment.

Wilbur N. has a high-pitched falsetto voice. Except for changes in intensity, it is markedly monotonous. Few inflections can be heard. He is deeply troubled by the voice and the reactions shown him by other people. He is a wrestler and varsity football player, as male as they come. He is unable to carry a tune or to recognize one or to find a given pitch but his auditory acuity is excellent. In but two sessions, we have been able to get him to produce a few very low pitched tones by alternately inhaling and exhaling spoken vowels and by using the technique termed the "vocal fry." We are certain that he is capable of a deep bass voice and that it will be forthcoming fairly soon.

Clyde A., a repairman, comes to our clinic each day to learn how to speak on esophageal air. In his neck there is a hole through which he breathes, for his larynx has been surgically removed due to cancer of the vocal folds. The windpipe is sealed off from his mouth so the only source of sound is that produced by the sort of burp from partially swallowed and then expelled air. He is very depressed and gives up too soon despite the fact that he has been able to say a few words and syllables. We may have to provide him with the vibrating buzzer called the electrolarynx. This, when pressed against his neck, will produce a monotone which he can then turn into intelligible speech by moving his lips and tongue in pantomimed speech. We hope we won't have to resort to this device because the resulting utterance is far from satisfactory, but any speech is better than being mute.

There are other voice disorders but you have read enough to help you understand the material that follows.

Pitch Disorders

There are four fairly common types of pitch disorders: (1) the habitual pitch level which is too high, (2) the monotonal or mono-pitched voice, (3) pitch breaks, and (4) the falsetto which is usually a disorder of both pitch and quality. There are also several less common ones: (5) the tremulous voice, (6) peculiar and stereotyped inflections, and (7) too low a pitch level in children or females.

Habitual Pitch Levels. The concept of a habitual pitch level must be clearly understood. Except in the case of monotones, it does not refer to a certain fixed pitch upon which all speech is phonated. It represents an average or median pitch about which the other pitches used in speech tend to cluster. For example, in the utterance of the sentence, "Alice was sitting on the back of the white swan," the fundamental pitch of each vowel in any of the words may differ somewhat from that of the others. Moreover, certain vowels are inflected—that is, they are phonated with a continuous pitch change which may either rise, fall, or do both. Of course, each inflection has an average pitch by which it may be measured, if the extent of the variation is also considered. If all the pitches and pitch variations are measured and their durations are taken into account in the speaking of the preceding illustration, we shall find that they cluster about a certain average pitch, which may be termed the "key" at which the speaker phonated that sentence. This may be determined experimentally through the use of the trained ear, as indicated in the chapter on speech tests and the reference by Gilkinson listed at the end of this chapter. It should be understood, of course, that different pitch levels will be used under different communicative conditions. Nevertheless, each voice can be said to have a habitual pitch and a habitual pitch range, in which most of the communication is phonated.

The pitch of the normal human voice presents many mysteries and much research needs to be done before we can hope to understand its abnormalities. We know that the voice of a young child is high-pitched when compared with that of the adult, and that in old age it tends to creep back again to higher levels. We know that the major pitch changes occur at puberty, the bottom of the girl's pitch range descending from one to three tones with an equivalent gain at the upper limit. Boys' voices usually drop a full octave and there is a less marked but noticeable loss at the upper end of the pitch range. Usually, but depending upon the onset of sexual changes, the voice changes occur in boys between the ages of thirteen and fifteen with the girls showing the same basic changes a year earlier. Occasionally, the change of voice has been known to occur very suddenly (usually when puberty comes late) but most frequently it takes from three to six months on the average.

Why do some people fail to make the normal pitch change? There are several reasons besides delayed sexual development. Some cases have voices which are high-pitched primarily because of infantile personalities, because they cannot or prefer not to grow up. This case study may help to make the point:

> Charles J. was first referred to the public-school speech therapist for his articulation difficulty at the age of twelve. He substituted *w* for *r* and *l*, *t* for *k*, and *d* for *g*. He had a marked inter-dental lisp. He sucked his thumb, cried easily. He preferred the company of very young children and still played with dolls at home. He was rejected and despised by boys of his own age and bore the nickname of "Sister." He was an only child, pampered and babied and over pro-

tected by an anxious mother. Although intelligent he had failed the third grade twice. He was absent from school a good share of the time for chronic headaches and stomach upsets. The articulation defects were very resistant to therapy and the child was not cooperative. Consequently, he was dismissed from speech therapy classes and referred to the school psychologist, who was unable to solve the home problem because of the mother's attitudes.

At seventeen he was again referred to speech therapy, this time at a college clinic. No articulation defects were present, but the voice was very high-pitched, rather nasally whiny, and weak in intensity. The secondary sex characteristics were present and he was quite fat. The personality was still infantile.

In such cases psychotherapy is the indicated treatment, although vocal training may be used along with it, either to make the psychotherapy more palatable or to help the person to make changes in the habitual pitch as he comes to accept and solve his psychological problem.

Another common cause of the high-pitched voice is tension. The tighter the vocal cords are held, the higher is the pitch of the tone produced. Tension in any area of the body tends to flow toward and focus in the larynx. Many individuals who, in their occupations, are compelled to speak very loudly will raise their voices to make themselves heard, and this raising also lifts the habitual pitch. Speech therapy will be of little avail unless the underlying cause of the tension can be eliminated or reduced. Some case presentations may help us understand the problem.

Joan P., a high-school senior, referred herself to the speech clinic after hearing a recording of her voice. "Why, I sound like a little first grader," she complained. "After hearing that voice I'll never dare talk to a boy again over the telephone. Please do something!" Analysis of the average pitch levels used by the girl showed that she phonated about the pitch of middle C, a level which is well within the normal range for females of that age. When the test recording was played back, she said, "That's funny. That's a little bit higher than I thought I talked but not so high as the other recording." We then made another recording, in front of a class, and this time the average pitch level did reach F above middle C. We explained to Joan that most females hear their recorded voices as seemingly higher in pitch just as most males hear themselves as possessing a deeper voice than they expect. We also explained the effect of tension and fear on the pitch level and the need for learning to adapt to the pressures of confronting a group. A series of experiences in making recorded talks to a group while trying to use the middle C habitual pitch of her conversational voice proved successful and no further difficulty was experienced.

Most of us tend to raise the pitch of our voices when communicating under fear or stress, or when trying to speak loudly. In examining a voice case, we must always be alert lest the case's uneasiness give us a false picture.

A boy of seventeen was referred to us as a monotone, and most of his speech was pitched at D above middle C. He tended to use loudness instead of pitch variations to give the meaningful inflections necessary in asking questions, making demands, and so on. For example, he would say this sentence with each syllable pitched at the one note, but saying the last word quite loudly. "Are you planning to GO?" The effect was often one of hostility, which he did not mean to convey at all. The voice quality was rather harsh. Most strangely, he was able to sing in a very high tenor voice and sing very well. A series of counseling interviews and examinations resulted in our refusal to accept him as a case for therapy at that time. A year later, he was re-examined and his voice was entirely normal, being pitched at B below middle C, with a range of an octave and a half, and normal inflections and quality. He had meanwhile started to shave.

As the foregoing case implies, pitch levels are dependent upon many factors. The case mentioned was slow in acquiring the secondary sex characteristics. His larynx, at the time of our first examination, was childlike and under-developed. Highly conscious of this, he had endeavored to compensate for the natural high pitch by speaking at the very bottom of his range.

Monopitch. We have never seen a case whose voice could be viewed as strictly monopitched, although we have known many whose voices were highly monotonous. All of them were capable of some pitch change and all of them had some inflection. The key characteristic was the narrow range of inflection and pitch change, often no more than one or two semitones. Also, these individuals often substitute a change in intensity for the pitch change and this creates the impression of deviancy. Many persons whose voices strike us as entirely lacking in inflection are merely those with stereotyped inflections. These are the ones whose voices fall after every pause, comma, or period. There is deadly monotony to be sure but not monopitch. Nevertheless these restricted, lifeless voices are miserable to listen to and they interfere with communication by sheer lack of variety.

The causes of monopitch are (1) emotional conflicts, (2) lack of physical vitality, (3) hearing loss, and (4) the use of habitual pitch levels too near the top or bottom of the pitch range. The role of emotional causation in producing the monotonous voice has been described by various authors and researchers. Diehl's[1] review of the literature indicates that individuals who are in states of depression, and schizophrenics, tend to show this type of voice. We have also found it in paranoid or suspicious individuals or those who are barely able to keep their emotions under control, as a defensive mechanism to prevent others from knowing how they feel.

Undernourished, sick, or fatigued persons also tend to show little range of pitch or inflection. They seem to have insufficient energy available for the normal melody of speech. Those who are very hard of hearing also present the picture of monotonous voice, although careful scrutiny often reveals certain stereotyped inflections, most of which are alike and yet unlike those of the normally hearing person. Finally, when the habitual pitch for any reason is either too near the ceiling or floor of the pitch range, we find a tendency toward monopitch. We need voice room to maneuver. If we cannot go downward, we do not go upward. Falsetto voices often show this feature.

Pitch Breaks. Most of us tend to think of the change of voice as occurring abruptly when it does occur, and the "pitch breaks" have been the subject for a good deal of humor in our culture. However, recent unpublished research has shown that most children, boys and girls alike, do have these sudden shifts of pitch as characteristic of the period of voice change, and also, some children as young as seven and eight can show similar sudden shifts of pitch. We also are prone to think of the pitch changes as always shifting toward the higher notes, but when this does occur consistently, it does so only toward the end of the puberal period. Voice breaks can be downward as well. See Curry (21).

The majority of the pitch breaks that do occur are generally an octave in extent in most children. They occur involuntarily, very

---

[1] Diehl, C. F. "Voice and Personality" in Barbara, D., *Psychological and Psychiatric Aspects of Speech and Hearing*, Springfield, Ill.: Charles C. Thomas, Publisher, 1960, Chapter 9.

suddenly, and the child seems to have little control over them, reacting at first with great surprise. The upward pitch breaks of boys,
according to Curry (21), start when the word spoken is pitched
below the habitual pitch of the moment. It often seems as though,
in the attempt to return to the level they feel most natural, they
overshoot their mark. In a few children the experience is so traumatic that they resort to a guarded monotone, and develop a very
restricted range.

The cause of the puberal pitch changes is not entirely understood,
though we do know that profound alterations in the organs of voice
occur at this time. The male larynx grows much larger and the vocal
cords longer and more suddenly; the female larynx increases more
in height than in width, and the vocal cords seem to thicken. The
male vocal cords lengthen about one centimeter, the females only
a third as much. At the same time the child is growing swiftly in
skeletal development. The neck becomes longer, and the larynx
takes up a lower location relative to the opening into the mouth. The
chest expands greatly, and perhaps some of the cause of voice breaks
is the greater air pressure which suddenly becomes available. The
following case may be illustrative:

> One of our cases was a boy who had been delayed markedly in
> physical growth until his sixteenth birthday, at which time a great
> spurt of development occurred. He grew six inches in three months
> and his voice seemed uncontrollable as far as pitch was concerned, so
> much so that he developed a marked fear of speaking and a profound
> emotional disturbance. Speech therapy was ineffective until he was
> taught by the speech therapist to fixate the chest and to use abdominal
> breathing as exclusively as possible. Immediately the pitch breaks
> disappeared and the technique tided him over the next six months, at
> which time he returned to his normal thoracic breathing pattern with-
> out difficulty.

The above case illustrated another of the characteristics of the
truly abnormal voice. Not only did he have many more pitch breaks
than does the average boy, but also he showed shifts of pitch which
were not of the usual type. Sometimes the break in pitch was of
fourteen semitones. The speech therapist can often distinguish a
pathological case who will not "outgrow" his adolescent pitch breaks
by listening to the type of pitch shift which occurs. Curry (21) cites
the following similar case from the German literature:

Case four is that of a 23-year-old girl with a mutation disorder; since age eight her voice had been continuously hoarse and accompanied by many involuntary breaks. These breaks from a higher to a lower pitch took place so rapidly that the voice was originally diagnosed as diplophonic (two-toned). In this instance, however, the apparent diplophonia is due to a rapid succession of different fundamentals rather than to different rates of vibration of the two individual cords. This case is of especial note because the difference between the two frequencies is not necessarily an octave.

Public-school speech therapists who have to make surveys of large populations of school children should recognize the fact that the control of pitch during puberal development can vary widely from day to day. Very often there is less control early in the morning than later in the day. We have also found that anger, excitement, fear, and other emotions may give a false picture of the severity of the problem. Laughter, especially if uncontrolled, will also produce an unusual number of breaks.

Too high a pitch in some individuals, either male or female, may be the result of failure to make the necessary transition to the adult voice. The social penalties upon the male with a voice pitched too high are severe in our culture. Indeed, an old name for this voice problem was the "eunuchoid voice." The penalties upon the female are less severe. An occasional male may even find a "baby voice" as attractive as a "baby face." Nevertheless, the high-pitched voice is rarely much of an asset. We have seen some marked tragedies resulting from the disorder. Personalities have been warped by social rejection; vocational progress has been blocked; self-doubts have destroyed the person's ability to cope with the demands of existence. There is nothing humorous about a high-pitched voice.

The Falsetto. This voice is one which is available to all of us. We may not be able to yodel but we can at least use the falsetto at will, both in speech and song. Authorities are not agreed as to the manner of its production but it is most easily produced when the throat and laryngeal muscles are fairly relaxed. Some individuals use only this particular adjustment of the larynx habitually in the production of voice and its oddness in speech can provoke much distress. It usually begins in puberty and is more frequently encountered in the male.

The causes of the habitual falsetto voice appear to consist of (1) emotional factors as a protest against sexual or social maturity, (2) use as a defense against pitch breaks, and (3) use as a method for preventing the hoarse or husky voice. The first of these presents a problem in counseling and psychotherapy in some cases and professional help may be needed.

R. James S., III, came to us with a very high-pitched falsetto whose only inflection was at the end of his phrases and sentences. He was a fat boy at eighteen and he was a boy rather than a youth. His divorced mother had spoiled and babied him for years and he was almost totally unable to cope with his freshman year in the university. She phoned him every evening and wrote to him every day. He refused to eat in the dormitory, to have a roommate, and often to go to class. In our examination, he wept easily and frequently and also in a falsetto. We recorded his voice, played it back to him, and then referred him to a psychiatrist. He dropped out of school and we lost track of him for a year. When he returned, he told us that he had continued his psychotherapy, had cut his ties with his mother, and was working as a janitor. His psychiatrist reported that he was now ready for voice therapy. Within a single week he found his deep bass voice. It was one of the easiest bits of therapy we have ever had. Had we attempted to work with Bob, as he had finally come to call himself, earlier, we are sure we would have been unsuccessful.

This case points up another significant bit of information. Abnormal voices can persist of their own momentum and habituation long after the original cause has ceased to exist. They perpetuate themselves by the reinforcement they get from successful consummation of communication.

In some of our cases, the falsetto appears to be the result of a defensive reaction against the traumatic experience of pitch breaks. It is not pleasant to have one's voice flop around, especially when this behavior provokes mockery and social penalty. By using the falsetto, one can prevent these breaks and some beginning adolescents use it for this purpose, only to find that they have lost the ability to find the normal adult voice. They fear to use the low-pitched voices we can teach them fairly easily and our problem is to help them realize that the pitch breaks can be controlled and prevented. We use a lot of negative practice in working with these individuals, deliberately practicing the pitch breaks and desensitizing them. Chanting and singing on the lower pitches is useful. These same basic principles are employed when working with a person whose falsetto is a defense against hoarse or husky voice qualities.

Other Pitch Disorders. The tremulous voice may be due to paralysis, to muscular dystrophy or other similar neurological disorders or to cerebral palsy on the one hand, or to fearfulness on the other. Referral to medical or psychological services is indicated. Females or children with very low-pitched voices should be referred to the physician before undertaking speech therapy. Often glandular and hormonal problems are present. Stereotyped inflections may be due to foreign-language influence, to psychological conflicts, or to hearing loss.

Intensity Disorders

Voices which are not loud enough for efficient communication are fairly common, but they seldom are referred to the speech correctionist. Imitation, overcompensation for hearing loss, and feelings of inadequacy leading to retreat reactions account for most of them. Many pathological reasons for such disorders are common, but they are frequently accompanied by breathiness, huskiness, or hoarseness, or other symptoms sufficiently evident to necessitate the services of the physician, who should rightfully take care of them.

One individual with a history of prolonged laryngitis, but with a clean bill of health from the physician, claimed that she was afraid to talk loudly because of the pain she had experienced in the past. Something seemed to stop her whenever she decided to talk a little louder. She constantly fingered her throat. She declared that she was losing all her self-respect by worrying about her inability to speak as loudly as she could. Use of a masking noise during one of her conferences demonstrated to her that she could speak loudly without discomfort. Under strong clinical pressure, she did make the attempt, but the inhibition was automatic.

When we speak we expose ourselves, and the louder we do it, the greater that exposure is. The insecure, withdrawn person finds even ordinary levels of intensity almost unbearably revealing. His very nature resists the display of self. Usually he has good reasons for his inhibited utterance although they may remain hidden until counseling makes them bearable and manageable. An emotionally healthy person enjoys a certain amount of display speech. One who is not finds it traumatic. And once again, we find that even when psychotherapy is successful, often there is need for voice therapy to enable the person to use an adequate vocal intensity.

Aphonia. This term refers to the loss of voice, to its absence. The person with aphonia is able to whisper but he cannot produce any tone. Only in severe organic conditions such as paralysis of vocal cords, or where the presence of the growths called vocal nodules prevents their closure, or when there are deep psychological reasons for loss of voice, do we have true aphonia. We more frequently meet cases of dysphonia where the loss of voice is intermittent. Here is such a case:

> Wilma's parents and grandparents had been schoolteachers and they desired her to follow their profession. Her college education had been financed on that understanding. But Wilma didn't want to be a school-ma'am. As soon as she entered college she became engaged to a young man and thought she might escape the horrible prospect of teaching by becoming a housewife. However, in her senior year, he suddenly de-cided to enter medical school, a decision which meant that she would have to support him by teaching for several years. She fought the de-cision but finally acquiesced. It was in her first week of practice teach-ing that her voice began to go. She would begin her sentences all right but after saying a few words, she could only whisper. At times longer words would be uttered with the first syllable voiced and the other syllables produced in pantomime. No organic cause was evident. She dropped out of school and he dropped her and we don't know what happened thereafter.

Spastic Dysphonia. In this disorder, we have a mixture of aphonia and a strained, tense, vocalized whisper. The person labors hard to squeeze out some voice. It sounds like the grunting speech of some-one performing tremendous strenuous muscular effort and trying to speak at the same time. The mountain labors and produces a mouse of sound. At times there are facial contortions almost as in the severe stutterer. Fear of speaking is present but usually not fear of words. This is usually of emotional origin and requires appropriate referral, but it is also to be found in the cerebral palsied or aphasic or some other type of central nervous system disease.

Indistinct Utterance. Indistinct speech is so frequently confused with intensity voice disorders that it will be discussed in this section. Many individuals possessing this type of speech phonate with suffi-cient intensity to be heard, but their intelligibility is affected by improper rate, indefinite articulation, and unprecise resonance.

These individuals are frequently asked by their auditors to speak more loudly. When this is done, the intelligibility is often decreased still further, owing to the masking of the high-frequency consonant sounds by the lower tones of the vowels. Fletcher[21] concludes from his experiments that consonants are generally harder to recognize correctly than vowels, and that *th*, *f*, *v*, and *z* are the most difficult to perceive at weak intensities. He also demonstrates that a small improvement in articulation produces a great improvement in intelligibility: "If the articulation shows an improvement of from 5 to 10 per cent, the intelligibility will show an improvement of from 20 to 38 per cent."

These indistinct speakers are therefore taught to emphasize their

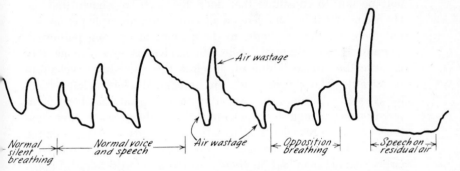

FIGURE 14. *Tracing of a Polygraphic Recording of the Breathing of a Person with Spastic Dysphonia*

consonants. The four continuants mentioned above as being responsible for most of the distortion are prolonged. The student is further taught to produce them with a more energetic airflow and a tenser lip or tongue. Since other research studies indicate that the stop consonants *p*, *b*, *t*, *d*, *k*, and *g* are among the least powerful of all speech sounds, these are also singled out for special attention. Sudden, precise, and energetic closures and openings are taught. At first it is wise to use prescored material in which only one or two of these sounds are underlined. Speech assignments and nuclei situations will carry the new attack into normal speech. Improving such general considerations as the student's posture, neatness, and self-respect often facilitates this more specific therapy.

[21] Fletcher, H. *Speech and Hearing*. New York: D. Van Nostrand, 1929, pages 266-289.

Disorders of Voice Quality

There are five major disorders of voice quality: hypernasality; denasality; the breathy, husky voice; the harsh or strident voice; and the hoarse voice. In addition, there is a peculiar throaty or guttural voice which is actually a low-pitched falsetto and it is treated accordingly in another section.

Hypernasality. This problem is not an uncommon one. It occurs primarily because the back door to the nose fails to close sufficiently. The contraction of the soft palate and pharyngeal muscles which elevate, spread, and squeeze the rear opening to the nasal passages may be said to constitute that door. Research has shown that the closure need not be complete on all sounds to prevent hypernasality but there are definite limits to the amount of opening permitted. Certain organic conditions reflect themselves in excessive nasality because they make it difficult to close this valve-like mechanism sufficiently. The person with an unrepaired cleft palate shows hypernasality; so does the person whose soft palate has been paralyzed or made sluggish by poliomyelitis or other disease. Investigations have also revealed that hypernasality tends to occur after the adenoids have been removed, a process which leaves a relatively larger channel than had previously existed due to the adenoid mass.

Hypernasality, when excessive, creates a voice quality which most listeners find unpleasant although the vocal yokel who loves hillbilly ballads may deny this. It has some virtue in enabling the speaker to get his message across in the presence of masking noise for it carries piercingly. Auctioneers and barkers at carnival side shows find it useful, if not ornamental.

Assimilation Nasality. Hypernasality may be general and exist on most of the vowels and voiced consonant sounds or it may be restricted only to the sounds which precede or follow the nasal consonants *m*, *n*, and *ng*. This latter type is termed assimilation nasality. Many speakers of general American English show some assimilation nasality in such a sentence as "Any man can make money." This is because of the need for alternate openings and closings of the velo-pharyngeal opening. In the word *man*, the passageway to the nose must be open on the *m*, closed on the *a*, and opened again on the *n*. It's easier just to leave the space open.

Also, even on a word such as *and,* we tend to prepare for the *n* opening, while we're still saying the *a,* and this may cause a premature
lowering of the soft palate, thereby producing the sound nasally.
The assimilation may thus be either forward or backward. Hypernasality of either type seems to be more likely to occur on certain
sounds than on others. High back vowels such as *oo* (u) and *o,* show
less hypernasality than do the lower front vowels such as *A* (e) or
a (ae) as in *cat.* The consonants *z* and *v* tend to show more hypernasality on them than do the other consonants. It is possible to have
much hypernasality without ever having any airflow coming out of
the nose because it is the resonation of the sound, not the air flow,
which creates the unpleasant voice quality. The louder the voice,
the more prominent the hypernasality appears.

There are other causes besides the organic for hypernasality.
Through imitation and identification, children can learn the excessively nasal voices of their parents or associates. Low vitality and
fatigue also tend to produce more of the problem, for it takes energy
to make the swift adjustments needed. Finally, whining children and
adults have whining voices; complaint prefers the trombone of the
nose. Certain stereotyped rising-falling inflections along with the
hypernasality tend to identify this causation. It is different from
that shown by the organic cases.

Denasality. This is the voice of the head cold, of the hay-fever
victim, of the post-nasal dripper, of the child with enlarged adenoids.
The nasal passages are occluded, perhaps by growths within the
nostrils, by congestion in the nasal cavities above the roof of the
mouth, or by adenoids in the rear passageway. Often some of the
nasal consonants are affected, the person saying "Mby syduhzziz are
killig mbe." The voice sounds are dulled and congested. Listeners
desire to clear their own throats or to flee. Again, as we have found
before, denasal voices may be maintained long after the cause has
ceased to exist.

The Breathy, Husky Voice. This disorder often coexists with other
problems. It may show itself in intermittent aphonia, in cases of
weak intensity, in conjunction with the hoarse voice. Its major
characteristic, as the name implies, is an excessive output of air
flow along with the phonation. Breathy voices are not whispered,
but they are aspirate in quality. Phonation is present but the rush
of air is obvious. At times, the huskiness accompanies the tone; at

other times the constricted hissing of the air precedes or follows the tone. There is air wastage. In some cases, a sort of gasping series of short inhalations throughout the person's speech produces the impression of huskiness. When this occurs, the phrases are short and choppy and the rhythm of utterance is disturbed. From this description it is obvious that there are different types of breathy voices.

The causes of the breathy voice may be either organic or functional. A paralyzed vocal cord may fail to join its twin at the midline for part of its length, thus leaving a gap through which the airflow may leak. A vocal nodule—a tiny corn-like growth on the edge of a vocal cord—may prevent complete closure. Certain

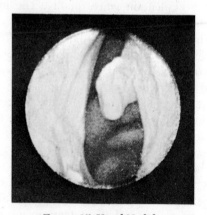

FIGURE 15. *Vocal Nodule*

diseases may inflame or swell the membranes of the vocal cords so that they vibrate inefficiently. Excessive strain may make them weak—as it does any muscle when overloaded too long. Whenever you meet such a disorder, you should first make sure that the person hasn't just been yelling too long at a football game or has a bad cold, and then, if the condition has persisted or is getting worse, the case should be immediately referred to a physician.

There are also other causes. We have known individuals whose breathy voices were being produced and maintained solely by improper habits of vocal attack. They always began voicing with a preliminary exhalation of air. We had to teach them to start speaking without this preparatory windup. Some persons use a breathy voice because of the fear of being heard or exposed. And a few of them employ it deliberately. The following case illustrates the latter point.

> Ruth, a rather plain high-school girl, was referred to us by her English teacher who reported that her voice was so husky she was unable to make herself heard in class. We examined the girl and discovered not only the huskiness but also a low habitual pitch level with certain inflections which were unmistakable. She could sing well and without any breathiness. A bit of sympathetic interviewing explained the situation. "The boys like this kind of voice," she said grinning. "I'm not too attractive, but a moose is a moose and they come when I call." We found out later that the boys called her "Hot-breath Harriet." We kept her secret.

The male has also been known to mistake asthma for passion.

The Harsh or Strident Voice. There are voices which are so rasping and piercing that they repel listeners. The basic characteristic of these voices is the presence of what is called the "vocal fry," because, perhaps, it sounds like the sizzling of bacon in the frying pan. It is hard to describe but fairly easy to produce. By opening your mouth and making a ticker-like, crackling sort of sound you can produce it and even slow it down until the separate clicks can be distinguished. When this vocal fry is fast, however, and accompanied by great tension, we have the basic quality of the strident or harsh voice. It is often accompanied by strain localized about the larynx and often this structure is pulled up almost into the position used in swallowing. If you will place the tip of a finger against your Adam's or Eve's apple and produce a very harsh voice you will know what we mean.

Along with these features we also find the presence of what is called the "hard attack." Normally, the vocal folds should be brought together almost simultaneously with the pulse of air pressure. In the aspirate or soft attack, as we have already seen, the vocal folds close *after* the air has begun to flow. In the hard attack, the folds are closed and held tightly prior to the breath pulse. To break them open and start them vibrating from this tight position requires extra effort. If you will squeeze and hold your vocal folds tightly closed and suddenly utter a vowel, you will hear the little strained click that indicates the hard attack. It is not a good way to produce voice; vocal nodules or contact ulcers may result from the strain.

The usual causes of the harsh voice are imitation, personality problems involving hostility and aggression, the need to make one-self heard in the presence of masking noise, and the use of improper pitch levels. We need not belabor the obviousness of the first two of these causes but some comment on the others is necessary. Strident voices seem to be able to make themselves heard more easily than normal voices even though the effect is often unpleasant. In this regard they are somewhat like hypernasality. They're harsh but you can hear them. Those of us whose professions demand constant speaking in noisy situations often develop them, and sound more aggressive than we are. One of the nicest persons we have ever known was a lady who was in charge of the woman's swimming classes at our university, and she sounded like a witch until she developed vocal nodules and had to have voice therapy as well as a change of jobs. The only way she had found to pierce the echoing noise of the splashing squealing girls was to scream at them harshly. One of our cases was a foreman in a noisy factory whose harsh straining voice finally gave out due to the formation of contact ulcers near the back ends of his vocal folds. Those of us who become teachers or speech therapists must remember to take care of our own professional tool, the human voice. It cannot be abused with impunity.

Finally, let us say something of pitch levels. Some persons, for one good reason or another, may lower their habitual pitch level nearly to its floor. If you will attempt to speak loudly at your own lowest note, you will find harshness and the vocal fry coming into your voice. You will find strain. Most of us, however, tend to raise our pitch level when we speak loudly. This too can lead to screaming stridency. It is possible to speak very loudly at your own natural pitch level, but some of us never discover this skill.

The Hoarse Voice. Acoustically, the hoarse voice may be said to be a combination of the breathy and the harsh voice quality disorders. In it you can hear the air wastage and also the straining vocal fry of the strident voice. When voices suddenly become hoarse, we look for evidence of over-use or abuse. Most of us have become hoarse from too much yelling at one time or another but not from praying. Usually with rest the hoarseness disappears. You've got to stop calling the pigs from the back forty, Ma. The same situation occurs as the result of a severe cold or laryngitis. Many boys develop a hoarse or husky voice just before puberty in an effort to assume the deep low tones of the adult male or to demonstrate their toughness. This too shall pass. But we wish to sound a strong note of warning about hoarseness. When it persists long after the abuse or laryngitis has disappeared, and there seems to be no apparent reason for its continuance, referral to a laryngologist should be made. Cancer of the larynx often shows its ugly head first in this form.

A hoarse voice may also be produced through ventricular phonation. By this term we refer to the vibration of the false vocal folds which lie above the true ones. It is uncommon but we have found it in some few bedeviled children who suffered many penalties. The following account by Voelker[3] may illustrate the problem.

One patient complained of dropping his voice at the end of sentences, and it was found that he did not lower his vocal-cord pitch but actually stopped using his vocal cords at the end of the sentence and substituted for them a ventricular vibration. An actor, with an excellent stage voice, complained of hoarseness only in conversation. It was found that in intimate and quiet conversation he used a ventricular voice to "save for his art" his stage voice. A youth was criticized by his parents for having a high and squeaky voice and acquired ventricular phonia in order to lower his voice to a normal pitch. Thus, instead of lowering his voice to a normal pitch, of perhaps 150 cycles, he lowered it to one of between 48 and 57 cycles. A similar case was found in which a man 31 years old, who had a deaf wife, became self-conscious about his yelling and outside his home developed phonation with the ventricular bands to subdue his voice. A college student raised the pitch of his voice to read aloud or to recite but used a ventricular tone in conversation. Sometimes it is found in careless conversation only. A 5-year-old boy was kidded by his playmates for having a high voice, and he lowered it by acquiring a ventricular voice. An 18-year-old youth, with a eunuchoid quality, substituted ventricular phonation for his weak and strident vocal cord voice and thought his new hoarse voice gave the impression of masculine virility.

In this chapter we have presented the various disorders of voice and their causes. In our next we shall describe their treatment.

1. Tape-record and analyze the voice of a person with poor pitch placement in singing.

[3] Voelker, C. H. "Phoniatry in Dysphonia Ventricularis," *Annals of Otology, Rhinology and Laryngology,* Volume 44, 1935, pages 471-472.

2. Hold a tone before a mirror but deliberately—manually, if necessary —raise the larynx and lower it. What happens to the voice under these conditions?

3. Speak a paragraph at the bottom and again at the ceiling of your pitch range and report the effects upon your intensity and voice quality.

4. Examine one of the old case folders of a voice case and summarize the diagnosis.

5. What is meant by "register" as it pertains to the voice?

6. Demonstrate clavicular breathing, air wastage, and opposition breathing.

7. Make a polygraphic breathing record of some person with cerebral palsy or of some severe stutterer.

8. Ask some otolaryngologist for permission to observe a laryngoscopic examination.

9. Prepare a large chart showing the location of adenoids or nasal polyps and discuss these before the class.

10. What are contact ulcers? See reference by Van Riper and Irwin. Summarize this information.

11. What is the effect of masking noise upon voice? Demonstrate.

12. Perform the activities listed on pages 150-151 in the reference by Hanley and Thurman and report your experience.

13. Demonstrate and discuss assimilation nasality.

14. Attempt to determine your own opitimal pitch range for speech. Report how you did so.

15. Write up a dialogue illustrating the diagnostic interview with a person who shows aphonia.

REFERENCES

16. Allen, B., and Peterson, G. E. "Laryngeal Inflammation in a Case of Falsetto," *Journal of Speech Disorders,* Volume 7, 1942, pages 175-178.

17. Bangs, J. L., and Freidinger, A. A. "Diagnosis and Treatment of a Case of Hysterical Aphonia in a Thirteen-year-old Girl," *Journal of Speech and Hearing Disorders,* Volume 14, 1949, pages 312-317.

18. Bartholomew, W. T. "The Paradox of Voice Teaching," *Journal of the Acoustical Society of America,* Volume 11, 1940, pages 446-450.

19. Curry, R. *The Mechanism of the Human Voice.* New York: Longmans Green, 1940.

20. Curry, T. "Hoarseness and Voice Change in Male Adolescents,"

Journal of Speech and Hearing Disorders, Volume 14, 1949, pages 23-25.

21. Curry, T. "Voice Breaks and Pathological Larynx Conditions," *Journal of Speech Disorders,* Volume 14, 1948, pages 356-358.

22. Fairbanks, G. *Voice and Articulation Drill Book,* Second edition. New York: Harper and Brothers, 1960.

23. Hanley, T. D., and Thurman, W. L. *Developing Vocal Skills.* New York: Holt, Rinehart and Wilson, 1962.

24. Hanley, C. N., and Manning, C. C. "Voice Quality After Adenectomy," *Journal Speech and Hearing Disorders,* Volume 23, 1958, pages 257-262.

25. Huber, M. W., and Kopp, A. E. *The Practice of Speech Correction in the Medical Clinic.* Boston: Expression Company, 1942.

26. Levin, N. M. (editor). *Voice and Speech Disorders.* Springfield, Illinois: C. C. Thomas, 1962.

27. Moses, P. J. *The Voice of Neurosis.* New York: Grune and Stratton, 1954.

28. Sokolowsky, R. R., and Junkermann, E. B. "War Aphonias," *Journal Speech Disorders,* Volume 9, 1944, pages 193-208.

29. Travis, L. E. (editor). *Handbook of Speech Pathology.* New York: Appleton-Century-Crofts, 1957, Chapters 22, 26.

30. Van Riper, C., and Irwin, J. V. *Voice and Articulation.* New York: Prentice-Hall, 1958.

31. Weiss, D. A. "The Pubertal Change of the Human Voice," *Folia Phoniatrica,* Volume 2, 1950, pages 126-159.

32. Williamson, A. B. "Diagnosis and Treatment of Eighty-Four Cases of Nasality," *Quarterly Journal of Speech,* Volume 30, 1944, pages 471-479.

33. Wilson, K. D. "Children with Vocal Nodules," *Journal Speech and Hearing Disorders,* Volume 26, 1961, pages 19-26.

CHAPTER EIGHT

Voice Disorders: Treatment

Motivation. Speech therapists who have watched professional singers working hour upon hour to perfect their tone, practicing scales, spending long hours with their voice teacher, sometimes envy that teacher. To find the same devotion in a person with a voice disorder is unusual. Even when the person has a falsetto or the husky voice due to severe vocal nodules, it is difficult to get him to work hard enough to hope for a favorable result. The reason for this state of affairs seems to lie in the relative lack of attention we pay to our voices. We listen to our thoughts rather than to the carrier waves on which they ride. In the expression of emotion, we are more concerned with the cargo of anger rather than the voice vehicle which carries it. In most communicative interchanges, the basic message is carried by the articulation rather than the tones, and unless the voice is so weak it cannot be heard, the fulfillment of communication generally rewards unpleasant voices as well as good ones. It is only in display speech such as that of the teacher or actor that a poor voice is a major handicap. Our society seems to be more tolerant of deviant voice than of deviant articulation or timing or language. For these reasons, then, it is always wise to explore the amount of motivation we can expect before undertaking therapy with our voice cases.

Identification of the Problem. One of the best ways we have found to motivate these cases is to have them hear their own voices on tape recordings, not once but over and over again. Once we put a schoolteacher with a very hypernasal voice into a booth, locked the door, and piped in her own recorded voice a bit amplified for fifteen minutes. From then on she worked very hard. We also have a delayed-speech apparatus which echoes what the person says about four seconds later. But best of all is a therapist who can imitate almost exactly the voice he hears. We train our own student therapists in this skill so that they can be the echo machine. Amplification, by means of one of the new binaural auditory training·units, can be very effective, especially if the therapist joins the person and first uses the abnormal voice, then shifts to a better one. The same effect can be had by having the person cup his hands to make a channel from his mouth to one ear, then the therapist alternately puts his echo and his normal voice into the other ear as they read in unison. At other times we feed a masking noise into the person's ears from an audiometer as he is speaking and then suddenly turn it off so the person hears his voice more vividly. Since much of the inability to hear one's voice comes from the adaptation to the usual conditions of phonation, almost anything which alters the usual conditions helps one to hear it as it is. Radio announcers long ago found that they could hear their own voices better by cupping one ear to alter the sound field. We use this device and occasionally employ a hearing aid to help the case identify his problem. It has been said that voice is monitored by bone conduction rather than by air-conducted sound, although the research on this is not definitive. However, we have often found that having the person plug his ears with his fingers makes it possible for him to hear his defective voice more clearly and to modify it.

Analyzing the Deviancy. We find that often the person is unable to recognize the deviancy in voice until he is trained in its analysis. One has to know what to listen for. One needs training. The therapist must train the case to do this analyzing, patiently providing examples of what is wrong, checking their occurrence in the person's voice. Let us give a description of this analyzing process as it would be done in hypernasality.

Recognition of Defective Quality. In order that the student may learn to recognize the unpleasant voice quality whenever it occurs in his speech, the vowels that are least defective should be used. The teacher should imitate these vowels as the student produces them, and then repeat them, using excess nasality. The student will readily recognize the difference. He should be required to produce these vowels first normally and then with excess nasality, carefully noting the difference. Lightly placed thumb and forefinger on each side of the septum, or the use of the cold mirror placed under the nostrils, will provide an accessory check of the presence of the hypernasality. The student should then listen to the teacher's production of his worst vowel, with and without nasality. If difficulty is experienced in recognizing this, the student can correlate his auditory judgments with the visual and tactual sensations received from the use of the mirror and finger-septum contact. Requiring him to close and open his eyes during alternate productions of the vowels as the teacher uses the mirror under her nostrils will soon provide adequate discrimination.

After some of this training has been successfully completed, the teacher should read a passage in which certain vowels are underlined and are purposely nasalized. The student should listen carefully, checking on a copy of the passage all vowels in which he hears the unpleasant quality. Many of the games and exercises used in the ear training of articulatory cases can be modified to teach the student better discrimination and identification of the good and bad voice qualities. Although at first the teacher will need to exaggerate the hypernasality, she should endeavor to decrease it gradually until the student is skilled in detecting even a slight amount of it. After this has been done, the student should read and reread a certain paragraph, making judgments after each word as to whether or not excess nasality occurred. These judgments may be checked by the teacher, and the percentage of correct judgments ascertained. This procedure will serve as a motivating device. The student may also be required to repeat series of words or isolated vowels, using the mirror under his nostrils and making his judgment of normal or nasal voice quality before opening his eyes to observe the clouding or nonclouding of the mirror. Much home practice of this sort can be used.

The same sort of self-scanning should be used with other voice disorders. Unless the person comes to hear what is wrong, he will not right it. There is one caution we wish to leave with you. Occasionally, a person may feel that he is becoming much worse as the result of the recognition training. All that has happened is that he has become more conscious of what has always been there before, but it is wise, early in treatment, to warn him that this may occur and that it is a good sign of improvement. Similarly, some of our voice cases may become rather emotional and rejecting of themselves as the defective voice becomes more apparent to them. However, if the therapist is able to share the problem, using the abnormal voice calmly and without anxiety, the person usually soon becomes desensitized to it. We have found it wise from the beginning examination to present the task as a joint endeavor. We explore its causes together, and together we work to modify the voice.

Discovering the New Voice. We have written earlier that each of us is the potential possessor of many voices. We can all vary our pitch, intensity, and quality pretty much at will, although few of us have ever felt that it was possible or necessary to learn a new habitual voice. When this necessity becomes apparent, as a result of the training in awareness, we might think that little further difficulty in procuring cooperation would be necessary. However, a storm of resistance usually arises at this point. This is what one of our cases said to us:

> Yesterday, when we made that tape recording of my new voice and I heard it, I felt all mixed up inside. I told you it sounded much better, and it does. Compared to my old voice, it's a great improvement. But it isn't ME! It just isn't. I sound like a phony or like an actor playing a part. I know it's better but I don't want to talk so strangely. I just couldn't keep my appointment with you today because I'm so upset about it. I'm even thinking of quitting. I know you said I'd get used to it but right now I don't think I ever could.

She got used to it and now it is the old voice which seems unbelievable to her. But this is a problem to be faced. The voice is closely integrated with the personality. Its inflections, volume, and quality have been used since childhood to express emotion. The old voice has a long history of being associated with basic feelings. It does not yield easily to modification, but it does yield. The important thing is that both the therapist and the person with the voice problem must anticipate this resistance and be prepared to cope with it.

Variation. One of the ways to overcome this built-in rigidity and resistance is to begin by exploring all the possible ways of producing phonation. We must together share in free variation, almost in tonal play, trying one vocal variation after another. Van Riper and Irwin describe this process as follows:

> First we can get the case to run through his entire repertoire of possible phonation, locating within it the desired target tones. Few indi-

viduals are entirely consistent in their abnormal voice. Some vowels, for example, may be less nasalized than others; in certain activities, such as sighing, no hard attacks or tension may make the tone strident; in shouting, no breathiness may occur; in humming, a higher pitch level may be used. By varying the postural, breathing, pitch, intensity, or quality factors we may be able to locate within the individual's own phonation the voice we need to use as a standard, as a goal.[1]

Let us view some of the specific ways by which we might help our voice case to do this varying of his phonation, this searching for a better voice. We shall describe this phase of our therapy for a pitch disorder, for an intensity disorder, and for one of voice quality, realizing that the techniques used are not mutually exclusive. Some of those used in finding a better pitch level can also be used to find a better voice quality.

Varying the Pitch Level.   Instead of listing some abstract principles, we present some actual casework:

T. J. was a nineteen-year-old boy with a high-pitched monotonal falsetto which was inconsistent in that occasionally nonfalsetto tones were heard although they too were spoken at the same high level. After the usual ear-training in identifying the problem, we had a session in which we demonstrated the following kinds of phonation and asked him to join us and to duplicate what we heard: (1) We asked him to do some vocalized donkey-breathing, alternately on inhalation and on exhalation, and very rhythmically. As we produced the model, we occasionally changed the pitch of the exhaled sound, using first the falsetto ourselves and then lower normal tones. Several of his tones were very good. (2) We asked him to retract his head as far as he could, then to bring it forward until it dropped down on his chest, producing a long sigh as he did so. We showed him and first did what he did so far as sound was concerned, then gradually let our own pitch fall as the sigh ended. He followed us and ended with a weak breathy but very low tone. (3) We showed him some stretching and yawning and asked him to join us, saying "Awwwww" in the middle of the yawn. (4) We placed some tissue paper over a comb and asked him to buzz it, using a prolonged *z* sound with his lips against the paper. The tone we used was of low pitch, and so was his. We then asked him to say *zzzeeezzz* and *zzzooozzz* and then *zzzzoooooo* as he buzzed the comb. This failed for he used a falsetto buzz. (5) We asked him to duplicate a vocalized clearing of the throat as he held his fingers in his ears. It was very low-pitched and without any falsetto. (6) We

---

[1] Van Riper, Charles, and Irwin, John V. *Voice and Articulation.* Englewood Cliffs, N.J.: Prentice-Hall, Inc., 1958, page 285.

then taught him the clicking vocal fry until he could sustain it for several seconds, then had him open and shut his jaws and lips during the fry phonation. In this activity we heard normal phonation along with the vocal fry. (7) We demonstrated head and jaw shaking from side to side while we produced various vowels of different pitches.

Varying the Pitch. The pitch of the voice usually varies with the intensity. By increasing the loudness, the tone will usually be made to rise in pitch. Even high-pitched falsettos will shift downward if a tone is first initiated very loudly, then gradually softened as it is prolonged. Pitch rises when the laryngeal musculature is tensed, and we can use this feature in therapy. Tension in almost any part of the body seems to be reflected and finds some focus in the larynx. By asking the person to pull upward on the seat of his chair, or to push down on the table, we can increase the tension of the vocal folds and raise the pitch of a sustained tone. This works best if the effort is applied in pulses. Conversely, if we wish to lower a pitch, we can begin by using strong muscular contractions and let go jerkily in a series of relaxations.

The self-perception of pitch is still mysterious. We still do not know why some individuals with excellent hearing seem to be unable to match a given pitch or to locate their own voices on a scale. They sing off key and do not know it. However, there seems to be some evidence that pitch perception is tied in somehow with body postures and kinesthesia. Even little children who have never seen a musical scale lift their heads and rise on tiptoe when they reach for a high note. When we try to sing very low, we tuck our chins in, lowering our heads. At any rate, we have found that, by having the case follow our head or arm or body movements as we show him how his pitches are rising or falling or being sustained, we can improve his faulty pitch placement. Here is a brief transcript of part of a session with such a person whose pitch breaks were driving him crazy.

Therapist: Now lower your head way down like this, then bring it up in three steps as we sing together doh-me-sol.
Case: doh-fa-la.
Therapist: O.K. You went up—but you took two big steps. Raise your head in smaller steps. Here, I'll hold your head and move it. . . .
Case: doh-fa-sol.

Therapist: That's better. The first and last were all right. You sang
do-fa-sol. It should be do-*me*-sol. Let's make the second
movement smaller. . . .

We stopped the transcript just in time. The case sang, "doh-la-
tee." This is patient work, this voice-retraining—but we have suc-
ceeded often when our first attempts seemed to reveal a hopeless
prognosis. With real motivation, surprising results may be had. In
this regard, we find that a prime motivation is the opportunity provided by a permissive therapist for the case's singing. These sour-
toned people love to sing and they've been penalized and frustrated
most of their lives because their "pear-shaped tones" turn out to be
lemons. So we let them sing a lot and do some voice therapy when
we can. Another similar method consists of pitch-writing. We take
the case's hand as he holds the pencil or chalk and tell him to go
up and down or hum or sing his own invented tunes. Then we trace
the variations and provide a graphic record.

Although the above method for teaching a new pitch level is most
effective, there are several others. One frequently employed uses the
vocalized sigh or yawn to produce the desired pitch. These sighs
and yawns must be accompanied by decreasing intensity and relaxation in order to be most effective. Another method employs excla-
mations of disgust or contempt in order to provide a lower pitch.
Still another makes use of the grunts and noises symbolic of relief or
feeding. Clearing the throat may also be used to provide a lower
pitch. These methods are often effective with true monotones when
the former stimulation or matching method fails. Many of the techniques included in the stimulation method are combined with the
biological-activity methods in order to provide the necessary stability of performance.

Varying the Intensity.   Since the majority of our intensity problems
consist of voices which are too weak rather than strong, our therapy
is usually designed to strengthen them. Where there is no organic
pathology such as vocal nodules, paralysis, or contact ulcers, we
can assume that the person does possess an adequate voice. Our task
is to help him find it. Often we discover that emotional insecurity
lies at the bottom of the problem and we must provide opportunities
for exploration and release of these feelings. These people often are
fearful of establishing close relationships and their barely audible
voices reflect this fear. A warm, permissive therapist can make the

vocal therapy itself a means of creating at least one nonthreatening relationship. Often the speech therapy is less important than the case's testing of the therapist's acceptance, but we use the vocal exercises as the pathway to reassurance. By extending the therapy to other communicative situations, the person comes to find that the world may not be as threatening as he had supposed.

But there are often habits involved too. Whatever the original cause of the weak voice, these people often show inefficient forms of breathing when speaking. They may habitually exhale much of the inhaled air prior to vocalization (air wastage), or make a series of small inhalations rather than one large one (staircase breathing), or speak on the very end of the exhaled breath, or speak while the chest is expanding (opposition breathing). A certain amount of air pressure is needed for adequate phonation and these methods of speech breathing make it difficult to speak loudly enough for communication. We seldom need to teach the person how to breathe; but there are times when we have to teach him to stop breathing in an abnormal way. Once he knows what he is doing wrongly and recognizes the moments of normal breathing which he always shows occasionally, the normal patterns will return.

Often, the problem may consist of the use of improper pitch levels. The person who speaks at the very bottom, or very top, of his pitch range, for any reason, cannot have normal vocal intensity. We may therefore have to change the habitual pitch. We have had cases referred to us as having weak voices who merely were fearful that if they spoke in their usual way, they would have pitch breaks upward into the falsetto. With these, it was necessary to work on pitch control and to ignore the intensity. Generally, intensity becomes louder as the pitch rises. By prolonging tones and then introducing rhythmic pulses of pitch rises which go higher and higher, the intensity of the pulses becomes louder and louder.

Certain voice quality changes can also increase the intensity. By making the voice less breathy or aspirate through the use of very sudden bursts of sound, the voice becomes louder. Increasing the nasality a bit also helps. We once solved the problem of a foreman in a steel mill who was constantly losing his voice and could barely speak above a whisper due to the constant strain to make himself heard. We trained him to speak with a nasal twang while he was on the job.

Also the duration aspects of voice should be explored. By prolonging the vowels a bit, the carrying quality of the voice can be improved. Most public speakers have learned this technique. Also, a slowing down of the rate and the use of longer pauses seem to aid intelligibility.

Some of these cases are difficult to hear merely because they speak with their mouths almost shut—because they do not articulate with any energy. Putting a stopper in any horn diminishes the loudness of its tones. We teach these people to uncork their mouth openings. Also, by making the plosives distinctly or by stressing the fricative consonants, we can compensate for the lack of vocal intensity. Many of the bad habits of utterance are due to excessive tension in the mouth, tongue, or throat, and by relaxing these focal points of tension, the voice becomes freer and louder. One of the common areas of excessive muscular contraction is the region just above the larynx and below the chin. The larynx is often raised almost into the position for swallowing. When a person habitually assumes this abnormal posture prior to vocalization, it is difficult to produce normal voice no matter what effort is expended. Again, we must identify this abnormal behavior and bring it up to consciousness so that it can be brought under voluntary control and eliminated. Voice should not be squeezed out. It needs an open, relaxed, natural channel. At times we have these persons talk while chewing to discover the normal function. Some of our voice cases have forgotten how to produce voice normally. We must show them.

A few of our voice cases, especially those who have some paralysis of the vocal folds, need more energy rather than less, and they need it in the right places. Certain pushing exercises with the arms or legs, or sudden contractions of the fists may aid if they are accompanied by phonation. Also we have found that certain large body postures facilitate louder and freer voices. One of our cases first found his natural voice while on hands and knees with arms extended forward and his head backward. Once he had found it, he gradually became able to produce it in any position.

Finally, we use masking noise to prevent self-hearing when we feel that the person can really produce normal voice but inhibitions prevent it. We ask such a case to continue reading aloud while we gradually introduce a masking noise from an audiometer or tape recorder into both ears. Usually, the person's voice grows much louder as the noise level increases. When we feel that sufficient change has occurred we suddenly shut off the noise and he hears himself speaking with a normal voice. One of the author's cases was "cured" when he suddenly emerged from a noisy factory and found himself shouting.

Aphonia. Aphonia, or the complete loss of voice, is usually due to overstrain, organic defects, or emotional causes. If the cause is overstrain, rest and silence, or, at the best, whispered speech, should be prescribed. Occasionally the case is required to use a different pitch level when his voice begins to return. If the disorder is due to pathology, medical and surgical care is necessary. If it is due to emotional conflicts, psychiatric treatment (or the type of treatment discussed under readjustment methods) should be administered. In any case, if voice retraining is used, it is merely an accessory tool.

Suggestion is frequently used with hysterical aphonias. Physicians often use a faradic current or ammonia inhalation or massage as the culminating procedures in a period of treatment marked by complete cessation of speech attempt and strong cumulative suggestion. In many instances, coughing is used to demonstrate to the patient that voice exists. Persons who have once had such aphonia are likely to have it again unless the cause is removed. In some instances, when the cause cannot be discovered, a relapse is prevented by having the individual perform some simple vocal ritual each day, such as prolonging each of the vowels for ten seconds.

Some quotations from an article by Sokolowsky and Junkermann[1] will illustrate some of the methods for treating hysterical aphonia:

> First, we administered breathing exercises in connection with a systematic speech and voice retraining . . . (using a humming breathing; speech attempt while "pressing together the hands of a nurse standing behind him";) . . . By means of this phonetic re-education we succeeded in restoring the voice to about 60 per cent of our aphonics, a rather meager result considering the relatively tiresome treatment which sometimes lasted several weeks.
>
> Induced by the publications of Muck and his extraordinary results we then tried his method—the introduction of a pellet or small ball into the larynx between the vocal cords, in order to bring about a

[1] Sokolowsky, R. R., and Junkermann, E. R. "War Aphonia," *Journal Speech Disorders,* Volume 9, 1944, pages 192-208.

sensation of being suffocated which superinduced a cry of fright. We
have to confess that our own results with Muck's ball were not very
encouraging.

As soon as the anamnesis pointed to a psychogenic aphonia and the
laryngoscopic mirror confirmed this assumption a short remark such
as, "You will be all right quite soon," or, "You will be getting your
voice back quite soon," was made. After that the patient was not permitted, so to speak, to "collect his wits." All manipulations such as
setting the head in proper position and pulling out the tongue were
carried out as quickly as possible, and accompanied by short, crisp
and somewhat commanding words. Then followed the deep introduction of the mirror and the attempt to obtain a vocal retching reaction.
After this was accomplished, it was brought into the consciousness of
the patient with short, crisp remarks, such as "Here we are," "Now
your voice is back," or "Do you hear your voice?" After that it required but relatively little effort (the mirror, of course, remaining
continually in the throat) to elicit from the patient the unpleasant gag-
reminding but nevertheless audible "ah."

Varying the Voice Quality.   Nowhere will we find resistance to
change as tenacious as in voice quality. A habitual voice quality
seems as much a part of the person as his nose and unconsciously
the case seems to say "Keep your therapeutic fingers off my proboscis!" It has been so closely associated with egocentric speech, with
emotional expression, with communication, that it is almost a basic
feature of the self. Even when the case hates her voice, a better voice
sounds so strange and artificial, she tends to sabotage any attempts
to change it. We have found it essential to verbalize this, to predict
the resistance and to help the case understand it. It is unwise to ask
the person to use new voices in communication, in social gesture, in
emotional expression until this phase of resistance has passed.

Accordingly, our first experimentation with change in voice quality should be attempted only in play, in fantasy, in imitation of
animal noises, or imitation of other people. The therapist must set
the appropriate models and he must be in command of almost as
many voices as a professional actor. We have trained our majors in
speech therapy in these skills so that they can provide these variations in voice quality. Too many beginning therapists try too soon
to get a better voice quality from their clients. First they must discover how many voices they own; first they must vary and play with
their voices.

This variation should first of all involve changes in pitch and intensity which are easier to accomplish. Then perhaps a falsetto, or a hypernasal voice can be attempted. Then a denasal or throaty (low pitched falsetto) or harsh or hoarse voice can be assumed.

After these gross variations, we have found it useful to go with the client into stores and to study and later to imitate the voices of various clerks. We help the person to learn the technique of silent echo-speaking, pantomime in sub-vocal form the speech of the person being heard. Then we use playlets or dialogues, taking various parts and adopting the voices most appropriate. Again the therapist must share the variation and set the models.

Out of all this variation training comes the firm understanding that voice change is possible. The experiences have been pleasant. The person realizes for the first time that he has not one voice but many —and that he has a choice!

Fixation. Once the person has come to identify his abnormal voice and has learned to vary it, our next task is to get him to locate and fix solidly his new voice. The process is at first a bit like target shooting. He may miss the bull's-eye of the new voice quality more than he hits it. His voice gun tends to wobble. New patterns of muscular contractions and of laryngeal or pharyngeal postures must be learned. It is the therapist's role to help him know how far off the mark his vocal attempts have been. Patiently the therapist makes suggestions, points out the extent of the difference between the voice produced and that desired.

In this process it is helpful if the therapist is able to imitate with some fidelity the case's various voice productions and also to present a model of the voice to be attained. We seem to use a tape recorder more often with voice cases than with any other of the speech disorders. Usually it is possible, even very early in treatment, to get a sample or two of the desired voice. This we isolate from the rest, make a loop of tape bearing the good sample, and use this as our target.

Every session at this phase of treatment begins with a playing of this model loop and we use it often to provide the bull's-eye. We also often make a tape recording which has on it, first a vivid sample of the abnormal voice at its worst, then a series of graduated and numbered voice samples which progressively come closer and closer to the voice desired which forms the terminal example. After the case becomes familiar with this "measuring tape," he is able, with fair consistency, to evaluate any vocal attempts in terms of its proximity to the desired new voice. Strong motivation is thereby procured.

Progressive Approximation. Let us say here again, that speech therapy is not a matter of exchange of one type of speech for another but a process of progressive approximations. Therapists who have only *good* and *bad* or *yes* and *no* in their professional vocabularies should exchange them for *closer* and *further* or *hotter* and *colder* as in the old nursery game. In voice therapy, we work with little shifts, and we reinforce with our approval those vocal attempts that come closer to the desired goal. This holds for disorders of pitch, intensity, and quality and for all types of variant human behavior seeking to modify itself.

To aid in getting this concept across (for the case too tends to make judgments in terms of black and white) it is well for the therapist to present models of these miniature modifications that change in the direction of the goal. It is the client's task to judge whether they approach or retreat from the goal. By using large changes first, and then smaller ones, the case's perceptions and discriminations are sharpened and he can then evaluate his own attempts with objectivity.

One of our favorite ways for using progressive approximation in voice therapy is to use a binaural auditory trainer. We then feed in the case's voice into one ear and our own voice into his other ear, thereby permitting simultaneous comparison. We usually begin by joining the case as he reads or phonates a tone, imitating him closely so both voices harmonize in unison, then gradually we change our own voice in small steps in the direction of the desired voice. Perceiving the difference, the case often shifts unconsciously to bring both voices together again, and so a progressive approximation has occurred. Often it is necessary for the therapist to rejoin the case and use the latter's voice again before attempting another shift. But careful training in this way, along with commentary, breaks for relaxation, and suggested corrections, can be very effective. There is also in this procedure a basic psychotherapeutic healing. The case is not alone. Some one is sharing his problem, someone is identifying with him who knows the path out of his troubles.

If no auditory trainer is available, the case may use his cupped hands to bring his voice to one ear while the therapist puts his mouth to the other. We have often used the Van Riper speech shoe (see figure 23) to present the gradual modification of voice monaurally.

Stabilization. New voices are weak and unstable. They need careful tending at first. We have found it wise to insist that the case use it at first only in the therapy sessions where we can concentrate on its motor and acoustic aspects and make it stronger therein.

Once we feel the case has the new voice fairly solidly and can use it consistently in therapy when he's listening to himself, we introduce masking noise into his ears so he can monitor it by proprioception alone, by feeling the vocal postures and muscle tensions. Often at first, this masking tends to create a regression to the old voice, so we introduce the masking noise gradually and intermittently. No one can ever come to use a new voice habitually if he must constantly listen to it. We have to use our ears to hear what others are saying and, indeed, to discover what thoughts we are verbalizing! Let's not burden the ears too much. It is also necessary to be sure that the case can use the new voice at his natural tempo or speed of utterance. It must not be labored or too careful. It cannot be confined to a monotone or chant. All these motor and acoustic variations need some attention.

Next we attempt to stabilize the new voice in display speech, and we like to make recordings of the new voice so the person can listen to them and feel good. Role playing, orating, readings, all can be used for this purpose. Often at this point we ask the person to give us a verbal autobiography, and to use the new voice while doing so. This should run for several sessions. We do this so as to help to identify the new voice with the self. The perpendicular pronoun "I" especially should become colored with the new voice. This provides an opportunity for some mild psychotherapy at the same time. However, as we shall see, we prefer at this stage to keep emotional expression fairly innocuous.

Next we like to stabilize the new voice in the thinking aspect of speech. We show slide films, provide problems, and ask the case to keep a running commentary going in the new voice. At times we even have him do a lot of free or controlled association, saying whatever thoughts that come. It is interesting to watch a case whispering and pantomiming in the new voice. We cannot hear it, but he insists that it is *there* and when we suddenly signal for him to vocalize, it appears. Pantomimic speech is close to thought.

When we feel definite progress has been made in the foregoing aspects of speech, we stabilize it in communication. We ask the case now to use the new voice outside the therapy sessions—but at first only when he talks to strangers. We do this to avoid the listener's shocked surprise that often greets a voice case when he confronts them with a new voice. The father of a young man who had never known anything but a high falsetto voice stormed into the bathroom one morning to find out what strange man was in the house at seven in the morning. The boy had only said something to the family dog.

Once the new voice has been used easily with strangers, it can be brought out in the circle of acquaintances and friends or family. It is wise to suggest that the person speak of his voice therapy casually or use it as a conversation piece. Most people are very interested. About this time (and perhaps we have elongated the process unduly in describing it, for at times we have changed voices in a single hour), the new voice becomes stabilized and is felt as natural as the old one had been. There will be a few momentary relapses, usually in emotional expression, but the task has been accomplished.

PROJECTS

1. Demonstrate before the class all the disorders of voice quality. Practice them until you can produce reasonably close facsimiles.
2. Interview some esophageal speaker and persuade him to speak about his new voice before the class. Contact the local Cancer Society.
3. Ask some actor or successful speaker to speak to the class concerning his voice training and usage.
4. Interview some instructor in the music department concerning methods for improving pitch discrimination and placement.
5. Using an electric razor against the throat, or an electro-larynx if one is available, demonstrate artificial speech.
6. Summarize the various methods for changing the pitch of the voice. List all techniques you can find.
7. Find someone who can yodel. Record his yodeling and his comments on how he does it.

8. Do some experimenting with the projection of the voice across the football or baseball field with some listener. What ways of increasing your intelligibility do you find?

9. Make a clay or plasticine model of the larynx showing some vocal nodules.

10. Bring some samples of breathing records of assumed abnormalities. Use a polygraph. You may find one in your hospital or police station.

11. Determine your pitch range, your habitual pitch, and the location of the falsetto on this range.

12. Demonstrate to the class Jacobson's method of differential relaxation.

13. Demonstrate the vocal fry and describe its contribution to harsh voice quality.

14. Demonstrate the chewing approach to voice therapy. See references.

15. Demonstrate the influence of head, neck, and tongue postures on voice production.

16. Demonstrate the "hard attack" and the "aspirate or soft attack" before the class and discuss them in relation to voice disorders.

17. Select some victim from the class and demonstrate, with commentary, the effect of pitch change and intensity change upon voice quality.

18. Demonstrate a continuing falsetto quality as you gradually shift from a high pitch downward to the bottom of your range.

19. What are the articulatory deviations associated with the denasal voice? Illustrate.

20. Play tape recordings of hypernasal and normal voices backward before the class to see if the class members can distinguish between the two.

REFERENCES

21. Adler, S. "Some Techniques for Treating the Hypernasal Voice," *Journal Speech and Hearing Disorders,* Volume 25, 1960, pages 300-302.

22. Babcock, M. "Speech Therapy for Certain Vocal Disorders," *Journal of Laryngology and Otolaryngology,* Volume 57, 1940, pages 446-450.

23. Bangs, J. L., and Freiding, A. A. "A Case of Hysterical Dysphonia in an Adult," *Journal of Speech and Hearing Disorders,* Volume 15, 1950, pages 316-323.

24. Beebe, H. H. "Practical Aspect of Chewing Therapy," *Folia Phoniatrica,* Volume 7, 1955, pages 193-200.

25. Berry, M. F., and Eisenson, J. *Speech Disorders*. New York: Appleton-Century-Crofts, 1956, Chapters 9 and 10.

26. Brodnitz, F. S. *Keep Your Voice Healthy*. New York: Harper and Row, Publishers, 1953.

27. ———. *Vocal Rehabilitation*. New York: American Academy of Ophthamology and Otolaryngology, 1959.

28. ———. "Vocal Rehabilitation in Benign Lesions of the Vocal Cords," *Journal Speech and Hearing Disorders,* Volume 23, 1958, pages 112-117.

29. Canfield, W. "Dysphonia Associated with Unilateral Vocal Cord Paralysis," *Journal Speech and Hearing Disorders,* Volume 27, 1962, pages 280-283.

30. Duncan, M. H. "Personality Adjustment Techniques in Voice Therapy," *Journal of Speech Disorders,* Volume 12, 1947, pages 161-167.

31. Fairbanks, G. *Practical Voice Practice*. New York: Harper and Row, Publishers, 1944.

32. Froeschels, E., and Jellinek, A. *Practice of Voice and Speech Therapy*. Boston: Expression Company, 1941, pages 248ff.

33. ———. "Some Important Links between Logopedics and Otolaryngology," *Folia Phoniatrica,* Volume 4, 1952, pages 1-8.

34. Hanley, T. D., and Thurman, W. L. *Developing Vocal Skills*. New York: Holt, Rinehart & Winston, Inc., 1962.

35. Hyman, M. "An Experimental Study of Artificial Larynx and Esophageal Speech," *Journal Speech and Hearing Disorders,* Volume 20, 1955, pages 291-299.

36. Jacobson, E. *Progressive Relaxation*. Chicago: University of Chicago Press, 1938.

37. Levin, N. M. *Voice and Speech Disorders*. Springfield, Ill.: Charles C. Thomas, Publisher, 1962, Chapters 9-12.

38. Loebell, H. "Voice and Speech Disorders in the German Army," *Quarterly Journal of Speech,* Volume 30, 1944, pages 259-261.

39. Marland, P. M. "A Direct Method for Teaching Voice after Laryngectomy," *Speech* (London), Volume 13, 1949, pages 4-13.

40. Moser, H. M. "Diagnostic and Clinical Procedures in Rhinolalia," *Journal of Speech Disorders,* Volume 7, 1942, pages 1-4.

41. ———. "Symposium on Unique Cases of Speech Disorders; Presentaof a Case," *Journal of Speech Disorders,* Volume 7, 1942, pages 173-174.

42. Peacher, G. "Contact Ulcer of the Larynx: A Clinical Study of Vocal Reeducation, Part III," *Journal of Speech Disorders,* Volume 12, pages 179-190.

43. ———. "Vocal Therapy for Contact Ulcer of the Larynx," *Laryngoscope,* Volume 71, 1961, pages 37-47.

44. Rubin, H. J., and Lehrhoff, I. "Pathogenesis and Treatment of Vocal Nodules," *Journal Speech and Hearing Disorders,* Volume 27, 1962, pages 150-161.
45. Thorne, K. " 'Client Centered' Therapy for Voice and Personality Cases," *Journal Speech Disorders,* Volume 12, 1947, pages 314-318.
46. Van Riper, C., and Irwin, J. V. *Voice and Articulation.* Englewood Cliffs, N.J.: Prentice-Hall, Inc., 1958.
47. Weiss, D. A., and Beebe, H. H. *The Chewing Approach in Speech and Voice Therapy.* New York: S. Karger, 1951.
48. Williamson, A. B. "Diagnosis and Treatment of Seventy-Two Cases of Hoarse Voice," *Quarterly Journal of Speech,* Volume 31, 1945, pages 189-202.

CHAPTER NINE

※※ Articulation Disorders: Nature and Causes

The usual reaction of parents or teachers to a child who shows errors in his speech sounds is to start correcting them immediately. If he says "witto" for "little," they tell him he's made a mistake and should say the word right. The speech therapist goes at the problem a bit differently. He begins by attempting to see the difficulty as a whole, to understand its nature, its causes. He tries to answer the questions: *"Why does the child have articulation errors?" "What are the errors?"* before he asks, *"What must be done to eliminate them?"*

The Causes of the Disorders of Articulation

We may begin our investigation of the past history of the person by attempting to determine the origin of the problem. Often, however, the information we can procure from parents in this respect is vague and unreliable, primarily because the majority of these difficulties date from the earliest years of a child's life. Nevertheless, in interviewing parents or the person himself we often find clues which help us greatly in formulating our therapy program.

One of our cases, a fifth-grade boy, whose lalling made his speech almost unintelligible, had received public-school speech therapy for three years without any apparent improvement. Intensive interviewing of his parents finally brought forth the information that at the age of three, he had sucked a styptic pencil which had burned his mouth and tongue severely. It had finally healed after about a month and the parents had forgotten the incident. Our examination of the child's mouth revealed no scar tissue but we found that he showed great fear when we put a tongue depressor into his mouth. After a preliminary course of treatment in which we had him insert stick candies and lift them with his tonguetip, tap them around, resist their pressure, lick them with an open mouth, the fear disappeared and he began to be able to lift his tongue tip in speech.

In the case just cited, the original cause of the lalling, namely, a conditioned fear of moving the tongue tip, was still present. There are many such causal or etiological factors: a transient hearing loss, an inability to perceive the sequences of sounds composing the defectively uttered words, poor phonetic discrimination, and many others. To attempt to help these children without paying any attention to the sources of their disabilities is to waste our efforts and to create a profound sense of failure or frustration. When such causes are still operative, we must identify and focus our efforts to eliminate them.

However, we must also remember that speech is learned and may be mislearned. Once it is learned, it is difficult to change since so much of it is automatic. In a child who learned "thoup" and thinks "thoup" and has said it in successful communication a thousand times, the errors will persist of their own momentum. We must try to discover why he learned the error in the first place. Over and over again, intensive exploration yields significant answers. We may find no *present* causes operating currently except for this momentum of habit strength, yet discover that once there were causes which initiated the problem.

Some of the causes of defective articulation may have been lost in the mists of speech development by the time the person comes to us. Some may no longer be effective, though at an earlier period they may have been highly potent. Certain factors may have created habits of defective articulation which persist long after they themselves have been removed.

A preacher who came to us for help with his lateral lisp had no organic abnormality, hearing deficiency, poor coordination, or any other of the usual causes of such a disorder. No one else in his family had such a defect. Finally, however, he recalled that during his second and third years of life he had a nursemaid who was his constant companion and who had no upper teeth at all. When listening to the recording of another lateral-lisper, a woman, he said, "That sounds just like Nana's voice. She was my nurse."

Frequently several factors may be found, each of which could help to create or perpetuate the defective sounds. At times the defective consonant is merely the product of bad teaching, and its continued presence is due to habit alone. In view of this picture of a wide range of symptoms and causes, we have felt it advisable to devote an entire section to the genesis and analysis of articulation errors.

In summary then, we must recognize that there are some causal factors which are responsible for the onset of the disorder, others that currently maintain the disorder. In any given case, we may expect to find not a single cause, but often several which may account for the occurrence and persistence of articulation error.*

Developmental Factors

Our last two chapters have stressed the importance of developmental factors. First we should explore the *maturation of articulation in the child.* Of greatest importance is the approximate determination of the onset of first words and phrases, for we must know immediately whether the articulation errors are merely the natural residue of speech which is still maturing or whether instead they represent fixed mislearnings of the standard sounds. The child of eight who had no intelligible speech until five, but who has been improving rapidly since, does not present the same picture as the child who began to speak at the normal time but whose errors have shown no change in six years. If we had a choice of cases, we would certainly prefer to work with the first, if swift progress in therapy is expected. We also need to know the kinds of models provided, the amount of speech stimulation, the ways in which the parents have tried to help the child, the parental attitudes toward his defective speech.

Illnesses and Disabilities. We must also assess the importance of illnesses or accidents, of abnormalities in physical growth or development. Are these speech disabilities the result of brain injuries? Are the articulation errors merely the reflection of poor coordinating

---

* In the Appendix at the end of this book you will find descriptions of the methods used for testing auditory memory span, phonetic discrimination, phonetic analysis and synthesis, tests of motor coordination, and the examination for organic abnormalities. See pages 472-484.

ability which shows and showed itself in walking as well as in talking? Is this case one of dysarthria or dyslalia? Did he suck, chew, or swallow in an odd fashion? Is there any evidence that might explain a persistent lateral lisp in terms of early temporary hearing loss— severe earaches, running ears, periods of seeming deafness? Was this person chronically sick during the speech readiness period? All these are important questions, all-important questions. They help us know the problem we confront.

Intelligence and Social Maturity. Similarly, we must know something about the child's *intelligence and social maturity*. Perhaps he is talking as well as his mental age and circumstances permit. Speaking involves thinking. Is this speech retardation appropriate to the degree of mental or physical retardation shown by the child? How socially mature is this case of our—or how infantile? Is he using his defective speech as a tool to control others? What needs for defective speech are present? A developmental history will help find the answers. Let us illustrate briefly, in terms of the case history, some samples of the significant information it can provide:

Parental and Family Influences

Names. If the names of the parents are foreign, the child's consonant errors might possibly be due to imitation of parental brogue, or to the learning of similar consonants belonging to another language. Thus, in one of our cases, the child who substituted *t* for *th* (ɵ), did so because he imitated his father's pronunciation of *th* words. The father's name (which gave us the first clue) was Molo Zymolaga.

Age. When the age of the parents seems somewhat unusual in terms of the child's age, certain emotional factors may be influencing the latter's speech development. Thus, Peter, age seven, had parents aged twenty-two and twenty-four, and (as we found out by following the clue) was an unwanted child, neglected, unstimulated, and untrained. His articulatory errors were easily understood against this background. Or, consider Jane, who astonished her forty-nine-year-old father and forty-five-year-old mother by being born. Their excessive attention and demand for adult speech standards too early drove the child into a negativism which made her reject their constant corrections and persist in her errors.

Speech Defect. Imitation is often a causal factor in articulation, but we must be sure that the symptoms are similar. All five children of a family living on an isolated farm had nasal lisps. Organically, they were perfect specimens, but their mother had a cleft palate. It is often wise to explore to ascertain whether or not the parents had possessed a speech defect in their own childhood, since such an event would affect their attitudes toward the child's difficulty.

Physical Defects. If the mother is deaf, we can easily understand how a child's articulatory errors would receive little attention from her. Here are two other items from our case history files which had significance in our understanding of the child's speech problem: a father whose tongue-tip had been shot off in a hunting accident; a "nervous" hyperthyroid mother so unstable that she screamed whenever the children made noise or mispronounced a word.

Emotional Conflicts. Conflicts between one parent and the other, or between parent and child, can arise in each of the other areas mentioned in the case history: handedness, religion, education, occupation, and so on. Other people living in the home or closely associated with the child may have significant harmful influences on the child's speech development.

Developmental History

Birth History. Severe birth injuries have malformed the mouth cavity and wrecked the alignment of the jaws or teeth. They sometimes produce, through their injury to the brain, not only feeble-mindedness but the unsure, trembling or spastic coordinations of cerebral palsy.

Physical Development. When we learn that a child was delayed in sitting alone, in feeding himself, in walking, we usually probe to discover whether the speech development was similarly retarded. Almost any factor that retards physical development also retards speech. Many articulation cases with sluggish tongues and palates have histories of slow physical development.

Illnesses. These have importance according to their severity and sequela. Certain illnesses such as scarlet fever may impair hearing. Others may so lower the child's vitality that he does not have the energy to learn the difficult skills of talking correctly. Prolonged illness may result in parental attitudes of overconcern or of overprotection. The parents may anticipate the child's needs so that he learns to talk relatively late. They find it difficult to "correct" the speech of a sick child. If illness occurred during the first years of life, the child may not have had the necessary babbling practice. Injuries to the tongue may make certain sounds defective. One child who had burned his tongue started immediately to lall and continued in this articulatory disorder long after the tongue had healed. Many children lose their speech after a prolonged illness with high fevers and find it difficult to master it again.

Mental and Educational Factors. It is often the unpleasant chore of the speech correctionist to help parents face the fact that their child is feeble-minded, and that his general retardation is not solely the consequence of his delayed speech. When we find such children, we usually postpone speech therapy until they have a mental age (on a nonverbal test) of from five to six years.

Failures in school subjects, especially in reading, may be a direct consequence of defective articulation, and remedial reading can frequently be combined with remedial speech. Children who fail in school are likely to be resistant at first to speech correction. If they have been penalized for their school failure, they may become so emotional over their speech handicap that their tension prevents new muscular adjustments of the articulatory organs. One of our cases made no progress in his speech until he was transferred to another grade. The hatred he felt toward his teacher constantly reflected itself in our work with him.

Play. Children adopt the consonant errors of their playmates as well as their grammatical errors. In one instance, children from three different families in the neighborhood acquired a lisp by identification and imitation of a dominant older boy. It is said that *s* and *z* are pronounced as *th* (θ, δ) in Castilian Spanish because a certain king of Spain lisped and his courtiers adopted his pronunciation of the sibilant sounds. Little tyrants in every child kingdom similarly impose their speech peculiarities upon their subjects.

Home Conditions and Emotional Problems. A knowledge of the home conditions, the tempo of life lived therein, the attitudes of its inmates, is often vital to the understanding of the articulatory problem. Parents may bedevil a child for his social blemishes merely because they are sensitive about their own. An unhappy home can make our speech correction difficult. The list of emotional problems given in the case history can give us some indication of the child's reaction to his speech defect. The child who is always fighting, hurting pets, setting fires, or performing similar aggressive acts must be handled very differently from one who withdraws from the challenges of existence. Articulatory disorders, even as stuttering, can be primary or secondary, according to the manner in which the child regards his difficulty. We have known lispers to substitute easier words for those which included sibilant sounds. One boy's speech was so halting that he was referred to us as a stutterer. Extremely maladjusted and antagonistic, he avoided speech whenever he could. Asked to recite in school, he would growl, "I don't know and I don't care." Investigation showed that he had been penalized severely by his classmates for his lisp. His breaks in fluency and his behavior problem disappeared simultaneously with his lisp.

Language Development. In exploring this area, we sometimes find not only that the child was delayed in the onset of the first words but also that he was a very quiet child showing little babbling or vocal play. Or we may discover that the normally developing speech was suddenly interrupted, that he regressed to gesture or jargon or even became mute. There may be in the history certain periods or episodes in which he seemed to fail to understand or be interested in the speech of others. The parents may tell of speech reversals and confusions in sentence structure. They may describe the picture of idioglossia in which the child invented his own names for things. One of our cases, for example, insisted that bed was *tubboo* and refused to call it anything else. Or perhaps, other children in the family may have done all the talking for the child or competed so successfully for attention and communication that he had no opportunity to learn normal speech. This may be one of the lonely children, the isolates. Or he may be a twin and prefers twinlingua to English. Or he may have been the teacher rather than the pupil, his parents learning to understand his mutilated speech. Indeed all the factors which we have described as being important in creating delayed speech may be said to be productive of sound errors. What we are saying is that these matters should be explored rather than ignored. It is not enough to examine the child's present picture; we must also know something of his past if we are to treat him intelligently.

Emotional Conflicts

Most of us go through the difficulty of mastering the standard speech sounds because we wish to identify with, communicate with, and control our parents or playmates. However, where these relationships are painted with unpleasant emotion, with penalty and frustration, with *pfagh,* our motivation falters. Why talk like big people if the speech they show is full of quarreling anger, reproach, or anxiety? Some children seem to feel, and with some reason, that it is better not to grow up too far. They keep a few infantile errors as a hedge against such identification. Homes that are full of trouble are not good schools for the teaching of normal speech.

The Troubled Child. Growing up in our culture means running a gauntlet of many penalties and frustrations. There are so many things one must and must not do. Most of us have tough skins on our souls and manage to make our way to a precarious maturity despite these blows and barriers. We know anxiety and guilt and hostility but we seem to be able to handle their burden fairly well. There are some children who do not. Some of them have suffered more deprivations and hurt than any child should be expected to bear. Some of them are just more vulnerable. In either instance, they possess within themselves the turmoil of anxiety, guilt, and hostility. It's hard to learn anything when we are overflowing with any of these acids, and it certainly is hard to learn those tiny speech sounds which flick in and out of the constant flow of audible speech. It's difficult to concentrate, let alone discriminate. To a love-starved child the mastery of an *r* sound has little attraction.

Speech Conflicts. In some children, the correction of speech errors has become traumatic. Children who have been mocked or teased unmercifully find it painful to touch, to confront the thing that has caused these unpleasantnesses. They repress and deny to themselves the presence of misarticulation. Social penalties placed upon relatively unconscious habits always make them hard to eradicate. The parent who scolds or ridicules a child for his articulatory errors may make it impossible for the latter ever to attempt to correct himself. We have known lispers to become so emotional over their errors that they could not make an intelligent attempt to produce the *s* sound in a different way. One girl smashed a radio with a mallet upon hearing a "comedy" program in which an articulatory defect was assumed for humorous purposes. Another fainted when she heard a recording of her speech. When we find these speech conflicts, we must do our utmost to desensitize the person to his errors. We must make not only speech, but the correction of errors a pleasant process.

Neurotic Profit. We have known a few children who used their defective articulation to get the attention they could achieve in no other way. We have known college girls who used baby talk to attract some gullible man. Here is another such instance:

> For over two years we worked with a cooperative girl who had what seemed like a fairly simple frontal lisp. She seemed to do her utmost; she obviously disliked the penalties which it evoked in her college classes, but she consistently failed to master the correct *s* and *z* sounds. We interviewed her at some length but were unable to discover any emotional blocking. Then her father visited us and said: "Dorothy always gets what she wants from me. If I say no, she just crawls up on my lap and puts her arms around me and talks baby talk. I'm a sucker, but she hooks me every time. That lisp of hers cost me $800 last year. Put it into a car she wanted."

Many of these emotional conflicts are discovered only after speech therapy is under way, although some of them may be uncovered in the initial interview. When resistance is strong or cooperation lacking, we always scrutinize our cases again for evidence of emotional conflicts. Usually we find other evidence of maladjustment to help us locate the emotional difficulties. Such children may show behavior and personality problems in school, on the playground, and at home which may help us assess the importance of these maintaining causes of articulation disorders. We also have psychological tests which can reveal them. The C-A-T (Children's Apperception Test),[1] the Rosenzweig Picture Frustration Test,[2] and the California Personality Scale[3] are instruments which we can use with children. For adults, the Thematic Apperception Test (T-A-T),[4] the MMPI (Minnesota Multiphasic Inventory),[5] and the Rorschach[6] are useful in indicating the need for professional psychotherapy.

Organic Abnormalities

The role of organic deviations in the production of defective articulation has always been a favorite belief of parents and teachers. All children who do not talk clearly are suspected of having a tongue-tie or shortened frenum, that little cord beneath the tongue which most of us visibly possess. Tonsils have been removed, teeth straightened, and tongues trained gymnastically because of this belief, even when these structures were within the normal range. Yet there are many persons possessing such organic abnormalities or deficiencies who speak well. Speech therapists are usually conservative in attributing the defective sounds to organic factors. They know that the matter is not so simple. It is possible to produce the speech sounds in many ways—as the ventriloquists can show us. It is possible to compensate. A perfectly good *l* sound may be produced with the tonguetip down or even outside the mouth. An adequate

[1] Bellak, L., and Bellak, S. "Introductory Note on Children's Apperception Test (CAT)," *Journal of Projective Techniques,* Volume 14, 1950, pages 172-175.

[2] Rosenzweig, S., Fleming, E. E., and Rosenzweig, L. "The Children's Form of the Rosenzweig Picture Frustration Test," *Journal of Psychology,* Volume 26, 1948, pages 141-191.

[3] Clark, W. W., Tiegs, E. W., and Thorpe, L. P. *California Test of Personality,* California Test Bureau, 5916 Hollywood Boulevard, Los Angeles, California, 1942.

[4] Murray, H. A. *Thematic Apperception Test,* Cambridge: Harvard University Press, 1943.

[5] Hathaway, S. R., and McKinley, J. C. *Minnesota Multiphasic Personality Inventory,* Psychological Corporation, 522 Fifth Ave., New York, N.Y., 1948.

[6] Rorschach, H. *Psychodiagnosis,* 4th edition. New York: Grune and Stratton, 1949.

f or *v* can be made upside down. We have known adults without a tooth in their heads who could produce every speech sound correctly. In our clinic cupboards we have tapes of men and women without tongues or with only half of their tongues who speak with intelligibility.

Do these observations mean that organic abnormalities play no part in causing or maintaining articulation errors? The answer is no.

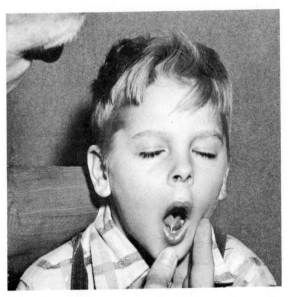

FIGURE 16. *Tongue Tie—Laller*

Only extra effort, only extra learning can overcome these obstacles. Many of our cases have not put forth this effort and no one has helped them learn the necessary compensatory movements required. It is important therefore that we examine our cases to ascertain the organic deviations which are present.*

Orthodontia and Surgery, Physical Therapy. In recent years, orthodontia has made great strides, and almost unbelievable changes in dental, palatal, and jaw structures have been accomplished. The speech-correction teacher should refer all children with marked

---

* An outline and description of the examination for organic abnormalities will be found in the Appendix, page 472.

mouth deformities to these specialists and should begin her work after the reconstruction has been carried out. Unfortunately, such reconstruction is expensive, and many cases cannot be taken care of in this way. Nevertheless, the speech-correction teacher should acquaint herself with the resources in the orthodontic field so that she will not waste months of effort in teaching compensatory movements to a child whose speech problem can be taken care of through surgery or the displacement of structures. Similarly, she should realize that palatal abnormalities are frequently associated with those of the jaws, and that orthodontic projection or retraction of the jaw can facilitate tongue contact with the roof of the mouth. Modern surgery also offers a wide variety of repair and reconstruction techniques. Scar tissue can be excised, and grafts can be made which will provide the necessary mobility. High palatal arches can be lowered, and the velum can be modified to almost any desired degree. Much of this work should be done early in childhood, and the speech-correction teacher is often responsible for seeing that it is done. Frequently, parents postpone such remedial work until too late, but they may often be convinced of its necessity by the teacher who points out the social maladjustment which such defects may produce.

Paralyzed structures occasionally can be helped by exercises, and a professional physiotherapist should be consulted in planning a remedial program if the physician's report indicates a possibility of success. Such remedial work usually consists of recourse to the more biological functions and the tying up of the specialized movement with gross muscular action. Spaced practice, well motivated by graphs of successes, is advisable.

Teaching Compensatory Movements.   As we have said, many cases showing severe organic defects cannot be helped by the orthodontist or plastic surgeon because of age or financial reasons. The picture is by no means hopeless, however, since all of the speech sounds may be made in various ways. The art of the ventriloquist demonstrates compensatory activity of the tongue for that of the lips and jaws. Many normal speakers have profound anatomical abnormalities, occasionally so marked as to excite wonder in the speech correctionist familiar with the ordinary production of the speech sounds. Perfect *t* and *d* sounds, for example, have been made by individuals so tongue-tied that they were unable to lift the tonguetip to contact the upper teeth. Inmates of prisons frequently learn to talk out of the side of the mouth—the one farthest away from the guard—with but minor jaw movements.

In order to teach compensatory or nonstandard ways of making any speech sound, it is first necessary to make a phonetic analysis in terms of the type of sound to be produced. For example, the pro-

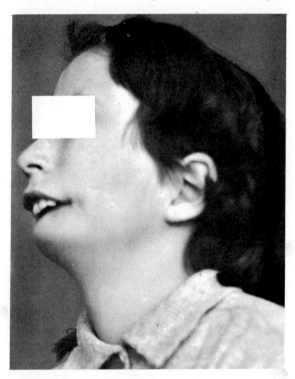

Figure 17. *Type II Malocclusion (Undershot Jaw)*

duction of an *s* sound requires the propulsion of a narrow stream of air past a cutting edge. The cutting edge should be placed at about right angles to the air stream in order to produce a clear *s*. The average person produces this narrow stream of air by placing the sides of the tongue along the side teeth, thereby cutting off all lateral escape of air, and by grooving the center of the tongue so that the air stream is projected directly past the cutting edge of the front incisors. Lacking these front teeth, or having them widely spaced, the person can get an equally good *s* by directing the air stream past the cuspids or bicuspids on the side of the mouth having the better teeth. This new procedure, however, is not quite so simple as the preceding sentence might imply. The tongue must adjust itself so that on one side it makes a larger occlusion and the groove is diagonal. The lips must plug the former opening and part at the appropriate side. Frequently the mandible must be moved sidewise so that the best upper teeth and lower teeth will be brought together. Thus the teacher must plan the type of compensatory mechanics necessitated by the particular mouth deformities involved. In this plan, the teacher should take into account or seek to minimize as far as possible the following factors: complexity of performance (the fewer adjustments, the better), ease of transition from other sounds, amount of facial contortion, distinctness of kinesthetic and tactual sensations, and the motivation and cooperation of the subject.

In teaching compensatory mechanics, then, the teacher should follow this general outline. (1) Note how the student articulates the defective sound. (2) Make a phonetic analysis to determine what the essential mechanics of the sound must be. (3) Discover what structures the student might possibly use to satisfy these requirements. (4) Give the student a thorough course in ear-training, stimulation, and discrimination along the lines of the program sketched in a future section. (5) Through manipulation, phonetic diagrams, mirror work, imitation, and random activity, try to get the student to produce a sound similar to that made by the instructor. (6) Once achieved, do not let the student move a muscle of face or body until he prolongs, repeats, and uses it in nonsense syllables many times. (7) Build up its strength through techniques suggested in the next section. (8) Do not worry about exaggerated movements used by the student in making the sound. At first, most students will use facilitating movements of other structures as a baby uses gross movements prior to specialization. We frequently encourage head and jaw movements or modifications of smiling, chewing, biting, and swallowing as accessory tools. These extraneous movements drop out as the new performance pattern becomes habitual. (9) Increase the speed with which the new performance pattern can be initiated. No compensatory movements will become habitual if they cannot be used quickly and easily. (10) Be careful to change the transition

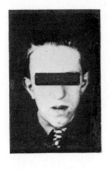
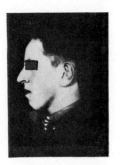
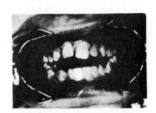
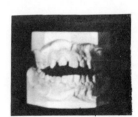
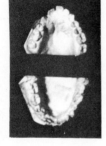
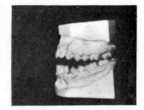

FIGURE 18. *Open Bite, of Fifteen-year-old.* Severe lateral lisper.

movement as well, working for new and quick patterns of change from one speech sound to another.

Acoustic and Perceptual Deficiencies

Hearing Loss. In our discussion of developmental factors we pointed out the necessity for exploring the histories of our articulation cases to determine whether or not temporary hearing losses might have occurred during the speech learning period. It is equally important, in examining our person with sound errors, that we ascertain if such hearing losses are still present. Certainly if a child cannot hear a sound with fidelity it will be difficult for him to produce it correctly. While we shall discuss this topic in more detail later, we should make clear at this point that some children have a loss of acuity which affects all the sounds of speech while others may hear certain sounds very well, yet be unable to identify the characteristic features of others. In high-frequency hearing loss, for example, the vowels and voiced sounds may be heard very clearly while the unvoiced sibilants such as *s* or *sh*, may be so faintly heard as to be nonexistent. Shouting at such a person will only amplify sounds which he can already hear and perhaps mask out those which he hears weakly.

Auditory Memory Span.   There are some children who find it very difficult to remember sounds even when they can hear them. Sounds disappear very swiftly once they are spoken. In the swift rush of conversation the life of a given consonant is very brief—much shorter than a fruit fly's. Most of us find it easy to hold a familiar sound in memory but have great difficult in hanging onto one which is strange. It seems to fade so fast. We even find it difficult to repeat a snatch of our own free babbling or jargon after a short period of silence. Most children with articulation errors do not have defective auditory memory spans. They can hold a sound as well as we can. But there are others who have much difficulty. They may remember the meaning but not the characteristics of the sounds which have been spoken. Indeed, often they cannot even recall how they have uttered their own sounds. We can readily see how such a disability would make it difficult to correct articulatory errors. Fortunately, it is possible to improve this deficiency through training.

1. Auditory memory-span drill. Teacher pronounces a series of digits or words. Student repeats them after intervals varying from 1 to 60 seconds. This assignment should be followed by the student's giving himself his own series, waiting the prescribed interval, and then repeating. Errors should be checked, and this procedure should be strongly motivated. The above drills can be carried out through phonograph records, the student being asked to write down the series.

2. Jabber-repetition. This consists, like the above, of stimulation and repetition. The teacher says certain nonsense words (polysyllabic) such as "wahwo-kadda-makeree-samma." The student repeats these after a certain interval, which should be gradually increased. As in the last assignment, the student should then give himself the jabber stimulation and attempt to repeat as closely as possible. The syllables may also be recorded phonographically for stimulation.

3. Student distorts certain speech sounds and then attempts to repeat

these distortions exactly. The teacher should illustrate using the "dark *l*" sound or the lateral lisp.

4. It is often wise to begin these assignments with the direction of the speech defective's attention to the duration of his sounds, since this feature is more easily recognized and judged. Thus the student is instructed to repeat after the teacher the nonsense word *laaaaaaalo*, seeking to keep the relative and total durations of the repetition as close as possible to those of the stimulation. Other similar nonsense words, including those which prolong the continuant consonants, are given. Phonograph records in which the duration can be identified are used in providing a checkup. The student should then give himself similar stimulation, and repeat it after an appropriate interval, while the teacher checks.

5. Assignments similar to the above but using inflections as the stimulus material are helpful in training the individual to listen to his speech.

6. The student is told to pronounce certain continuant consonants or vowels (both in words and by themselves) five times, prolonging the consonant or vowel slightly each time. The same type of assignment may be used for inflected vowels and consonants. The teacher checks. Written material may be used for this, such as *sso, ssso, sssso, ssssso*.

7. The student, using a stage whisper, prolongs, inflects, or distorts certain vowels or continuants. He then repeats vocally, as closely as possible.

8. The student should be given frequent self-listening periods, in which he makes a sound and listens closely to it. Not more than two or three words should constitute a period, and the student must be extremely alert. Later in the treatment it is wise to have the student use these periods for judgments of correct sound production.

Difficulties in Phonetic Discrimination. It is not enough merely to be able to recall a given sound. We must also learn to distinguish it from others. Each sound, like each Chinaman, has its own distinctive features. To some of us, all Chinese look alike, and we probably look alike to them. As we become acquainted and familiar with specific individuals, we discover that there are great differences, and we wonder why it took us so long to see them. Some of the people with whom we work find a similar difficulty in recognizing the differences between sounds. They have not learned to look or listen to the distinctive differences. Some of them can tell these differences when the sounds are paired and compared in isolation yet show a remarkably poor performance when defective sounds are incorporated within the sentence. The distinctive characteristics seem to get lost in the flow of speech much as individual faces in the photograph of a crowd seem much alike. At any rate, we find such difficulties in phonetic discrimination and when we do, we must take steps to provide the necessary training. Many of the ear-training techniques to be described in our next chapter are devoted to the improvement of phonetic discrimination.

Difficulties in Phonetic Analysis. In our discussion of how children learn to talk we have stressed the importance of vocal phonics, of learning to recognize that words have heads and tails and middles. Lumps of sound are difficult to analyze for errors. Words are little melodies of successive phonetic notes. If one of those notes is sour, it should be corrected, but all of us have heard singers who cannot carry a tune, who blithely flat or sharp a pitch and never know it. They sing "Home on the Range" with gusto but not with precision. Only through the reactions of others do they come to realize that they do not sing well. When queried, they cannot analyze their tunes to locate the miss-sung notes. A similar difficulty exists in the articulation problem of some of our cases. They find it very difficult to analyze words into their component sounds and so they have trouble in correcting their errors. In helping these individuals specialized training in vocal phonics is essential.

Poor Motor Coordination

Motor Deficiencies. Articulation cases are occasionally seen who could truly be called the "slow of tongue." They can scarcely protrude the tongue even in the expression of impudence without having it loll around and droop over. Sometimes these poorly coordinated movements seem to be localized about the mouth. The tongue, jaw, soft palate, all are sluggish. But in most of these clumsy-mouthed individuals the other coordinations are similarly affected.

Not all articulation cases are thus poorly coordinated, but those who are so handicapped must be given therapy devoted to their needs. In earlier speech correction, tongue exercises had the status of a religious ritual. All speech defectives were given rigorous training in this routine. In modern speech correction, the emphasis on tongue exercises has almost disappeared. Yet for certain of the "clumsy-tongued" individuals with whom we work, modern forms of these exercises are very valuable.

A good many diseases and defective neuromuscular conditions reflect themselves not only in muscular incoordination but also in distorted speech. The speech correctionist is often able to refer them to the physician they need. The student of speech correction should therefore be able to recognize the general symptoms of paralysis, both flaccid and spastic, and pronounced neuromuscular incoordinations. Besides the tests mentioned in the references, other simple activities which may demonstrate poor coordination are: walking a straight line; extending arms above head and dropping them suddenly; beginning with hands resting on knees as one sits in a chair, alternately touching nose with forefinger of each hand; standing first on one leg and then on the other, with eyes closed; skipping; standing on tiptoe for five seconds.

It is possible to get an excellent estimate of the sluggishness of the articulation apparatus by measuring the rate of jaw movement. Maximum rates are achieved in about ten seconds, but several short practice sessions should be used to ensure understanding of the task. Demonstrate the opening and closing of the jaw with a clicking of the teeth on the closure. Instruct the case to imitate you as rapidly as possible, and count the number of clicks in five seconds. Be sure not to create fatigue. Jenkins[7] gives the following norms for this diadochokinesis of the jaw in number of jaw closings *per second:*

AGE	NUMBER OF JAW MOVEMENTS PER SECOND	
	Males	*Females*
7	3.5-3.8	3.7-4.0
8	3.6-3.9	3.8-4.0
9	4.0-4.4	4.0-4.3
10	4.1-4.3	4.2-4.3
14	4.9-5.1	5.0-5.2
15	5.1-5.3	5.2-5.4
Adults	5.2-5.4	5.4-5.6

The tongue seems to be of greater importance in articulation than the jaw. We therefore cite the research of Blomquist,[8] who found

[7] Jenkins, R. L. "The Rate of Diadochokinetic Movement of the Jaw at the Ages of Seven to Maturity," *Journal Speech Disorders,* Volume 6, 1940, pages 13-22.

[8] Blomquist, B. L. "Diadochokinetic Movement of Nine-, Ten-, and Eleven-Year-Old-Children," *Journal Speech and Hearing Disorders,* Volume 15, 1950, pages 159-164.

that children of nine years averaged 4.6 jaw movements for the syllable *tuh* (tə); 4.6 for the syllable *puh;* and 4.0 for the syllable *kuh.* When these syllables were combined in the nonsense word *puhtuhkuh* (pʌtəkə), children of nine could utter the word 4.5 times per second. At eleven years of age, the corresponding figures were *p*:5.3, *t*:5.2, and *k*:4.7. Lundeen[9] tested diadochokinetic rates for ten consonants, finding the following order (from fast to slower rates): *t*,

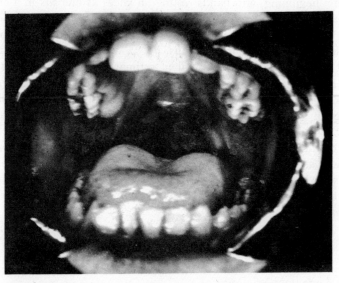

FIGURE 19. *Mouth of a Child Who Had Suffered a Severe Lye Burn.* The tongue is being lifted as high as possible. Despite this handicap, the child had learned compensatory movements sufficient to give him perfect speech.

d, p and *b*. These are the sounds which can be repeated most quickly; then follow *f* and *v*; and slowest of all were the sounds *s*, *g*, and *z*. We have found that training in diadochokinesis is extremely valuable with most articulation cases who are slow in it.

Lest the student come to the improper conclusion that all articulation cases need muscle training, we cite the research of Mase[10]

[9] Lundeen, D. J. "The Relationship of Diadochokinesis to Various Speech Sounds," *Journal Speech and Hearing Disorders*, Volume 15, 1950, pages 54-59.

[10] Mase, D. J. *Etiology of Articulatory Speech Defects.* New York: Columbia University Teachers Contributions to Education. Number 921, 1946.

who found no group differences between articulatorily handicapped and normal speaking of school children either in five tests of diadochokinesis or in rail-walking, a general motor-skill activity. But when we deal with an individual case we want to know whether or not he needs help and training in his motor skills.

Here are some tests to measure the rapidity of the articulatory structures:

A. "As soon as I give the signal repeat what I say very slowly and carefully: 'Puh-puh-puh.' . . . . Now, I am going to say it five times but this time as fast as possible. Now, let's see how fast you can say it five times. Ready—go!" (Examiner times the five trials.)

B. and C. Repeat the above, but use first the syllable "tuh" and then the syllable "kuh."

D. Repeat the instructions above but use the nonsense word "puh-tuh-kuh." Children of from seven to nine years should, according to Rainey's research, be able to utter this word at least once per second.

From Mase's monograph (21) we select the following alternate tests, citing the means of his fifth- and sixth-grade boys:

E. With mouth open, subject is to move his tongue repeatedly from left corner to right corner. Examiner counts total number of cycles in two trials of ten seconds. Norm: 23 cycles.

F. Subject is required to say "Daddy" as many times as he can in each of two five-second trials. Examiner totals both trials. Norm: 25 times in ten seconds.

It would seem important to have tests for accuracy as well as speed of movement, but so far as accuracy of the tongue or jaws is concerned, little research has been published.

We often find persons who articulate fairly well when speaking slowly but whose errors increase terrifically with each increase in speed. Some of these children are just slow-moving children, whose tempo of living should be an unhurried one. Most of us make slips of the tongue when we try to talk at a rate far beyond that of our usual speech and so do they. Geared up by competition for speech, by impatient listeners, by parents who themselves talk very swiftly, these children race their speech motors beyond their normal capacities and so they fail to articulate. By measuring the diadochokinesis (the speed of repetitive movement) of the tongue, lips and jaw, and by observing the general rate of other motor behaviors, we can determine the importance of this factor.

Accuracy.   We have spoken of the clumsy tongue. By this we mean that the coordinations of that member lack precision and accuracy. We see this very clearly in the speech of cerebral palsy or other forms of dysarthria. The child finds it difficult to curl up the tip of the tongue, to swing it from side to side, even to hold it fixed in an outthrust position without trembling. He may find the location of contact points within the mouth to be very difficult even when he watches himself in the mirror or attempts to touch the spot stroked by the examiner's tongue depressor. He overshoots or undershoots. He cannot maintain a necessary posture. It wobbles. These phenomena are not found in all articulatory cases but when they are present, they must be considered in therapy.

Lack of Differentiation.   When the baby first lifts his tongue, he probably lifts his legs and curls his toes. When he cries, he cries with his whole body. Later, we find less gross bodily movement involved. What has happened? Essentially the child has learned to differentiate the finer movement from those larger ones out of which it emerged. We find this process of differentiation in all motor skills, in handwriting, in playing badminton, in speaking. In our consideration of all the aspects of speech we must not forget that one of the most fundamental is the motor aspect. Accordingly, we should scrutinize our cases to determine whether there has been a failure in differentiation. When the child lifts his tongue, does he also lift his jaw? When he lifts his jaw, does he also round his lips? Does he still show an infantile swallow in which the tongue is protruded? We have worked with college students who could not produce an *r* or *l* sound without lifting the jaw and pursing the lips as in sucking. This is a disability almost as important as the inability to move the forefinger without moving the arm. What happens usually in these cases who cannot lift or click the tongue without moving the jaw is that they do not lift the tongue and the speech becomes lalled and slurred. It is important for good articulation that the tongue be able to move independently of the lips and jaws.

Training in Motor Coordination.   Since we frequently find, in these persons with motor disabilities, that other motor activities are also slow, imprecise, or undifferentiated, it is often necessary that we begin our training first with the larger motor skills. It might seem odd to the observer to discover the speech therapist teaching children to dance, to swing, to balance, to do rhythmic calisthenics. But the clumsy body often carries a clumsy tongue. Fortunately, as general bodily coordinations improve, so too do those of speech.

It is often necessary however to work directly on the coordinations of tongue and lips. Tongue exercises have in the past been much abused. Only a relatively few of our cases need them. But there are some. They are the ones whose tongues do not move with the speed and precision demanded by good speech. They can assume only the simplest tongue positions. Therefore, they raise the front or middle of the tongue instead of the back, and protrude it rather than lift it. It is difficult for them to curl the tip or groove the tongue. Tongue exercises are useful and necessary for these cases.

The exercises that follow are given in a form suitable for adults where we may be direct in our therapy. For children, it will be necessary to cast the same activities in the form of games. The principles governing the use of tongue exercises are as follows:

1. Learn to recognize the movement as part of some familiar biological movement such as chewing, swallowing, coughing, or others to be mentioned later. Practice these basic activities.

2. The finer movements should be taught first in conjunction with larger movements, then alone.

3. The movement should be used with increasing speed, strength, and accuracy.

4. The movement should be combined with other movements (breathing, phonation, and so on) used in speech.

5. The emphasis in this training should be on the activities (lifting, thrusting, drawing, tip-curling, and grooving) and the contacts (upper gum ridge, lower teeth, interdental, palatal) and the positions actually used in speech, rather than random and generalized tongue movements.

6. Not only the tonguetip, but the blade, middle, and back of tongue should be exercised.

7. In any drill period, use a few from each of the lists of exercises under each major activity heading rather than complete one section at a time.

8. Avoid fatigue and hurry. Identify movement by imitation or mirror observation rather than by oral description. Identify contacts by stroking or pressure. Identify new positions in terms of their variation from other well-known positions.

9. After movement is well learned, combine it with production of other speech sounds.

10. Compare, contrast, and combine the various movements.

Habit Strength

Perhaps the most important maintaining cause of articulation disorders is habit strength. Both a lateral lisp and the substitution of the *f* for the *th* sound are learned reactions. They have been overlearned; they are part of the warp and woof of the person's language. They have been practiced so much that they operate automatically. Used in controlling others, in exchanging messages, in thinking, in the display of self, in the expression of emotion, they have received a tremendous amount of reinforcement along the way. Such learned responses persist of their own inertia, their own momentum. They resist extinction and change.

Error Consistency. And yet, so potent is the constant stimulation of the standard speech of other speakers, we usually find that some of these articulatory errors are still not stabilized completely. When we analyze the several errors in a given speaker's utterance, we usually find several which are not as strongly fixed as others. They are used inconsistently. In some words, which we term "key words," the standard sound is used instead. Also, we find correct sounds occurring under certain conditions: slow speeds, in isolation, in oral reading, in nonsense syllables, in echoed utterance, in certain consonant combinations. These infrequent instances of the normal production of an error sound indicate that these errors are not completely learned and that these particular ones should respond more easily to speech therapy. To start working with a child on one of several defective sounds without scrutinizing the relative consistency of his errors is obviously unwise. Motivation increases with successful progress. Why should we start with the errors which might be most resistant to treatment? Let's work with these which are sometimes spoken correctly.

Articulation Errors: Their Nature

Terminology. By definition, articulation disorders are those in which the abnormality in speech is due to the presence of defective, nonstandard speech sounds. As we have seen earlier, there are many terms used to describe them. Such labels as "lisping," "lalling," "baby talk" are in common use although they fall far short of being precise.

If we say that a person lisps, we mean only that certain sibilant sounds are defective. It is an acoustic label. If we say that a person lalls, the term refers to defective sounds produced by an inactive tonguetip—a label based upon motor coordination disability. Baby talk—or infantile perseveration as it has sometimes been called— refers to a pattern of errors reflecting incomplete maturation. More- over, lallers may lisp and baby talkers may lisp and lall. Even if a rose is a rose is a *wose,* it would seem wiser to find some other way of regarding the disorders of articulation than by trying to place them in these conflicting categories.

The speech therapist solves the dilemma by examining the child, listing the sounds which are defective and simply describing their errors. Some workers in this field, needing a label to satisfy parents, colleagues, or their own egos, use some five pound words to indicate the sounds which are defective. You will remember *sigmatism* and *rhotacism.* Most of us are content to list these sounds and to describe their errors.

More commonly used are the terms *dyslalia* and *dysarthria.* These refer to the presumed etiology or causation of articulatory error. The first refers to disorders of functional origin where the causes may be due to mislearning, imitation, emotional conflicts, or the like. Dysar- thria implies that the defective articulation is due to brain or nerve damage. A child with a partially paralyzed tongue or with cerebral palsy is said to show dysarthric errors. In adults who formerly spoke well but who have contracted multiple sclerosis or muscular dys- trophy we find dysarthria rather than dyslalia. It must be remem- bered that these are etiological (causal) terms and that they do not describe the errors. A person with dyslalia can show the same acoustic error on the *r* sound that a person with dysarthria will portray.

Sounds Most Frequently Defective.   It is probably significant that the sounds most frequently misarticulated are those last mastered by all of us in the course of speech development. The *r, s, l,* and *th* sounds are those most commonly defective, both as single sounds or in blends. The vowels are the least defective. Indeed, when we find defective vowel sounds we usually have a tough problem to solve.

Severity of the Disorder.   One of the first things we do when exam- ining a person with an articulation disorder is to make some estimate of its severity. In line with our original definition of a speech defect we attempt to assess its features in terms of its conspicuousness, its effect upon intelligible communication and the amount of emotional maladjustment. We need to know how others react to it and how they view the problem. We try to ascertain the degree to which it would interfere with social and scholastic success. Will it or has it affected the ability to read, to participate in group activities, to earn a living? How aware is this person of his errors? Does he have a distorted self-image as well as distorted speech sounds? Does the severity change with different conditions of communication? Is this the sort of speech that would evoke penalties or produce frustration? Is there evidence of anxiety, guilt, or hostility? What is the big picture?

Number of Defective Sounds. We do not remain content with this over-all scrutiny; we must also do a careful analysis of the speech itself. Our first item in such an analysis is the determination of how many speech sounds are defective. A crude measure of severity consists of this very counting. The more defective sounds the person has, the more severe a problem he possesses. Each additionally defective sound adds to the conspicuousness, to the unintelligibility, to the probability that the case has experienced penalty and frustration. One of the crude devices we have to predict the successful maturation of articulation or to prognosticate the success of therapy is to determine how many different speech sounds are defective. The fewer, the better. When a child comes to the speech therapist with eight or nine sounds misarticulated, we know that we have a real job before us.

Type of Error. Although the above principles are generally true, we must also consider the type of error since certain errors are more difficult to eradicate than others. Distorted sibilants as in lateral lisping or the distorted r and l sounds as in lalling may be very resistant to therapy even when they are the only errors present. Some of the sounds used by our cases as replacements for the standard sounds are much more difficult to change than others. An interdental lisp, for example, is usually easier to work with than is a nasal or lateral lisp. The child who substitutes a t for the k should have less trouble in conquering that error than if he substituted the little cough-like glottal catch. It is necessary, therefore, to scrutinize the error sounds.

Phonemic Approximations. It is very important that we analyze the actual sounds used by our cases as replacements. Unless we are careful, we may fail to detect that the error is a distorted approximation of the standard sound. Few children ever say *wabbit* for *rabbit*. The initial sound they make is usually a bilabial *r* with rounded lips. Often as a child makes progress in mastering a new sound he proceeds through a whole series of gradual approximations, one different distortion after another, all of which progress in the direction of the standard sound. They seldom jump from the error to the correct sound; they make progressive approximations. If the therapist is not alert, these little shifts may be unnoticed and unrewarded. A child can make progress even if his standard sounds are not being produced perfectly by modifying his errors in the direction of the correct sound. When a new case comes to us, we can use this analysis of approximation distortions to tell us how far he has to go.

Phonetic Analysis. Speech therapists tend to make their phonetic (phonemic) diagnoses more accurately than a mere listing of defective sounds would permit. They also want to know the type of phonetic error. If the *k* is defective, is it distorted or omitted? Is some other sound used in its place? Is the utterance defective because other unnecessary sounds have been added or inserted?

These are some of the questions the speech therapist must ask himself in sizing up an articulation problem. He must analyze the phonetic errors in terms of substitutions, omissions, insertions, and distortions. The child who says, "Tally taw me tee-tawing" is substituting the *t* for the *s*. We record this: t/s. The child who says, "Oh ook at the itto doggy" is omitting the initial *l* sound but substituting an *o* for the final *l*. We would record this as: −l(I) and o/l(F). The letters in the parentheses indicate the location of the error. We use *I* (for "initial") if the error is found at the beginning of words, *M* if in the middle, and *F* if in the final position. The minus sign (−) indicates that the sound has been *omitted;* the plus sign (+) represents an *insertion* such as the pronunciation of "blue" as "brrlue" (+r); the diagonal represents a *substitution;* th/s equals a frontal lisp; *distortions* are substitutions of sounds foreign to our language, and we use adjectives or symbols to describe them.

A lingual-frontal lisp is a substitution: (th/s). Let us analyze a lateral lisp which has distortions. We have no unvoiced *l* in our language. Welshmen do, and much of their speech seems lisped to us. One common variety of our lateral lisping is the use of a whispered *l* for the *s*. If you will attempt to say "LLLLLLee the LLLLLun" and whisper the *L* sounds, you will be saying "See the sun" with a lateral lisp. These are distortions, and so we write them: S (I, lateral-emission), or more simply: −s−(I). If the *s* were laterally emitted in every position of the word, it would be recorded: −s−(I,M,F). If the student has mastered the International Phonetic Alphabet with its modifying marks, he can record many of the distortions accurately, and as substitutions. For example, it is difficult to record on paper the *l* which is produced by holding the tonguetip

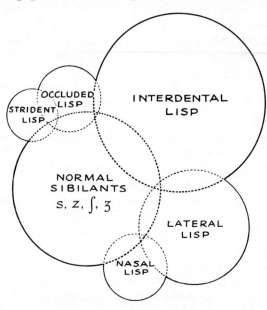

FIGURE 20. *Types of Sibilant Errors.* Where circles intersect, blends and distorted approximations or combinations of errors are found.

down and using the middle of the tongue for making the contact against the palate. It seems to be a distortion. The best we could do is to call it "a dark *l*" or a "retracted l."

An alternative method for recording distortions is by the use of intersecting circles representing the sounds nearest to the error. Many distortions are actually homogenous blends of two standard sounds. The diagram in Figure 29 illustrates the various distortions by the intersecting arcs. For example in the intersected area of the circle (ǝ), for *th,* and the large circle for *s* represents a very common error, much more common than the substitution of a pure *th* for the *s.* Few children really say *thoup* for *soup;* instead they use a replacement sound which is this combination of *th* and *s.* You can duplicate it by protruding your tongue slightly and still trying to prolong a *ssss* sound. It has the characteristics of both. It is a distortion.

To summarize, we cannot understand or diagnose an articulation case without making a *phonetic* analysis of his speech in terms of (1) the sounds which are defective; (2) the type of error in terms of substitution, omission, insertion, or distortion; and (3) the location of the error within the word (initial, medial, or final). This sort of analysis is not academic. It has vital importance for therapy. It helps us answer such questions as: "With what sound or sounds should we begin? Does the case ever make the sound correctly? How much ear training will be required?"

> One of our student speech therapists gave an articulation test to a boy of seven and came out with the astounding summary that although he had thirty-two defective sounds, his speech was perfectly intelligible. When we checked her findings we found that the child actually was doing only one thing incorrectly: He was *forming* the final sounds of every word but he was not pronouncing them audibly. The student therapist had been right in finding that thirty-two sounds were defective, but this actually had no significance or importance. Our therapeutic task was clearly to teach the child to strengthen his terminal sounds.

To show you what a brief report of a typical phonetic analysis would be like, we submit this one of an eighteen-year-old college student whose tongue had been badly cut during the first grade of his schooling:

Name of case: K. J.   *Examiner:* Leith   *Date:* 1/4/53   *Rapport:* OK

Summary of errors:

> y/l(I,M); o/l(F)
> w/r(I,M); -r(F)
> t/ch(I,M,F)
> -s-(Lateral, I,M,F)
> -z-(Lateral, I,M,F)

Why are these sounds defective? Besides a phonetic analysis such as we have described we also need a *kinetic* analysis. It is important to know which sounds are being mis-uttered, but we need also to know how they are being produced. The label "lisp" is a *phonetic* term; the modifying adjectives "lateral," "occluded," "interdental," or "nasal" are *kinetic* terms. They describe how the error is being made. They refer to the *manner of production.* The term "lalling" is such a kinetic or kinesiologic term. It refers to the type of speech produced when the individual characteristically makes most of his speech sounds without raising the tip of the tongue from the floor of the mouth. It tells us only that this tongue position is at fault. If you were told that a child was a *laller,* all you could guess about his actual speech would be that certain of the consonants which normally are made with an elevated tonguetip would be defective. You could be sure that the *r* would be defective; the *l* probably would be poor, and perhaps the *ch* and *j* or even the *t, d,* and the sibilants. Those would be the probabilities but you could not be certain. Only by analyzing the manner of error-production could you know what the person is doing incorrectly.

Each of the speech sounds can be incorrectly produced in several ways. The most frequent error of such *stop-plosives* as *k* and *g* seems to be due to (1) the wrong location of the tongue contact. Other errors include (2) the wrong speed in forming the contacts; (3) the wrong structures used in contacts; (4) the wrong force or tension of the contacts; (5) too short a duration of the contacts; (6) too slow a release from contacts; (7) the wrong mode or direction of release; (8) the wrong direction of the air stream; and finally (9) sonancy errors in which voiced and unvoiced consonants are interchanged. Examples of these errors are now given for illustration:

1. The child who says "tandy" for "candy" is using a tongue-palatal contact, but it is too far forward.
2. A breathy *k* sound (xki) for (ki), results when the contact is formed so slowly that fricative noises are produced prior to the air puff.
3. A glottal catch or throat click (ʔæt) for (kæt) is often found in cleft-palate cases. They make a contact, but with the wrong structures.
4. Insufficient tension of the lips can result in the substitution of a sound similar to the Spanish *v* (ɸ) for the standard English *b* sound.
5. When the duration of the contact is too short, it often seems to

be omitted entirely. Thus the final *k* in the word *sick* (sɪk) may be formed so briefly that acoustically it seems omitted (sɪ).

6. Too slow a release from the contact may give an aspirate quality to the utterance. "Kuheep the cuhandy" (kʰip ðə kʰændɪ) is an example of this.

7. The lowering of the tonguetip prior to recall of the tongue as a whole can produce such an error as "tsen" for "ten" (tsɛn) for (tɛn). In this error the case is not inserting an *s* so much as releasing the tongue from its contact in a peculiar fashion.

8. Occasionally the direction of the air stream is reversed and the plosion occurs on inhalation. Try saying "sick" with the *k* sound produced during inhalation, and you will understand this error.

9. The person who says "back" for "bag" illustrates a sonancy error.

Most of the errors in making the *continuant* sounds are caused by: (1) use of the wrong channel for the air stream (using an unvoiced *l* for the *s*), (2) use of the wrong construction or constriction ("foop" for "soup"), (3) use of the wrong aperture (a lateral lisp), (4) use of the wrong direction of the air stream (nasal lisp, inhaled *s*), (5) too weak an air pressure (acoustically omitted *s*), (6) the presence of nonessential movements or contacts (*t* for *s*, occluded lisp), and (7) cognate errors (*z* for *s*, or vice versa).

Most of the errors in making the *glide* sounds are produced by combining the types of errors sketched above. They may be generally classed as movement errors. They include: (1) use of the wrong beginning position or contact ("yake" for "lake"); (2) use of the wrong ending position (fɪʊ) for (fɪr); (3) use of the wrong transitional movement in terms of speed, strength, or direction (rweɪd) for (reɪd); (4) the presence of nonessential contacts or positions (tjɛloʊ) for (jɛloʊ); (5) cognate errors (wɛn) for (hwɛn).

It is necessary to analyze any given articulation error according to the above scheme so as to understand its nature. It is not sufficient merely to start teaching the correct sound. We must also break the old habit. Many of our most difficult articulatory cases will make rapid progress as soon as they understand clearly what they are doing wrong. Insight into error is fundamental to efficient speech correction.

To show you how we would record the results of a *kinetic* analysis, let us present the summary report of both the phonetic and kinetic procedures:

Name of case: P. T.   *Examiner:* Wensley   *Date:* 2/5/53

Rapport: Good

	Phonetic		Kinetic
Summary of errors:	k/g	(I,M,F)	Confusion of voiced and
	t/d	(I,M,F)	unvoiced sounds; cognate
	f/v	(I,M,F)	or sonancy errors.
	s/z	(I,M,F)	Ditto: Vocal cords silent.
	θ ð	(I,M,F)	" " " "
	w/r	(I,M)	" " " "
	-r	(F)	Uses lip glide instead of tongue glide. The *r* position was made but it was unvoiced.

This case mastered all of his errors at once except the w/r. He was taught the concept of cognates: that there are pairs of sounds, articulated in much the same way but one is voiced or sonant while the other is unvoiced or surd. He learned that the *v* was made by having his vocal cords vibrate as he made the lip-teeth position for an *f*. He found out that the *s* was a whispered *z*. By feeling both his own and his clinician's throat as the pairs of sounds were produced, he learned to discriminate between them. By holding his fingers in his ears as he shifted from a prolonged *ssss* to a prolonged *zzzz* he learned to recognize one sound from its twin.

Under What Conditions Do the Articulation Errors Occur? In studying any articulation case it is also necessary to discover the circumstances in which the errors occur. Some of our lispers have difficulty with their sibilants only when emotional. We worked with an exasperating case who never made an error when speaking at a normal rate of speed but who became unintelligible when hurried. Some children can utter words perfectly when repeating from a model and yet substitute, omit, and distort their speech sounds in spontaneous speech. Some children who can produce every consonant correctly in isolation or in nonsense syllable will seem to be unable to use them in meaningful words. All of these observations point to the necessity for studying the articulation errors in terms of the type of communication being used. The importance of these factors in therapy is obvious. It would be silly to spend a lot of time drilling a child to produce the *r* sound in nonsense syllables if he has always been able to do so. For these reasons, we examine each error in terms of the following: (1) type of communicative situation, (2) speed of utterance, (3) kind of communicative material, (4) discrimination ability. Here is a typical summary report:

> Our analysis of the conditions under which articulation errors occurred is as follows: Jackson substituted θ/s (I,M,F) and ð/z (I,M,F) consistently in swift, emotional speech, swift nonemotional speech, when carefully trying to speak correctly in oral reading, and when repeating single words after the examiner. One exception occurred: he said "six" correctly when repeating it carefully. He made the same errors on nonsense syllables when they were spoken at fast speeds but had good final *s* sounds occasionally when the nonsense syllables were spoken slowly. He produced good isolated *z* sounds when prolonged with teeth closed. The *s* was only occasionally good in isolation, even with strong stimulation by examiner. He is always able to hear the error in another's speech but does not seem to be able to hear his own except on isolated words.

The only reason for such diagnostic procedures is that they may help us in therapy. In the above case, the therapy plan called for the teaching of the *z* sound prior to the teaching of the *s*. A great deal of discrimination ear training was used. Recordings and auditory training units which enabled Jackson to hear his own *z* and *s* at high amplification were used. The *s* sound was first taught by isolating it from the key word *six* and no attempt was made to have oral reading or conversation employed in therapy until the new sounds were thoroughly habituated. The *s* sound was used in the final position of nonsense syllables (*ees-oss-oos*) and in the final position of familiar words (*house, glass, ice*) before it was taught in the initial position (*see, sandwich, sick*). By analyzing the conditions under which errors occur, we are able to treat our cases much more efficiently.

Now let us present a complete articulation test report which will combine the *phonetic* analysis, the *kinetic* analysis and the conditions under which errors occur.

A Typical Articulation Test Report

Name of case: *Examiner:*   *Date:*

Summary of errors: t/k (I,M,F)   Except in slow nonsense syllables repeated after examiner. Wrong location of contact.

Name of case: *Examiner:*   *Date:*

d/g (I,M,F)   Same as above, but said "go" correctly. The case can hear these errors when imitated by examiner at both slow and fast speeds, but cannot hear his own errors except in slowly spoken nonsense syllables.

t/s (I,M)   Except in slow production of isolated sound after strong stimulation by examiner. Can always hear own error except in fast conversation. Doesn't realize no contact is needed.

-s (F)   Makes no attempt to produce it. Evidently does not hear it as a part of the word when it comes in the final position.

Organic factors: High narrow palatal arch, but teeth are normally placed and tongue assumes good lateral contact with the teeth in making the z sounds. Makes the contacts for defective k and g sounds too far forward and with blade of tongue. When he tries to produce a genuine t *or* d he uses the tonguetip against the upper teeth.

Motor coordinations: Excellent in every respect.

Emotional factors: Not particularly sensitive. Will try persistently to follow instructions even when failing. Mother says he will try to say a word correctly for his father but not for her. "I'm too impatient, I guess." Boy seems to be mature for his age.

Developmental factors: Had been seriously ill the majority of his first year and a half. Onset of speech at 32 months.

Perceptual deficiencies: Very poor phonetic discrimination except for isolated sounds. Auditory memory span O.K. Poor ability to analyze component sounds of words. Could not recognize "mouth," "shirt," or "nose" when they were sounded out phonically.

Prognosis: Good.

Articulation Testing

Finding the Articulation Errors.   The conductor of a large symphony orchestra is said to be able to hear any mistake made, whether by piccolo or bass viol. Some speech therapists of long experience and training also have this gift. They can listen to the conversation of an articulation case and come up with a detailed presentation of each error, how it was made and under what conditions. Most of us are not so adept. We must arrive at the same result by a systematic testing program.

Screening Tests.   In the public schools where large numbers of children enter the elementary grades each year, the speech therapist has found that she must screen the children to find those with speech problems. Most of those she does find have articulation errors and so, as quickly as possible, she examines them, not at this time to analyze the articulation problems presented, but merely to locate them. She must identify those children from the others with normal speech or other types of speech disorders. Analysis will come later.

Some of the common methods used in this initial screening are these: (1) The naming of objects or pictures selected so as to include all the most difficult speech sounds. (2) The repetition of test sentences such as "This girl thinks that the cowboys on the television are real," or a series of sentences, each designed to test the errors on just one sound such as the following: "This is my thumb. I put it in my mouth; but I don't bite it with my teeth." (3) Serial speech responses such as counting, naming the days of the week, naming the colors on a chart. (4) Repeating nonsense syllables or sounds in isolation or nonsense words. (5) Conversation and questioning. There are other methods but one or a combination of these mentioned will serve as a quick method for finding those children who have articulation errors.

Diagnostic Testing

Articulatory disorders, as we have defined them, are characterized by errors of sound substitution, addition, omission, and distortion. Each speech correctionist devises his own procedure for giving the articulatory examination. Even when students have been trained according to one standard technique, they find it necessary to make modifications to fit the individuality of each case they examine. For this reason, we have described various procedures under each of the types of articulation tests and have provided word lists, sentences, and reading passages which the student may use as he sees fit. His task is to determine the nature, number, and characteristics of the articulatory errors as they occur in the case's speech.

Spontaneous production of a speech sound may be tested in several ways, two of which are most commonly used. These are the naming of pictures and the answering of question riddles. For both, a common set of objects or activities is used, the names of which include all the speech sounds in all three word positions. Such a list, with the sounds classified according to manner of articulation, is given in the appendix, see page 482. The words are chosen from the lists given in *A Reading Vocabulary for the Primary Grades,* by A. I. Gates, and therefore are suited to small children as well as to adults. The technique of administering this test is simple. After gaining rapport, the teacher points to the picture and asks the child to name it. Or, for example, when using the question riddle to get the sound of voiceless *th* in the final position, she says, "Watch me bite my finger. What did I bite my finger with?" Pictures representing the words in the text list may be cut from old magazines, and every teacher should have such a scrapbook.

The same word list may be used in administering the part of the articulatory analysis which requires the subject to repeat after a model provided by the teacher. The teacher merely asks the child to listen carefully, to wait a moment until the teacher lifts her finger as a signal, and then to repeat what the teacher has said. In addition to the word lists, it is often wise to use nonsense material such as *tho, otho, oth* to determine if a child can follow a model when the effects of training are minimized. Nonsense pictures may be drawn and named with nonsense words containing the sound to be tested. The speech correctionist may also ask the child to repeat "monkey-talk" words.

Both the spontaneous production of the various speech sounds and the student's ability to repeat them after stimulation can be tested by having the student read material that has been organized to include all the speech sounds in all three positions within the word. In addition to the word lists given, the reader will also find individual sentences, one for each of the speech sounds. A continuous passage, "My Grandfather" (see page 484) may be used for this purpose when only a little time is available. (See appendix.) The Templin-Darley Tests of Articulation[11] provide both screening and diagnostic tests complete with pictures and word lists and they include norms against which any individual child may be rated and a scoring method which helps us determine the consistency of the errors. It is a test which every speech therapist should know.

Key Words. One of the important reasons for checking the occasional use of the correct sound is that it gives us a crude measure of error strength. If two sounds are misarticulated but, on further analysis, we find that one of them has several key words (that this sound is inconsistently misarticulated) while the other is always incorrect, we would feel that the first would be more amenable to therapy. The error is less stable, less strongly habituated. Since we usually concentrate on one or two sounds of the four or five which might be defective, we would pick the one which is more inconsistent, the one which occasionally is said correctly.

Key words are also useful in actual treatment because they provide for the person a model in his own mouth for the sound we seek to teach him. We can use these key words to help us perceive the characteristics of the standard sound, both acoustic cues and the postures and movements required for their production. They can be used in discriminating error words from normally spoken words. The new sound can be isolated from them. Key words are also useful in that they help us measure the progress of therapy. As the person improves they increase in number. Many words may still be misarticulated but if the number of correctly spoken ones increases, we know we are moving toward our goal and so does the person.

Error Consistency. As we begin to search for key words, we also find something else. We find that some sounds are always misarticulated in the same way: the child always says *t* for *k*; but we also find that other sounds may have two or three different replacements.

---

[11] Mildred C. Templin and Frederic L. Darley. *The Templin-Darley Tests of Articulation.* Bureau of Educational Research and Services; Extension Division, State University of Iowa, Iowa City, Iowa.

One may be a substitution; another may be a distortion. We have worked with children who sometimes substituted a *t* for an *s*; in other words they had an interdental lisp; on still others we found some lateral emission of the air; and on certain blends such as in the word *school* they omitted the *s* sound entirely. When we find such multiple errors for the same sound, we are happier than when only one replacement exists. It means that the error is not fixed and stabilized, that it is still in a state of flux, that it is malleable and can be changed. Similarly, we find that when a child uses a single error for several standard sounds, saying "one-two-twee-toh-tie-tih-teben" we've got a tougher problem to solve.

Deep Testing. It is for these reasons that, once we have located the major defective sounds, we often do some deep testing. If we discover in our initial testing that the person misarticulates the *l* sound, we then explore many utterances which include *l* words in many phonetic combinations. There are two chief ways of going about this business of deep testing. First, we check to see if the person can say these sounds in isolation or in nonsense syllables, with and without strong stimulation. Next, we put the sounds into phrases and sentences which are constructed so as to facilitate the production of the correct sound. Finally, we have the person say a host of words including the usually defective sound, hoping that among them we will find some which are key words. This deep testing usually produces some key words and it certainly gives us a measure of the consistency of the error.

Assimilation. In constructing these test sentences and in selecting our large number of test words, we use the principle of *phonetic assimilation*. This term refers to the fact that any given sound is influenced and affected by the sounds that precede and follow it. If the sound which precedes an *l* sound is one which required the lifting of the tonguetip, then the *l* sound will more likely be uttered with a tongue-lifting movement. The *t* and *d* and *n* sounds, for example require such lifting. Therefore, when the *l* sound follows these, it is more likely to be spoken correctly as in *bottle*. The same tendency exists if these sounds follow the *l* sound, as in *belt*. If we can surround an *l* sound with two of these tongue lifting sounds, it often is produced correctly and can be used as a key word.

Unfortunately, we do not have at this time a complete compendium of sentences and word lists which employ this principle of phonetic assimilation for deep testing. Each therapist must contrive his own. Perhaps we can at least provide a model, one which we used yesterday with one of our cases who had a defective *l* sound. In our deep testing we asked him to say the following, and the words italicized are those he said correctly.

Assimilation sentences:

1. Ted *lit* the candle. (Note the fact that the *d* preceded the *l* in the second word as well as in the word candle.)
2. The cat likes the *bottle*. (*t* and *l*)
3. The baby can *lift* the funnel. (*n* and *l*)
4. His *left* hand grabbed the *weasel*. (*z* and *l*)
5. The mice liked to *sleep*. (*s* and *l*)

Assimilation Words. Note that in these we use the assimilative blends not only at the beginning but also in other positions of the words.

slab, slack, slain, slam, slang, slant, slap, slave, slay, sleep, *sleet,* slept, slice, slick, sly, slight, slim, *slime,* sling, slip, slit, sliver, slobber, slope, slot, slouch, slow, *slug,* slum, *slung,* slur, sly.

Nell, *Nile,* null, nail, teal, till, tail, tell, toil, toll, deal, doll, dull, dial, drill, droll, drool, sale, seal, silly, cell, soul, soil, snail, *snell,* steal, still, stall, stale, stole, stool, style.

build, bailed, belled, bald, bold, boiled, child, drilled, drooled, filled, *foiled,* fooled, failed, felled, filed, heeled, hold, hailed, howled, killed, called, curled, cold, cooled, coiled, *kneeled,* nailed, sealed, sailed, sold, soiled, tilled, told, built, belt, bolt, dealt, fault, dwelt, felt, guilt, halt, jilt, jolt, *quilt* melt, malt, smelt, *knelt, pelt, silt,* salt, moult, *stilt.*

eels, ills, oils, ails, awls, owls, boils, bills, bails, bells, balls, bowls, boils, *deals,* dolls, dials, duels, fills, fails, fools, files, fouls.

salt, tilt, steals, stills, stools, stalls, *styles,* strolls, tills, tails, tells, tools, towels, toils, kneels, nails, seals, sells, sails, soils, souls.

battled, cattle, tattle, bottled, mottled, noodle, doodled, totalled, titled, *diddled,* fiddled, unless, unlike, unload, unleavened, inlet, outlet, *cutlet, starlit,* only, *kindling.*

These are only a few of the possible words which we could use for deep testing for the *l* sound errors. The person we tested was convinced that he could never say the sound correctly. We asked him to count the words we had underlined as having been spoken correctly, and we were off to a good start in therapy with real motivation. Often in deep testing we find that unfamiliar names can be used as key words or that asking the person to repeat foreign place names after us will provide them, possibly because they have not been spoken before with error. Diagnostic testing should always employ deep testing.

Summarizing the Diagnosis. At the end of the examination it is always necessary to put all our information together in a systematic and meaningful way. Only when this is done is it possible to get a clear picture of the case with which we will be working. If a therapy plan is to be constructed which has a real chance for success, the information gained from the examination must be organized. The following form can be used for this purpose:

Diagnostic Case Summary

Case: *Age:*   *Grade:*   *Address:*   *Phone:*

Type of disorder:
Results of Articulation test:
Phonetic errors: *Manner of error production:*   *Conditions:*
Phonetic transcription of conversational speech:
Intelligibility:
Key words (Underline sound usually defective):
Case history data:
Intelligence:
Hearing:
Emotional conflicts:
Motor incoordinations:
Organic abnormalities:
Perceptual deficiencies:
Attitude toward prospective therapy:

In order to demonstrate what an actual summary would look like we present the following example:

Diagnostic Case Summary

Case: Robert Johnson   *Age:* Ten   *Grade:* Fifth   *Referral:* by teacher
Informant: Mother   *Examiner:* Jackson   *Date:* March 2, 1953
Previous Therapy: None.   *Type of Disorder:* Articulation
Articulation test results:

```
    t/k    (I. M. F)    -k  (F)
    d/g    (M. F)       -g  (F)
    w/l    (I. M)       -l  (F)
    o/l    (F)
```
All *l* blends (sl, pl, etc.) have the *l* omitted. All *k* and *g* blends defective. Occasionally defective *r* (I) distorted by lip protrusion.

Manner of error production: This case tends to anchor the tonguetip on the lower gum ridge and produces the acoustically correct *t, d,* and *n* as well as the defective sounds by raising the blade of the tongue instead of the tip.

Conditions under which errors occur: Case can produce the *k* in isolation (kə) but only with strong stimulation and at slow speeds. The *g* can be produced in isolation and in nonsense syllables in all positions by repeating after the examiner and without need for strong stimulation. Case also uses *g* occasionally in his conversation. Fails consistently if excited or hurried. Omissions of both these sounds in the final position are most prominent in swift conversation. Discrimination of correct versus incorrect sounds as made by examiner is good. Self discrimination is poor. Child cannot produce or discriminate a good *l* sound even with strong stimulation. Error on this sound always occurs.

Intelligibility: Generally good. Occasionally when speaking swiftly or excitedly some difficulty in understanding a word or two was experienced by examiner. Other children and his parents and teacher understood him readily.

Key words: The following words were produced correctly: "OK" "go" "gum" and "li—" (like).

Case history data: No foreign language background; parental speech and attitudes toward child, good. No evidence of imitation as a factor. Birth history normal. Developmental history: child experienced great difficulty in sucking; bottle fed with large opening in nipple required; digestive troubles during first two years of life; much crying, "little babbling." Normal physical development. Usual childhood diseases were mild. Cut tonguetip with paring knife at 22 months; no permanent injury or scar tissue; intelligence normal: Binet IQ at eight years was 108; good student and excellent reader (silently); well-adjusted child with no pronounced emotional conflicts or behavior problems; interests normal for his age; first words spoken at 13 months and was speaking in "long sentences" by his second birthday; parents tried to correct child by demanding he repeat his difficult words after them but this method failed and no further attempts have been made except by the kindergarten teacher who also had no success. Child is aware of the fact that he does not talk correctly but is not too concerned. Some teasing to which he reacted by laughing and making his speech even worse.

Hearing: Audiometric examination reveals no hearing loss.

Organic examination: No abnormalities. Palatal arch fairly high but within normal variation. No frenum interference.

Motor coordinations: Large muscular coordinations adequate for his age norm. However, child seems unable to move tongue independently of jaw except at very slow speeds. Tongue thrust and strength seem normal. Tongue curling and lifting are accomplished with great difficulty. Cannot sustain half-lifted tonguetip in a fixed position. It always returns to lower gum ridge, or teeth.

Perceptual deficiencies: Auditory memory span normal; cannot discriminate *w* from *l* and made one error on *t* and *k;* cannot locate or recognize own errors in conversation or in single words; vocal phonics very poor: could integrate only two stimulus sounds (sh-oe); failed consistently in trying to integrate three sounds. Has little conception of words as sound sequences. Poor rhyming ability. Hears words as "chunks of sound."

Attitude toward prospective therapy: Fifteen minutes of trial therapy were administered in which discrimination of *t* from *k* was attempted. Child seemed interested. Cooperative. Rapport easily established. Should be a good case if motivation can be achieved.

How then should we treat Robert Johnson? Our final goal of course is to have him pronouncing correctly all of his defective sounds as unconsciously and automatically as other children do. But what are the sub-goals which lead to this final result? The therapy plan for this case should answer these questions. It is phrased in the form of the report to the therapist who was planning to help the boy.

. . . In addition to the preceding case summary, we are providing a tentative therapy plan which may assist you in organizing your treatment. We cannot, at this time, be certain that it will be adequate to the child's needs. Actual therapy alone will indicate the modifications necessary, but it should provide a framework for those changes.

Therapy Plan for Robert Johnson

Each therapy session, we feel, should be partly devoted to building a stronger foundation of essential skills and abilities and partly to the unlearning of an articulation error and the mastery of the correct sound which it replaces. Accordingly, we suggest that each session include some activity aimed at achieving each of these goals:

1. Convincing the child that it is essential that he achieve better speech.
2. Improving his ability to move the tongue independently of the jaw; increasing his precision and control of tongue postures. Also try to free tongue lifting from lip-rounding.

3. Teaching him to recognize the location of the upper gum ridge as an important landmark in speech production not only for the *l* but also for the *t, d* and *n* which are so often dentalized. Get him to explore the geography of the mouth so that he can distinguish the posterior focal articulation points needed for *k* and *g*.

4. Improving his vocal phonics. Much training is needed here if he is ever to learn to recognize his errors or to master the correct sound in words.

5. Ear training to help him (a) locate his errors within his utterance; (b) to discriminate between the correct sound and his error; (c) to recognize and identify the essential characteristics of the new sound to be learned; and (d) to receive enough strong stimulation with the isolated new sound to permit mastery.

6. As soon as the child shows real success in the ear training activities and you feel that Robert has shown improvement in tongue coordination and vocal phonic ability, we suggest that you devote a good share of each therapy session to teaching the new sound in isolation. However, this new sub-goal should not replace the five previously mentioned. They must receive a due portion of the therapy time.

7. When the boy can produce the new sound easily upon request, you should proceed to strengthen it, first in isolation, then in nonsense syllables or nonsense words. This strengthening should form the dominant part of the session at this stage, but again each of the preceding sub-goals must be reviewed in any therapy session.

8. Once Robert can make the new sound swiftly and easily in nonsense material you should begin to help him learn to incorporate it within meaningful words. The transition must be carried out with care using such techniques as signal practice and reconfiguration. Concentrate first on a few key words and continue on these until thoroughly mastered. Then proceed to the correct pronunciation of many words, using them in meaningful situations.

9. Finally, help him to use the new sound habitually, employing such techniques as negative practice, alternation of correct and incorrect sounds at swift speeds with rewards or token penalties by the use of checking devices in actual communicative situations. The child must be able to recognize his mistakes and to cancel them with correctly spoken words before you start working with one of his other defective sounds. This must be done without prompting on your part or reminder by others.

We suggest that you begin first with the *g* then the *k*, then the *l* and finally the *r* and the blends. You will probably find that careful training on the *g* will produce swift or even spontaneous mastery of the others. If it is possible, therapy should be individual, though group therapy can be employed, especially in the latter stages of the treatment. Since the boy's motivation to speak correctly is not very great, you will no doubt be forced to cast many of the therapeutic activities in the form of games or experiences suited to his age and intelligence. With good rapport, you may be able to work directly on the problem once he recognizes it. We feel his prognosis is very good. We doubt that any fewer than two therapy sessions per week for at least a semester will produce the desired progress.

PROJECTS

1. Find colored pictures in magazines for the words of the short-form screening test as given in the Templin-Darley Tests of Articulation. Cut these out, paste on individual cards, and assemble.

2. Devise loaded sentences each of which includes one of the following sounds in the initial, medial, and final word positions: *th, s, l, r,* and *k*. Use simple words.

3. One of your articulation cases distorts the vowel *r* sound as in *bird* and *father* because he fails to produce the rear elevation in the contour of the tongue. The high tip elevation is correct, however. Prepare a list of assimilation words which may help the back part of the tongue to rise. Note: the *k, g, ng, o,* and *oo* sounds use an elevated rear portion of the tongue.

4. Prepare three sentences, each of which contains an *s, l, r, th, f,* and *k* sound for use in quick screening of children.

5. Purchase a collection of miniature objects: foods, animals, etc., which, when named, would cover all the sounds usually in error.

6. Find or draw a picture which shows an activity scene sufficiently complex to enable you to ask questions which will evoke responses containing all these sounds: *s, l, r, th, f,* and *k*.

7. Prepare a list of questions about the child's body which will evoke responses containing the *s, l, r, th,* and *g* sounds. Example: "What do you bite with?"

8. Prepare a questionnaire which would elicit the necessary information concerning hearing loss.

9. Study the C-A-T and describe or demonstrate it to the class.

10. Make one ink-blot of your own similar to those used in the Rorschach and administer to five of your acquaintances. Report to the class the varied interpretations of your five subjects.

11. Select several items of the Oseretsky tests and administer them to a subject before the class.

12. Test five acquaintances by asking them to say these words backward: *cash, face, curl, naps.* Illustrate the process by giving them first this

example: "nose equals n-o-z; if we reverse this word, we say z-o-n which makes zone." Try to analyze their difficulties in terms of auditory memory span, phonetic analysis or phonetic synthesis.

13. Administer a portion of the Boston University Speech Sound Picture Discrimination Test to some child and report your findings.

14. Test three of your acquaintances to determine the diadochokinetic rates of *puh* and *tuh* and *kuh*. Which can be spoken fastest? Which is the slowest?

15. List under each of the following headings the types of structural abnormalities you might look for in the organic examination: lips, tongue, teeth, palate.

PERIODICAL REFERENCES

16. Artley, V. A. "A Study of Certain Factors Presumed to be Associated with Reading and Speech Difficulties," *Journal Speech and Hearing Disorders*, Volume 13, 1948, pages 351-360.

17. Beebe, H. H. "Auditory Memory Span for Meaningless Syllables," *Journal Speech Disorders*, Volume 9, 1944, pages 273-276.

18. ———, and Kastein, S. "Psychogenesis in Interdental Sigmatism," *Journal Speech Disorders*, Volume 11, 1946, pages 191-192.

19. Bilto, E. W. "A Comparative Study of Certain Physical Abilities of Children with Speech Defects and Children with Normal Speech," *Journal Speech Disorders*, Volume 6, 1941, pages 187-203.

20. Carhart, R. "Hearing Deficiencies and Speech Problems," *Journal Speech Disorders*, Volume 8, 1943, pages 247-253.

21. Goodstein, L. D. "Functional Speech Disorders and Personality: A Survey of the Research," *Journal Speech and Hearing Research*, Volume 1, 1958, pages 359-376.

22. Hansen, B. F. "The Application of Sound Discrimination Tests to Functional Articulatory Defectives with Normal Hearing," *Journal Speech Disorders*, Volume 9, 1944, pages 347-355.

23. Karlin, I. W., and Strazzulla, M. "Speech and Language Problems of Mentally Deficient Children," *Journal Speech and Hearing Disorders*, Volume 17, pages 286-294.

24. Kronvall, E. L., and Diehl, C. F. "The Relationship of Auditory Discrimination to Articulatory Defects of Children with No Known Organic Impairment," *Journal Speech and Hearing Disorders*, Volume 18, 1954, pages 335-338.

25. Lundeen, D. J. "The Relationship of Diadochokinesis to Various

Speech Sounds," *Journal Speech and Hearing Disorders,* Volume 15, 1950, pages 54-59.

26. Metraux, R. W. "Auditory Memory Span for Speech Sounds," *Journal Speech Disorders,* Volume 7, 1942, pages 31-38.

27. Milisen, R., "A Rationale for Articulation Disorders," *Journal Speech and Hearing Disorders,* Monograph Supplement 4, 1954, pages 6-17.

28. Morrison, S. "Measuring the Severity of Articulation Defectiveness," *Journal Speech and Hearing Disorders,* Volume 20, 1955, pages 347-351. (Dec.)

29. Perkins, W. H. "Methods and Materials for Testing Articulation of (s) and (z)," *Quarterly Journal of Speech,* Volume 38, 1952, pages 57-62.

30. Pronovost, W. L., and Dumbleton, C. "A Picture-type Speech Sound Discrimination Test," *Journal Speech and Hearing Disorders,* Volume 18, 1953, pages 258-266. (Sept.)

31. Roe, V., and Milisen, R. "The Effect of Maturation Upon Defective Articulation in Elementary Grades," *Journal Speech Disorders,* Volume 7, 1942, pages 37-50.

32. Sayler, H. K. "The Effect of Maturation Upon Defective Articulation in Grades Seven Through Twelve," *Journal Speech and Hearing Disorders,* Volume 14, 1949, pages 202-207.

33. Snow, K. M., and Milisen, R. "The Influence of Oral versus Pictorial Presentation upon Articulation Testing Results," *Journal Speech and Hearing Disorders,* Monograph Supplement 4, 1954, pages 30-36.

34. Spriestersbach, D. C., and Curtis, J. F. "Misarticulation and Discrimination of Speech Sounds," *Quarterly Journal of Speech,* Volume 37, 1951, pages 483-491.

35. Templin, M. "Norms on a Screening Test of Articulation for Ages Three through Eight," *Journal Speech and Hearing Disorders,* Volume 18, 1953, pages 323-331.

BOOK REFERENCES

36. Berry, M. F., and Eisenson, J. *Speech Disorders.* New York: Appleton-Century-Crofts, 1956.

37. Bryngelson, B., and Glaspey, E. *Speech Improvement Cards.* Chicago: Scott Foresman & Company, 1941.

38. Johnson, W., Darley, F. L., and Spriestersbach, D. C. *Diagnostic Manual in Speech Correction.* New York: Harper and Row, Publishers, 1952.

39. Van Riper, C. *Case Book in Speech Therapy.* Englewood Cliffs, N.J.: Prentice-Hall, Inc., 1953.

40. ———, and Irwin, J. V. *Voice and Articulation.* Englewood Cliffs, N.J., Prentice-Hall, Inc., 1958.
41. West, R. W., Ansberry, M., and Carr, A. *The Rehabilitation of Speech.* New York: Harper and Row, Publishers, 1957.

CHAPTER TEN

Articulation Disorders: Treatment

The treatment of disorders of articulation may be viewed in terms of the following outline. Once he realizes that he has a problem, the person with an articulatory disorder needs training in (1) minimizing those causal factors which still maintain the disorder (this we have described in the preceding chapter); (2) identifying the error and the standard pattern of the sound; (3) scanning and comparing his own utterance with this standard; (4) varying his utterance until correct sound production is achieved; and (5) stabilizing and habituating the new correct ways of speaking so that they can be used automatically.

The Child Must Be Convinced that He Has a Problem Which He Must Solve. This is not so easily done. Owing to sheltered environments and the tolerance of associates who have become accustomed to the speech difference, many speech defectives grow to adulthood without ever having been made aware of their speech disorder, although it may be so noticeable that it shrieks its presence whenever its possessor opens his mouth. If friends and acquaintances will not mention it, certainly the average stranger will not. We seldom hear ourselves speak. Instead, we listen to our vocalized thinking. And so the speech defective himself has little chance of becoming fully aware of the nature or frequency of his errors.

Although many articulatory cases are thoroughly aware of their speech disorder, they do not seem to recognize all of their errors; and there are other cases who seem totally unaware of any speech difficulty. Small children, especially, need to be convinced that they have sound substitutions, additions, omissions, or distortions before they will cooperate or respond to treatment. The older ones must learn to recognize error whenever it occurs. A vague, generalized feeling that something is wrong with the speech will not provide sufficient motivation for the type of retraining that is necessary.

Teachers frequently ask whether or not it is advisable to work upon the child's speech in view of the self-consciousness and embarrassment which might be produced. The answer to this question is that the quickest way of getting rid of these errors is to make the child aware of them. The habits should be broken before they become fixed. Moreover, it is perfectly possible to work on a speech defect without shame, and if the teacher makes the child understand that a certain skill is to be learned and a problem is to be solved, no insecurity will be created. If she adopts a calm, unemotional attitude herself, empathic response will ensure a similar attitude in the child.

There are various ways of teaching an articulatory speech defective to recognize his errors, and some of them are given in the next paragraphs. One mother patiently corrected her child on every mispronounced word for three successive days, and he responded by refusing to talk at all for a week. With small children, no such nagging is necessary or advisable. The teacher should select five or six common words in which the child uses the error and should try to create in the child the feeling that in these words he is doing something incorrectly. She may tell him that there are other troublesome words, but she should set up as the first definite project the correction of these five or six. By narrowing the disorder to such a slender nucleus, the task is made easier and specific. The child must learn to recognize these words as "wrong words" and must come to realize that in these words he is likely to use "wrong sounds."

Sample Exercises for Teaching the Child to Recognize His Errors

1. The teacher reads a story to the child in which the five or six error words are used many times. The first time she reads it, she imitates the child's errors, cupping her ear every time she does so. The child is asked to do the same thing. The second time, the teacher reads it correctly except for one word. The child is asked to cup his ear when he hears the one error.

2. The teacher reads a list of words among which are included the

error words. The child repeats all but the error words after the teacher, who pronounces the error words twice, first correctly, then incorrectly.

3. The child tells a story or recounts some experience and the teacher rings a bell whenever she hears the child mispronounce one of the error words.

4. One of the error words that is the name of a certain object is selected. The teacher draws two pictures of the object and asks the child to scribble over one of them. The teacher then names the two pictures, pronouncing the scribbled one with the child's error, and pronouncing the other one correctly. She then tells the child a story, sometimes using the word correctly and sometimes incorrectly. The child is asked to hold up the appropriate picture. The child then tells a story while the teacher holds up one picture, usually the scribbled one.

Sample Exercises for Teaching the Older Child or Adult to Recognize Errors:

1. The student silently reads prepared material which illustrates the error, thus: "He thaw/saw the bird fly to the netht/nest." The teacher then reads it aloud.

2. Have the student write from dictation, putting down in phonetic spelling the errors which the teacher purposely makes.

3. Teacher speaks a word five times, once with error. Student signals when error occurs. The same assignment can be made but with the teacher saying the word correctly only once out of five trials.

4. Same as above but with student immediately imitating teacher's error. (*Note.* Speech penalties are more effective than any other penalty.)

5. Using material with *s* words (or other error-sound words) underlined, have student (1) make judgment as to error occurrence as he reads; (2) pause after attempt on *s* word while teacher imitates and asks for judgment of right or wrong; (3) pronounce the *s* in three different ways, raising finger for the incorrect pronunciations; (4) repeat each *s* word three times, making judgment as to which attempt was the best; (5) repeat *s* sound five times before proceeding, while teacher makes judgments for each; (6) prolong *s* sound and make judgment.

6. Use the same assignments as above but (1) reading lists of words, one at a time; (2) saying prewritten speech; (3) using conversation.

7. Student uses telephone and teacher interrupts conversation by hanging up immediately upon occurrence of error.

8. Teacher requires student to do something absurd (such as going to mirror, shaking head, and saying "Oh, oh") after each error.

9. Student confesses and points out own errors each time they occur.

10. Student imitates own error whenever it occurs, exaggerating it.

Design of Therapy. What do we do in teaching a person to speak the standard speech of his culture instead of using a distorted facsimile thereof? How do we correct the incorrect? Essentially we have here something more than a mispronunciation such as *suh-jest* for *suggest*. A person can eliminate such an error immediately once it is called to his attention and the correct model presented. But in misarticulation, we find that calling attention to the error is not enough. We must also teach this person how to produce the standard speech; he seems unable to do so voluntarily or upon demand. He may try to do so but the result is still unacceptably far from our standards of utterance. Therapy then is a learning process. We must teach and the case must learn how to talk as others do.

The Learning Process. Earlier, we have emphasized the motor and acoustic aspects of speech, and, in mastering an articulation error such as the substitution of a *th* for an *s,* we are forced to deal directly with movements and sounds. The changes which must occur must be new patterns of muscular movement which produce new sounds, at least so far as the case's utterance is concerned. Accordingly, the learning process requires goal-setting in terms of target sounds or movement patterns. The clearer the perception of the goal, the faster the learning. But locating targets is not enough. We must also try to hit the bull's-eye; we must try and try again. But this too is not sufficient. We must know, after we shoot, how far away from the center our arrows have hit. We must be able to scan our misses if we are to correct our aim. We must know the *amount* of error if we are to reduce that error. We may need help in varying our postures or the speed and direction of our movements so that we won't continue to make the same mistake. Finally, we need rewards, not only for the final hitting of the bull's-eye but also for shooting, for coming closer. We need also to learn to hit the target consistently.

Operational Levels. The mastering of a new sound so that it can be used in all types of speaking may be viewed in terms of four successive levels: (1) the isolated sound level, (2) the sound in a syllable, (3) the sound in a word, and (4) the sound in a meaningful sentence. This is the staircase our cases must climb. Once they have reached the top step of this staircase they find a wide platform on which they must explore the communicative, thinking, social control, and egocentric functions of speaking, using the newly mastered sound in each.

With such a concept, it is possible for both therapist and case to know just where the latter is at each moment during therapy, and to know what has been achieved and what remains to be accomplished. There is no excuse for unplanned therapy, for random activity or busy-work when a child or adult is unable to talk as others do. The therapist has many responsibilities when working with an

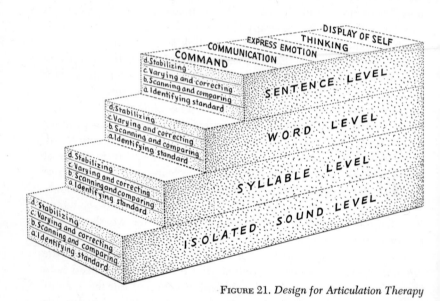

FIGURE 21. *Design for Articulation Therapy*

articulation case. She must establish a close relationship; provide many rewarding reinforcements; create situations in which learning can occur; and provide models not only of the correct utterance but also of scanning, comparing, varying, and correcting processes. But she has one other responsibility of paramount importance: She must know where the case is, where he has been, and where he has to go in therapy. And she must help the case to know too.

The Focus of Therapy. Since the essential error consists of a defective sound, it is upon this that we must focus our therapy. Let us repeat: It is the defective *sound* which is in error. It is the misarticulated, nonstandard sound which spoils the syllable, spoils the word, spoils the sentence, and spoils whatever type of speech is being used. In whatever context it occurs, the acquisition and use of a standard sound must be our goal. The child's playmates say to him, "What's the matter with you? You talk funny. Say it this way!" and they provide him with an entire sentence to attempt. The child fails. Parents and teachers focus their therapy on the word level. "Don't say wabbit," they command. "Say rabbit!" The child fails again, or if, by chance, he does say it correctly, there is no transfer to any other *r* word and there are thousands of *r* words he must use. The speech therapist usually focuses her efforts on the sound first, and then on the syllable, for she knows that these are the foundation stones of standard speech. Once a lisper can make a good *s* in isolation, in various nonsense syllables, and has learned how to incorporate it in a few words, he has acquired the tools needed to conquer all *s* words. He need not learn each one individually.

How shall we proceed in focusing our therapy upon the defective sound? Here we have two schools of thought. The one, represented by Backus and Beasley (see Reference 46) and others, insists that the correction of the defective sound must always occur in meaningful communication, in conversation. They begin at the functional level, and work downward through the sentence, word, and syllable levels until the defective sound is reached, identified, and corrected. Correction, they feel, must always occur in a communicative context.

We have no quarrel with these workers. Skillfully administered (and it is often difficult to do it this way), this sort of articulation therapy can be very successful. Indeed we often use this method with the milder types of cases, i.e., with those who are able to acquire the new standard sound with a minimum of stimulation. However, we feel that immediate and direct focusing upon the isolated sound or syllable has much to recommend it. It defines the target immediately. A new sound when mastered can spread very quickly to many syllables, many words, and not just those used in structured conversation. A child who learns to use the *th* sound in "Thank you" in a pretended picnic in the therapy room may remember to say the phrase correctly when his father gives him a dime to spend but he may have more trouble saying "birthday" or "think" or "bath" than those who have learned immediately to say "th." There are transfer problems in all types of articulation therapy. The second school of thought, then, begins by attempting to teach the child to master a new sound as an isolated sound or in a nonsense syllable. The majority of speech therapists seem to prefer this approach.

Therapy at the Isolated Sound Level

All of the continuant sounds such as *s, l, r,* or *th* can be produced in isolation since they are easily prolonged. Plosives such as *k* and *g* and affricates such as *ch* can be uttered only syllabically, and so when we teach these in isolation, we begin usually by using the schwa (or neutral vowel) uh (ə) or (ʌ) to create syllables such as *kuh, guh,* and *chuh.* We work on only one or two target sounds at a time. When too many quail flush at once, most marksmen miss. We shoot better when we have our sights focused on a single target.

The First Targets.   Those children who have but one error sound present no difficulty so far as targets are concerned, but those who have many errors do. With which sound or sounds shall we begin? No set rules can be offered but the following items should be considered when selecting the target sound. Of several defective sounds, we would select the one which (1) would have the most key words, (2) have the simplest coordinations, (3) is mastered earlier by most children in their speech development, (4) can be spoken correctly after a bit of trial therapy, (5) have been especially penalized by others. The therapist has to use her judgment as to the importance of each of these factors. At times it is possible to work on pairs of similar sounds, such as the *s* and *z*, or the *k* and *g* at the same time since they are cognates, having similar motor patterns. The lateral lisping errors and distortions of the *l* and *r* sound seem to be the most difficult. If the person can produce the sound as a *single* (*l* as in *lack*) but not as a blend (*bl* as in *black*) we might begin with this blend if there is much need to give the child some early success.

Identifying the Standard Pattern.   Many a child has persisted in his articulation errors merely because he has never really known the features of the standard sound. He has never heard it in isolation. The correct sound has always been buried in the fast flowing words, sentences, and communication of other people. The child has learned to listen for meanings, not for sounds, and so, even though he hears a standard sound flick by, he does not really attend to it. Hidden as these sounds are in the torrent of fast moving speech, they have little stimulus value. This is the first task of the speech therapist: to help the child to identify the standard sound through ear training.

Ear Training. If a child is to know what his target is, he must learn to cock his ears in such a fashion that he can locate and identify the standard sound he must learn to make. He must learn to analyze the speech he hears in terms of its sounds rather than meanings. He must come to know the characteristic features of this new target sound. The lisper must learn to listen with strange ears, to recognize the high pitched hiss of his therapist's *s*, to observe how she makes it. He must know when it is distorted and when it is right.

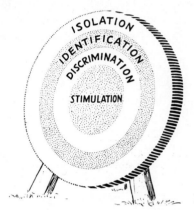

Figure 22. *Ear Training*

In helping such a person to acquire the concept of a standard sound, one against which he may later match his own utterance, we have four basic sets of techniques: (1) isolation, (2) stimulation, (3) identification, and (4) discrimination. All these are designed to define the target. They provide the model which he must match. Without such a model, how can he correct himself?

Please note that this is ear training, not mouth training. In this necessary perceptual defining of a standard pattern, the ear training period, we do not ask the child to attempt the new sound. Not yet. First let us be sure that he internalizes the model. In this first phase of therapy for articulation cases, the emphasis is all on listening. It is ear training.

Isolation Techniques. We have pointed out that, as long as a sound is lost within a word, it cannot be heard or felt with any clarity. The word configurations must be broken up so that the correct sound can be heard by itself. One adult declared that he had sincerely tried to hear the sound that his teachers said he used incorrectly, but, when they pronounced the words, the part in which he was interested was gone before he could perceive it. This adult could make the sound at will when he said it separately, but was unable to use it in familiar words. To the child speech defective, spoken words are lumps of sound. Indeed, he hears them as single sounds rather than as sound sequences. The older methods of teaching reading, in which children learned to sound out their new words, probably helped the articulatory cases much more than the new methods, which stress the acquisition of whole words. It is possible for an articulatory case to learn new word-wholes in which the correct sound is used, but it is much more economical, in terms of time spent in remedial work, to teach him to disrupt the incorrect word-wholes, to recognize the error, and then to integrate the correct sound into a sequence that is acceptable. He will then be much more likely to recognize his errors, and he will be able to master new words by himself.

A few illustrative exercises in isolating sounds from their contexts may be given. The individuals concerned were lingual lispers—hence the use of *s* as the sound illustrated. Any other sound may be used in the same exercises, and many other similar exercises may be easily invented.

Sample Isolation Techniques for Children

1. The teacher hides, in different places about the room, nine or ten pictures of various objects, one of which begins with the *s* sound. The moment the child finds this picture, he can run back to the teacher and ring a bell.

2. The teacher gives the child an old catalogue and a pair of scissors. A box is shown the child, and he is told that when he gets five pictures whose names begin with the *s* sound and one picture whose name ends with that sound, he can open the box and have what is in it. He does so and gets the jelly bean.

3. The child is covered with a bath towel and told to play Jack-in-the-box. The teacher tells him that she has three funny word keys, only one of which will open the box. The word key that fits has the *s* sound in it. The child is to jump and throw off the towel and say "boo" when the

teacher uses the proper key. The three keys are nonsense words or sound sequences such as *mo-bo-to-pay, ka-pa-la-tha,* and *ro-ssso-fa-ta.* The length of the nonsense word key and the location of the *s* sound within the word may be varied to fit the needs of the child. Word keys may be simple monosyllables at first.

4. The teacher arranges five boxes on a table and tells the child that she is going to put a word in each box. He is to watch and point to the box in which there is a word with an *s* sound in it. The teacher may use word lists first and then progress to interesting sentences.

5. The teacher sounds out words and asks the child to locate the appropriate picture, putting all *s*-word pictures in a special envelope.

Sample Isolation Techniques for Adults or Older Children

1. Student reads silently, underlining all *s* sounds (not only *s* letters). He reads the passage and notes how many he missed in silent reading.

2. The teacher and student read from the same material (or recite sentences previously agreed upon), the teacher omitting all *s* sounds and the student speaking them, or, in the earlier stages, the student reading and omitting all *s* sounds and the teacher speaking them. Thus:

    STUDENT: Thi . . can . . ertainly run fa . . t.
    TEACHER: ss   ss   ss

3. The student should make a list of words in which the *s* symbol refers to some other sound (as in *measure* or *his*), and also a list of words in which other symbols are sounded as *s* (*ice, extra*).

4. The student sho·ld talk while having pencil and paper before him, writing the symbol *s* each time it occurs in the teacher's speech. This can also be done for each t·me it occurs in his own speech.

5. Pause for a count of five after each occurrence of the correct or incorrect *s* sound in his speech. Repeat, pausing prior to the sound.

6. Teacher stimulates student by omitting, prolonging, or repeating *s* each time it occurs. Use reading material in which the *s* sounds have previously been underlined.

Stimulation Techniques. It is not sufficient to isolate and identify the correct sound during the preliminary period of ear training. The student must be stimulated with the sound so thoroughly that it may almost be said to ring in his ears. Every available agency should be used to provide this stimulation. Parents, friends, and classmates can help. Through various devices, the speech defective's attention to the sound must be focused and heightened. He must become aware of it not only in isolation but also as it occurs within spoken

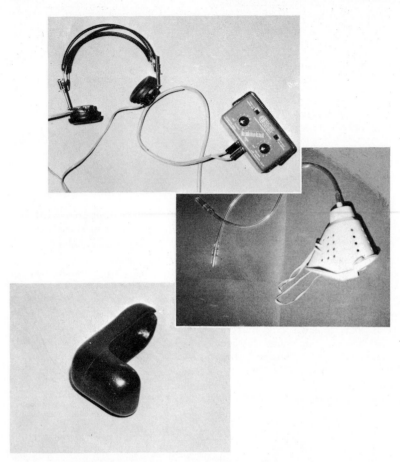

FIGURE 23. *Self-hearing Aids.* (*1*) *Ambco Binaural Auditory Trainer.* (*2*) *Voice Master.* (*3*) *Speech Shoe.*

words. If there is any law governing speech acquisition, it is the law of adequate stimulation.

Obviously, many of the techniques used in isolating the correct sound may be modified to provide adequate stimulation. The adult should be required to listen carefully and discriminatingly to variations in intensity and rhythmic presentation of the stimulus. He can be required to write the symbol simultaneously with the teacher's utterance. He may signal his perception of the presence of the sound within a jumble of nonsense material. Phonograph recordings may be used, and so also may such tongue twisters as "Sally sold silk and satin at the store on Saturday." The student, of course, does not pronounce these sentences. This is the period for ear training. He merely listens, or writes from dictation.

A correct attitude on the part of the speech defective is of the utmost importance to the success of this auditory stimulation. Koepp-Baker[1] gives this advice to his adult articulatory cases:

> When your clinician produces the sound, over and over again, for you, it is highly important that you pay the strictest attention. This listening must not be a passive act, but a highly active one. You must be listening—not just sitting. It would be much the same kind of listening you would do if you were studying a piece of music being played by an orchestra or single performer, to determine the nuances, variations, and subtleties of execution. Should you grow tired, inattentive, or disinterested, tell the clinician at once, for auditory stimulation is of value only when you are fully participating in the process of listening.
>
> As you listen, try to determine exactly in what way the sound which you are hearing differs from all other sounds of speech and in what way it is like them. Remember that your ability to detect the slight differences in sounds which give them their identity will develop slowly. At first you will hear nothing of any significance. *As you learn to listen discriminately,* you will discover much you have missed before.
>
> Do not be misled by the fact that your clinician *seems* to be doing all the work during the auditory stimulation period. His part is relatively simple and makes no great demands of him. On the other hand, your task of actively listening far transcends his in importance. All that really happens occurs in you. What you do during these stimulation periods determines the extent of any improvement to occur in your speech habits. Psychologically, the most important thing which will ever happen during your speech training is happening as you listen. Don't be fooled. Listening is hard work—and of greatest importance.

The cooperation of adults may usually be enlisted by such direct reasonable appeals, but younger children must be motivated to listen by the interest inherent in the activity itself. It is always wise to call for some type of performance to indicate the efficiency of the student's reception of the stimulation.

---

[1] By permission of the author, from *A Handbook of Clinical Speech*, Ann Arbor, Mich.: Edwards Brothers, 1936, Volume 2, pages 346-347.

Sample Stimulation Techniques for Children

1. Procure a calendar mailing tube or similar device. Hold one end to child's ear as he winds a string upon a spool. The moment the teacher stops making the sound, he must stop winding.

2. The teacher, parents, or classmates act as animals, machines, or objects which produce the sound. The child may be asked to tell a story in which these objects are mentioned, and, whenever he mentions them, the teacher makes the sound. Little dramas may be invented in which the child, for example, pretends to be an automobile with a flat tire in need of air, and the teacher is the station attendant who fills the tire with hissing air.

3. Certain objects are set aside as demanding the hearing of the correct sound before they can be touched. Such rituals appeal to children and compel attention.

4. A secret signal is arranged between the child and the parent or teacher. Whenever the child makes it, the parent or teacher must respond by a prolonged *s* sound.

5. A certain room in the home is set aside as a room which the child cannot enter until he knocks three times and hears the *s* sound.

6. Alliterative sentences using the correct sound in the initial position of most of the words are used as commands or requests. The child performs the activity.

7. Nursery rhymes, jingles, and even tongue twisters may be read to the child.

8. One minute of each hour is set aside as the *s* minute. Some associate of the child must pronounce the sound for a full minute. The child or teacher records the time in a little book.

Sample Stimulation Techniques for Adults or Older Children

1. The teacher prolongs or repeats the correct sound, using variations in rhythm or intensity. The student follows the type of stimulation by drawing a continuous line or separate lines on a sheet of paper, using dips to indicate decreases in intensity and crests to show increases. Rhythms may be indicated by spacing.

2. Phonograph records which carry variable durations of the correct sound can be played. The student is requested to time each of the durations until he makes a perfect score.

3. The teacher dictates to the student, prolonging all the *s* sounds.

4. The teacher holds a conversation with the student, interjecting the correct sound between all words.

5. Two students, one of whom is the lisper, sit side by side, with their eyes closed. The teacher produces a prolonged *s* sound as she slowly walks away from them. They indicate by raising their hands when they can no longer hear the sound.

Identification Techniques. As we have said, it is necessary to make the correct and incorrect sounds very vivid if the child is to learn to discriminate them in his own speech. The techniques for isolating and recognizing the sounds do a great deal toward this end, but they need to be supplemented by other methods which give the sounds their identities or personalities. This identification is largely a process of observation of the sounds' characteristics, in terms of both audition and mechanics. It is also a process of association.

Each correct sound and the error must come to have an individuality and an identity. Many people fail to realize that before we can have discrimination we must have identification. All good teachers of speech correction give personalities to the sounds with which they work. They give them names, traits, and even faces. From such identification comes recognition; from recognition comes discrimination; from discrimination comes success.

Sample Identification Techniques for Children

1. It is always well to begin the identification by giving names to the correct and incorrect sounds. These names are frequently those of objects which make noises similar to that of the sound in question. Thus *th* is called the windmill sound; *s*, the snake or goose sound; *ch*, the train sound; *r*, the growling-dog sound; *k*, the coughing sound; *f*, the spitting-cat sound. Many others are easily invented, for literalness is not nearly so important as repetition of the name.

2. Many teachers of speech correction find it advisable to give faces to certain sounds. These may be drawn on cards and used for stimuli. The faces can illustrate some of the more simple mechanics of making the sound. Thus *f* has a face with the upper teeth biting the lower lip; *s* is smiling; *th* is barely protruding a very red tongue; *l* seems to be looking for peanut butter, with his tongue exploring the roof of his mouth. Mirror work also helps.

3. It is wise to associate the sound with a symbol, either in script or printing. Children readily understand that the snake sound looks like a snake, and that it is entirely natural for the sound with the lip-biting face to wear a sweater bearing the monogram *F*. Hiding cards with such symbols around the room and requesting the child to find them, during which

time the teacher keeps repeating the sound, will prove useful. So also will be the technique which calls for the child to pick out the symbol, whose sound the teacher speaks, from a pile of cards.

4. Little stories, frequently repeated, about the sounds will often produce associations which will help identify them. No one can tell just what will best identify the sound for any one child, but once the child shows a clear and strong reaction of emotion or curiosity, that association should be remembered.

5. It is not well to get too many traits associated with any one sound. Not the number of traits, but their pertinence, interrelationship, and contrast to the traits of the error give them their value. It is important that the teacher work for close coordination of the associations with any one sound. The sound of *s* should bring to mind immediately the snake, the symbol, the smile, and the story of how the snake hissed when the filling-station man turned the air hose on him. It should also bring to mind that the little red tongue is never between the teeth as it is with the *th* sound.

Sample Identification Techniques for Older Children and Adults

1. Identification for the adult can also be enhanced by giving names to the correct and incorrect sounds. Thus, for one adult lateral lisper, the correct sound was always referred to as the "whistled hiss," while the incorrect one was called the "old sloppy shush." Derogatory adjectives which need not be truly descriptive are often used. The auditory characteristics of the sound also may give rise to the names used. Consequently, we speak of the "high-pitched" and "low-pitched" *s* sounds, the "whispered *f*," and the "sounded *v*." They may also be identified by names descriptive of the shape of the lips, the position of the tongue, or the use of the nasal opening. The teacher should always bestow some name on both correct and incorrect sounds. Other traits and characteristics of the sound are thereby given a nucleus about which to cluster.

2. Phonetic diagrams, palatograms, and models of the articulatory positions characteristic of the correct sound and the error may be used as identifying agents. The student should be examined in his production of the incorrect sound, and his performance should be described in detail. He should examine the teacher's mouth as the teacher produces the correct sound and the error. Observation in the mirror is also useful. A tongue depressor may be inserted within the mouth to probe and investigate tongue positions. A slender-handled throat mirror may be employed for those sounds in which access to the speech organs is difficult. From all these data, the student should finally attain an integrated picture of what the teacher does when she makes the correct and incorrect sounds. It is often wise to insist that the student write out a complete

description of this picture. Even though phonetically accurate descriptions are not obtained, the procedure has identification value.

3. Since adults and older children have associated incorrect sounds with the printed or written symbols, it is often necessary to use nonsense symbols to represent the new sound. All of the characteristics of the correct sound should be associated with this rather than with the old symbol. The student must be taught that his task is to learn a new sound rather than to change an old one, that the new sound has characteristics that he must discover, and that, for the time being, he should use a new symbol to represent this new sound. Typical nonsense symbols for several of the speech sounds will be found in the section of this chapter concerning methods for strengthening new sounds.

Discrimination Techniques. The final step in ear training is that of discrimination, and, if the preceding types of ear training have been carried out, it should not be difficult. Discrimination consists of comparing and contrasting the correct and incorrect sounds, both in isolation and in incorporation within regular speech. Selecting, matching, and signaling techniques are used. They are employed even when the student discriminates successfully, for the practice is valuable in itself.

These discrimination techniques frequently call for an ability which many untrained teachers do not possess—the ability to mimic or produce a reasonably accurate imitation of the student's error. While such substitutions as *f* for *v* or *t* for *k* make no great demands upon the teacher's histrionics, the imitation of a lateral lisp, dark *l*, or gutteral *r* often present great difficulties. Nevertheless, the teacher may be assured that a little practice will soon bring about an approximation so close to the student's error that it will serve well enough for the usual discrimination exercises. In a sense, all preceding steps are pointed at facilitating this auditory discrimination, for it is the essence of the necessary ear training of which we hear so much. Without the ability to differentiate correct sound from error, the student becomes discouraged, the treatment becomes blind drill, and the teacher wishes she had taken up library work.

Sample Discrimination Devices for Children

1. *Selection.* Show the child an object such as a cake of soap. After a short review of the identifying characteristics of the correct sound and error, the teacher pronounces a series of isolated sounds or nonsense syl-

lables, such as *k, p, th, s, f, r, n, s, f, th,* and requests the child to hand her the object when he hears the sound that starts the word when it is made correctly, but to hide it when he hears the sound that starts it when it is made incorrectly.

2. *Selection.* The teacher and student begin the game with ten tooth-picks each. The teacher holds up a series of pictures, one at a time, pro-nouncing the name of each. In naming one of the pictures she uses the child's error. If the child recognizes it, he can demand the picture and one toothpick. If he fails to recognize it, he loses a picture and toothpick.

3. *Matching.* The teacher produces two sounds, declaring that they begin words which name objects in the room. The student is required to find three objects for each sound.

4. *Matching.* The child is blindfolded and sits with his hands out-stretched on the table in front of him. He is allowed to pull only one hand away at a time. The teacher names one hand as possessing the cor-rect and the other hand as possessing the incorrect sound. She then pro-nounces the sound name of one of the hands, rapping it lightly with a pencil as she does so. This helps to speed discrimination and the children enjoy it.

5. *Signaling.* The teacher asks the child to ring a bell and to rap the teacher's hand whenever the teacher uses the wrong sound. The teacher then tells a story, occasionally using the error. After every signal the teacher repeats the word correctly.

6. *Signaling.* The teacher reads a list of *s* words with her back turned to the child. The moment the child signals, she must pronounce the next word using the incorrect sound. If she fails, the child gets some small re-ward.

Sample Discrimination Devices for Older Children and Adults

1. *Selection.* The teacher tells the student that she will pronounce a series of thirty isolated sounds, some of which are correct and some in-correct. The student is given a sheet of paper on which the thirty num-bers are printed and is asked to encircle those numbers in the series on which the teacher used the correct sound. The teacher then pronounces the sounds and checks up on his discrimination.

2. *Selection.* The teacher pronounces three nonsense words such as *pa-sa-no-see.* She tells the student that each word will contain two cor-rect sounds, two incorrect sounds, or one correct and one incorrect sound. She teaches the student to recognize the three types, then dictates ten or twenty of them, which he is to write phonetically or in any way he wishes, classifying them according to type.

3. *Matching.* Using the symbols taught the student in the identification exercises, the teacher dictates a list of words, occasionally using the error.

The student is asked to write down the symbol corresponding to the sound used.

4. *Matching.* The teacher slowly reads a newspaper article, occasionally using the student's error. The student is asked to name each correct and incorrect sound, using the names taught in the identification exercises. He must interrupt the teacher to do this naming.

5. *Signaling.* The student is asked to raise his right hand the moment he hears the correct sound and to raise his left when he hears the error. The teacher pronounces a series of nonsense syllables, slowly at first, but with a gradual increase of speed.

6. *Signaling.* The teacher reads tongue twisters, occasionally using the error. The student is asked to rap on the table the moment he hears the error. If his response does not occur until after the teacher has said the next two words, he has failed. The procedure is continued until he collects five successes.

Scanning and Comparing. The second major phase of therapy also involves ear training but now the case is to listen to himself. It is training in *self-hearing* rather than in listening to the speech of others. By this time, he should have acquired a clear concept of the target sound. Now he must scan his own speech so that the differences between his own utterance and the standard sound will be made clear. Most of our cases have no idea of how they sound. Many of them do not even hear their errors. This is quite natural. When we speak we have to use our ears to find out what we are saying. Only rarely do we think before we speak. When we were babies, babbling in the crib, we listened to the sounds we were making and found joy therein. But once we learned the magical power of speech in sending messages, in formulating thoughts, in controlling others, we stopped listening to the sounds that emerge from our mouths. We had to keep our ears relatively free for receiving the *thoughts* of others and for scrutinizing our own meanings to see if they were well expressed. Perhaps this is why articulation errors persist. We do not hear them.

Somehow we must open up the invisible channel between the person's ear and his own mouth. We must help him to locate his errors whenever they occur. We must give them new vivid stimulus value. When the laller says a defective *r* sound, some hidden signal must be triggered off somewhere within the skull. Usually the therapist has to do the signaling first, pointing out when the error has occurred. We have found that it is wise to make these therapist signalings pleasant experiences to prevent the child from hearing echoes of past penalties. Here is one example:

> T: Today we're going to try to help you know whenever you lisp because you've got to know when you do if you are to stop lisping.
> C: OK.
> T: Fine. Here's a gong. It makes a fine sound when you bang it like this . . . Now tell me what I'm doing as I'm doing it and if you ever hear yourself lisp like *thith,* instead of like *thissss,* you can give it a wallop. All right. Here we go. Tell me what I'm doing.
> C: You're putting the penthil in your mouth.
> T: Huh?
> C: Oh, you're putting the penthil (*Bangs the gong*) in your mouth. Wow, what a big noith!
> T (*Takes hammer away and rings the gong herself*): Noith . . . (*Banging gong*). It should have been noise. No, don't try to say it right yet. Just bang it when you hear it wrong.

The preceding example illustrates how we can use this training in self-hearing at both sentence and word levels. The following one illustrates the process at the syllable and sound levels.

> T: Let's play a follow-the-leader game. Do what I do and say what I say, and if you can notice when you say a sound wrong and can clap your hands before I can say, "Oops! Hey nonny nonny!" I'll go over and put my head in that waste basket. Understand?
> C (*Enthusiastically*): Sure.
> T (*Raises hand*): Bah-bah.
> C (*Raises hand*): Bah-bah.
> T (*Shakes her foot*):Moogie-moogie.
> C (*Shakes his foot*): Moogie-moogie.
> T (*Touches nose*): Nnnnnnnnnnnnnnnn.
> C (*Touches nose*): Nnnnnnnnn.
> T (*Wiggles fingers*): Sobba-sobba.
> C (*Wiggles fingers*): Thobba-thobba.
> T: Ooops! Hey nonny nonny. Hah, I didn't have to put my head in the basket then.
> C: I catch you nekth time.
> T (*Raises hands above head*): Allee-oh.
> C (*Raises hands above head*): Allee-oh.
> T (*Pulls ears*): Fff-a-sss.
> C (*Pulls ears*): Fff-a-th . . . There one. (*Claps hands.*)
> T (*Puts head in basket*): You got me. You said fff-a-th instead of fff-a-sssssss.

It is possible to teach a child to recognize his own errors most easily when the process is pleasant rather than distasteful.

Recalling, Perceiving, and Predicting Errors. In this training in self-hearing, we operate in a time dimension. At first the child recognizes his errors only after they have occurred; next, when they are occurring; finally he can predict them. The wise therapist understands this natural sequence of recognition and uses it. She signals her perception of the child's error at first only after an interval sufficiently long to let him listen to what his mouth has produced. Here are some examples:

> T: Repeat each of these sounds twice before telling me if you've made a mistake: mmm. . . .
> C: mmmm . . . mmmmmm . . . it's OK.
> T: Right! Now this one: rrrrr
> C: rrrrr . . . rrrrr . . . it's OK too.
> T: Yes. Now this one: ssss
> C: Th. . . . Th . . . no, thath wrong.
> T: Now let's do it in a syllable. Try this one: llleee
> C: Llleee . . . Llleee. Thath all right.
> T: Now this one: oossss
> C: ooossss . . . ooosssss. Thatth wrong. Hey, wait! ooosss. It ith OK . . .
> T: Now this word: coop.
> C: coop . . . cooop. Good one.
> T: Now this one: soup.
> C: thoup . . . thoup. . . . I got that wrong.
> T: Now this sentence: (*Illustrating the action*) I pat my face.
> C: I pat my fayth. . . . I pat my fayth. Hey, I thaid fayth wrong.
> T: Yup. You're beginning to catch almost all your mistakes. Pretty soon we'll teach you how to say that *sss* sound correctly.

In the simultaneous perception of the error as opposed to this delayed perception, one very effective device is to have the therapist read or speak in unison with the case with her mouth to his ear. If at the moment he makes an error, she signals by making the correct sound very loudly, or by stopping her own speaking, or by some other stimulation, he will be brought to notice it instantly. Another device is to have the child record some sounds, syllables, words, or sentences, a few of which contain the target sound, and then to require the child to say them again in unison with his own recorded speech. The therapist turns up the volume of the playback very loudly at the moment of error. There are many other ways.*

In predicting errors, the therapist provides sample utterances on each of the various levels and then asks the child to predict whether or not he will make an error on them when he says them. Here is one example:

> Therapist: I'm going to say three sounds: first, *mmmmmmmmm;* second, *ssss;* third, *ffff.* In a moment I'm going to ask you to say them but first you tell me on which one you think you might make a mistake: *mmmmm . . . sssss . . . fffff.*
> Case: On the latht one.
> Therapist: OK, let's see. Try them.
> Case: *mmmm . . . th . . . ffff.* Oh it wath the thecond.
> Therapist: All right. Now let's try these syllables: *eepoo . . . ommee . . . issah.*
> Case: Oh, it wath on the latht one.
> Therapist: Right! Now try these words: *house . . . ham . . . heavy.*
> Case: *Houth* ith the one.
> Therapist: Good. It should have been "house."

All the various exercises for isolating, identifying, and discriminating the correct sound in the therapist's speech can also be used to help the child recognize the errors in his own speech once he has a clear concept of how the correct sound is spoken.

Teaching the New Sound. Once we have been able to establish a clear perception of the standard sound and have opened up the circuit of self-hearing so that the child can recognize and identify his errors, we are ready for the next step: learning to produce the new sound. As we have said earlier, this mastery of a new sound must be accomplished on all levels: isolated sound, syllable, word, sentence, and function, but we have found it most efficient to teach it first in isolation by concentrating on its motor and acoustic aspects. There are five different ways of approaching this task. The new sound may be taught by (1) progressive approximation, (2) by auditory stimulation, (3) by phonetic placement, (4) by the modification of other standard sounds already mastered, or (5) by using key words. Each of these will be described in detail.

Varying and Correcting. Whichever approach is used—and there

---

* Further examples of delayed, simultaneous, and predictive recognition of errors may be found in Van Riper and Irwin, *Voice and Articulation* (74), pages 134-141.

are times when we must try first one then another—the person must go through a process of varying his utterance. Change must occur in the way he shapes his tongue, in the acoustic patterns which emerge from his mouth. One of the basic problems confronting the therapist at this stage of treatment is to provoke such variation. Long-practiced habits are very resistant to change. Often before we can hope to get our case to have a fair chance of hitting his target, we must get him to try new postures, new attacks, new movement patterns. Variation must precede approximation. By this we mean something similar to what happens when a person learns to shoot an arrow at a target. When he shoots and misses, he first must know where the arrow has hit, and next he must vary his aim or stance so that his second shot will have some chance of hitting a different part of the target, preferably a spot closer to the bull's-eye. But he must vary and he must try to correct. This same process occurs in articulation therapy. We must get our lisper to try and try again, but to try differently each time so that he comes closer and closer to producing the desired standard sound. Variation must precede approximation.

Progressive Approximation. This method is a trail-blazing method. The therapist joins the case and makes the same error the case makes. She then shows the case a series of transitional sounds each of which comes a bit closer to the standard sound until finally the standard sound is produced. Each little modification the case makes which comes a bit closer to the goal is rewarded. Those variations which move away from the target sound are ignored. Through this process, the *degree* of error is constantly determined and new attempts are aimed at reducing the amount of deviation. The uniqueness of this approach is that it resembles the way that infants seem to acquire normal articulation. They do not suddenly shift from saying *wabbit* to *rabbit;* instead they seem to proceed through a series of gradual and progressive approximations as McCurry and Irwin[1] have described. This also is the process known to psychologists as "operant conditioning." Instead of asking the person to exchange a correct sound for his incorrect sound, we help him to shift gradually from where he is to where he has to go. Let us observe some progressive approximation therapy.

---

[1] W. H. McCurry and O. C. Irwin. "A Study of Word Approximations in the Spontaneous Speech of Infants," *Journal Speech and Hearing Disorders,* Volume 18, 1953, pages 133-139.

Therapist: Now cup your hands like this so they make a channel from your mouth to your right ear. I'm going to talk into your left ear like this. (*Therapist cups her hands and speaks a sound into the person's left ear.*) Now we're going to try to make the new sound. Say *ssssssss.*

Case: *thththththththth.* Thath no good.

Therapist (*Still talking into his left ear*): OK, let's do it again. This time I will join you and make the same sound so that we're in tune even if it is wrong. But then I'll change it just a bit and you try to follow me. I'm not going to change it all the way to the correct *sss* but I'll pull back my tongue a little and that will make a different sound. Try to follow me. But we'll start with your sound. Say *sssss.*

Case: *thththththththth*

Therapist (*In unison*): Ththth. (*And then she makes a slight variation in the direction of the standard sound and the case varies his sound also.*) Start with your old sound and let's try to shift a bit further like this. . . . (*Therapist illustrates the change the case has already made and a second change that comes even closer to the* sss.)

We feel that progresive approximation is the best of the five main methods for teaching a new sound. It permits reward for modification instead of reserving it for final attainment of the goal. It helps the identification of therapist and case. It reduces the task. It encourages variation. Even very resistant cases seem to move under this regime. We have found it very efficient.

Nevertheless there are times when other methods are to be preferred. For example, if a child can make the new sound fairly easily with direct stimulation, we find it easier merely to ask him to imitate us as described in the auditory stimulation method. Again, some cases seem to be unable to perceive tiny variations in auditory experience. They are not at all ear-minded. They have better visual or proprioceptive imagery than auditory imagery. With these we prefer to use the phonetic placement techniques. Finally, there are some children who have been so long defeated in attempts to correct themselves that it is better to use the modification of sounds they have already mastered.

Auditory Stimulation. This method relies upon simple imitation and demand. An example might run as follows:

TEACHER: Now, Johnny, I'm going to let you have your first chance to make the snake sound, *sss.* Remember not to make the windmill sound, *th-th.* This is the sound you are to make: *sss, sss, ssssss.* Now you try it.

If the ear training has been adequate, this simple routine, in which the wrong sound is pronounced, identified, and rejected, then followed by the correct sound given several times, will bring a perfect production of the correct sound on the first attempt. Occasionally it will be necessary to repeat this routine several times before it works, and the student should be encouraged to take his time and to listen carefully both to the stimulation and to his response. He should be told that he has made an error or that he has almost said it correctly. He should then be encouraged to attempt it in a slightly different way the next time. No pressure should be brought to bear upon him, and a review of discrimination, stimulation, and identification techniques should preface the new attempt. He should be asked to make it quietly and without force. The procedure may be slightly varied by asking the child to produce it in a whisper. After the sound has been produced, the teacher should signal the child to repeat or prolong it and to sense the "feel" of it. The attempt should be confined to the isolated sound itself or to a nonsense syllable beginning with it.

Phonetic Placement. The phonetic placement method of enabling a speech defective to produce a new sound is the old traditional method. For centuries, speech correctionists have used diagrams, applicators, and instruments to ensure appropriate tongue, jaw, and lip placement. Children have been asked to watch the teacher's tongue movements and to duplicate them. Observation of the teacher's mouth in a mirror has also been used. Many very ingenious devices have been invented to adapt these techniques for children, and often they produce almost miraculous results. Unfortunately, however, the mechanics of such phonetic placement demand so much attention that they cannot be performed quickly or unconsciously enough for the needs of casual speech. At best, they are vague and difficult to sense or recall. The positions tend to vary with the sounds that precede or follow them, and to teach all of these positions is an almost impossible task. Frequently dental abnormalities will make an exact reproduction of the standard position inadvisable. Many speech correctionists produce the sounds in nonstandard ways, if, indeed, there is a standard way of producing any given speech sound. Despite all of these disadvantages, the phonetic placement methods are indispensable tools in the speech correctionist's kit, and, when the stimulation method fails, they must be used. They are especially useful in working with individuals with hearing defects, and they certainly help to identify the sound.

Excellent diagrams and descriptions of the various speech sounds may be found in the texts to which references are given at the end of this chapter. The speech correctionist should have these texts available and should know the mechanics of articulation thoroughly enough to interpret the diagrams and assume the positions illustrated and described. The teacher should be able to recognize any sound from its description and diagram.

In using methods of phonetic placement, it is necessary that the speech defective be given a clear idea of the desired position prior to speech attempt. If an adult, he should study diagrams, the teacher's articulatory organs in position, when observed both directly and in a mirror, palatograms, models, and the written descriptions of the mechanics whereby the sound is produced. Every available device should be used to make the student understand clearly what positions of tongue, jaw, and lips are to be assumed. It is frequently advisable to have the student practice other sounds that he can make easily, using diagrams and printed descriptions to guide his placement. This will familiarize him with the technique of translating diagrams and descriptions into performance.

Various instruments and applicators are used to help the student attain the proper position. Tongue depressors are used to hold the tip and front of the tongue down, as in the attempt to produce a *k* or *g*, or they may be used to touch certain portions of the tongue and palate to indicate positions of mutual contact. Tooth props of various sizes will help the student to assume a proper dental opening. Thin applicators and wedges are used to groove the tongue. Curious wire contrivances are occasionally used to insure lateral contact of tongue and teeth. Small tubes are used to direct the flow of air. The old texts by Borden and Busse and by Scripture provide examples of these instruments. In our experience, they are more dramatic than useful. Enforcing a certain tongue position through some such device produces such a mass of kinesthetic and tactual sensations that the appropriate ones can seldom be attended to. Usually, the moment the instrument is removed the old, incorrect tongue position is assumed, because, as Travis puts it:

> If a child used *p* for *f* from pressing lips too tightly together, a thick stick or finger was stuck between the lips so that they could not

close tightly. As far as the child is concerned, he is still making *p* regardless of whether a stick or finger was stuck between the lips or not. A sound cannot be broken up into its component parts, as into lip movements or tongue movements. It is a unit, a whole, and can be learned only as such.[2]

If these devices and instruments have any real value, it seems to be that of vivifying the movements of the tongue, and of providing a large number of varying tongue positions, from which the correct one may finally emerge. Many individuals have difficulty in realizing how great a repertoire of tongue movements they possess, and instruments frequently enable them to attempt new ones.

Tongue Exercises. The same result may be attained through various articulation exercises. Although the value of tongue, lip, and jaw exercises has been questioned and denied by many workers in the field of speech correction, they can be said to be useful in teaching the student to manipulate his articulatory apparatus in many new and unaccustomed ways. Too many articulation cases have only one or two stereotyped tongue movements in their speech repertoire, although they may have many more in their functions of swallowing, laughing, chewing, or sneezing. They need to learn how adaptable the tongue really is. Whenever possible, the articulatory exercises given should proceed out of the movements used in the biological functions or in babbling. The old, formal tongue exercises are of much less value.

When the correct sound has been produced (and frequently a lot of trial and error must be resorted to before it appears), the speech defective should hold it, increasing its intensity, repeating it, whispering it, exaggerating it, and varying it in as many ways as possible without losing its identity. He should focus his attention on the "feel" of the position in terms of tongue, palate, jaws, lips, and throat. He should listen to the sound produced. Then he should be asked to leave the position intact but to cease speech attempt, resuming it after a long interval. Finally he should let the tongue assume a neutral position on the floor of the mouth and then attempt to regain the desired position. Sounds produced by phonetic placement are very unstable and must be treated very carefully or they will be lost. Strengthen them as soon as possible and keep out dis-

---

[2] L. E. Travis, *Speech Pathology.* New York: Appleton-Century-Crofts, 1931, page 193.

tractions. After a successful attempt, one should insist that the student remain silent for a time before taking part in conversation. This will permit maturation to become effective.

Modification of Other Sounds.   Another special method of teaching a speech defective a new sound is that which involves the modification of other sounds, either those of speech, those that imitate noises, or those that imitate other functions, such as swallowing. These methods are somewhat akin to those of phonetic placement, but they have the advantage of using a known sound or movement as a point of departure for the trial-and-error variation which produces the correct sound. The modification method may take many forms, but in all of them the sequence is about the same. The student is asked to make a certain sound and to hold it for a short period. He is then requested to move his tongue or his lips or jaws in a definite manner while continuing to produce his first sound. This variation in articulators will produce a change in the sound, a change which often rather closely approximates the sound that is desired. An illustration of this method may be given. A lateral lisper is told to make the *th* sound and to prolong it. Then, while continuing to make the sound, he is required to draw in the tonguetip slowly and to raise the whole tongue, slowly scrape its tip upward along the back of the upper teeth, and finally bring it to rest against the alveolar ridge. The *th* sound will change as the tongue rises, and a rather good approximation to the desired *s* will be produced. If this is combined with ear training and stimulation, it will be found to be very effective.

There are many of these modification methods, and each speech-correction teacher invents others. The student should go through the references given at the end of this chapter and collect examples appropriate to each of the commonly defective sounds for his notebook. The text by Nemoy and Davis (71) is especially useful in this regard. Most of these techniques have been used by all speech correctionists for decades, and they are part of the standard equipment of any worker in the field.

We shall now provide some supplementary methods for getting the articulation case to produce the correct sound. The student should be warned not to use them indiscriminately. They have value only in their ability to get the child to make the sound in a new way, in varying his attack on the desired sound. The essential task remains the same: to give the articulatory case a clear auditory, kinesthetic, and tactual picture of the sound.

S and Z Sounds

1. Have the child protrude the tongue between the teeth so as to produce the sound *th* in the utterance of such words as *saw, glass,* and *rose.* Have him think of *th.* Then when he is thinking of producing the *th* for the *s,* force the tip of his tongue inward with a thin instrument such as a thick blunt toothpick. The result will be an *s.* The principle involved is that the child's thinking the *th* drives the air over the tip of the tongue. The value of directing the child's attention to the tip of his tongue when he is producing sibilant sounds is that he will eventually feel the current of air being emitted over it.

2. Have the child protrude the tongue as in the preceding exercise, and form the sound of *th;* but as this is formed, have him slowly and gradually withdraw the tongue and, while still attempting to make the *th,* scrape the tonguetip along the back of the front teeth and upward. The result will again be an *s,* which he should be asked to match with the *s* produced by the instructor until an adjustment is made which gives an excellent lispless *s.*

3. Have the child begin by forming a *t* in a word like *tea.* Have him pronounce it with a strong aspiration (*tuh-hee*), with a strong puff of breath after the explosion of the *t,* before the vowel begins. Then, instead of this sudden explosion or puff, take away the tip of the tongue from the teeth-ridge slowly. This will give the sound *ts.* Hold onto this sound and you will have the *s-s-s-s.* The child must not think he is saying *ts* as in the word *oats* or he will use his usual pronunciation. Keep him rehearsing the steps of this procedure till they are fixed in his mind, before showing him that he is making a good *s.*

4. Have the child hiss, seeking to raise the pitch of the hiss until it approximates that held by the instructor. Often it is wise to tell the student to experiment with the tonguetip positions during the production of his hiss, not before. Sometimes the instructor should change his hiss from the faulty one used by the student through several degrees until the correct *s* is made.

5. Have the child go through some brisk tongue exercises with special stress on the grooving of the tongue. The tongue should be grooved and protruded and the air should be blown through this groove. From this protruding position the tongue should be drawn back slowly while the blowing is continued, concentrating the attention meanwhile on the tip of the tongue. Sometimes use a thin stick or instrument to help the groove.

6. If the child can make a good *z* sound, take such a word as *zero* and ask him to listen carefully and to feel where his tongue is when he whispers it, prolonging the first sound. This is the sound which must become the child's model.

7. Put upper and lower teeth together. Ask child to stroke (with tongue) the back of his upper teeth as he blows a stream of air.

8. Put upper and lower teeth together and press lips tightly together. Keep teeth together but part lips to let a small hiss escape.

K or *G* Sound

1. Ask child to repeat the sequence *puh-tuh-kuh* in unison with the teacher. Teacher should give several samples first.

2. Ask child to imitate the teacher as she coughs up an imaginary wishbone in this fashion, *kuh-kuh*.

3. Ask child to anchor tongue against lower teeth and hold hand in front of his mouth so he can feel the puff of air as he imitates his teacher.

4. If the child can make the *ng* sound, ask him to do so and then give a little puff of air against his hand or a feather held in front of his mouth.

5. Ask the child to say *uhkuh* in a strong whisper.

6. Explore the child's vocabulary to see if he can say any word in which the word ends with a good *k* sound. Then ask him to repeat it many times and repeat the last sound, imitating the teacher, thus: *sick-kuh-kuh*.

7. If child can say *guh* ask him to whiper it because the (kʌ) is a whipered (gʌ).

8. Press underneath child's chin and ask him to say *kuh* in a whisper as you release the pressure suddenly.

9. Tell the child about two Australian birds, one a big one that has a long tongue that moves up and down and that always says *tee-tee-tee* and the other that doesn't have any tongue at all that you can see move and that always says *ook-ook-ook*. Ask the child to imitate both birds.

L Sound

1. Give strong stimulation through humming or singing the nonsense syllables *lay, lee, lie*, then ask child to hum or sing.

2. Give tongue-lifting and -lowering exercises, first in silence, then while blowing, then while whispering *ah*, then while saying *ah*. Gradually lift tongue higher and higher until it finally makes the contact at the right place.

3. Form mouth for *ah*. Keep whispering it softly as you place tongue

in firm contact with upper gum ridge. Then suddenly say the *ah* loudly as the tongue is released and a long *l* is subsequently made.

4. Practice this sequence very swiftly: *tah-dah-nah-lah*.

5. With a match or tongue depressor stroke the back of the upper gum ridge until child touches it with tongue. Ask him to stroke the spot with his tongue. Ask him to stroke it as he says *ee*.

6. Practice making the sound using a mirror and a wide-open mouth.

SH Sound

1. Tell the child to round his lips and flatten his cheeks and "slush" the air out between his teeth.

2. Ask the child to make an *s* sound and pull back the base of tongue with a pencil stuck between the teeth.

3. Ask child to make a *th,* then to pull back the tongue, shutting the teeth and continuing to blow.

4. Ask child to whisper an *er* sound, holding it for some time during which he gradually brings his teeth together.

5. Ask child to round lips and raise tongue and shut teeth as he whispers a prolonged *ee*.

6. Put spoon in mouth, rim up. Ask child to shut teeth over handle and to produce the *sh* sound.

7. If child can say "measure" have him whisper it and prolong the sound.

8. If child can make the *ch* sound, have him "let it leak out," prolonging it rather than releasing it suddenly.

9. During the production of an *s* sound, pull tongue one-half inch toward the back of the mouth.

F and V

Tell the child that today he is to have his first chance to make the new sound. Then say, "Now watch me. See how I bite my lower lip. Can you bite your lip in the same way? Now let's look at ourselves in this mirror. Don't bite hard, just lay the teeth on the lower lip. See how I do it? Now let's hold our mouths like that and suck in some air. All right. Now, don't move your mouth but blow some air out, like this, *f-f-f-* [give strong stimulation]. Now do it again and make this sound in a whisper *fuh, fffuh, fffuh.*" Give child a little rest then some new trials. Then have him say *fuh* whenever you raise a finger. Spend some time talking about the new and old sounds, showing him how they differ. Tell him that the new sound may feel wrong but that it "sounds" right, and that he must *listen* rather than feel.

1. Ask child to hold lower lip against upper teeth, with a finger laid crosswise, then to blow.

2. Ask child to smile broadly as he tries the sound.

3. Have child bite far down beyond the upper lip (toward the chin) as he blows.

4. By holding a feather against the mouth, show child that *p* is a puff of air while *f* or *v* is a gradual stream of air.

R Sound

1. Ask child to say *l*. Then with the depressor gently push the tip of the tongue back until you can insert the depressor between the tip and teeth ridge or until *r* sound results.

2. If this fails and the child can say *z*, ask him to make the sound and continue it while the jaw is dropped until the teeth are separated about one inch or until *r* results.

3. Have the child imitate you as you trill the tonguetip. Then use this trill to precede the vowel *ēē*.

4. Spread the sides of the child's mouth with your fingers; ask him to produce a prolonged *n* sound, then to curl the end of his tongue backward as he continues making the sound.

CH (tʃ) Sound

1. If child is able to make the *t* sound and the *sh* sound separately, these sounds can be combined to make a good *ch*. The *ch* sound is a combination of these two sounds. Have the child form his teeth and tongue as for the *t* sound, and then say the *sh* sound instead. You might also have him say *she* by first forming the *t*.

2. Tell the child to pretend to sneeze. Often a child who cannot follow instructions about tongue and lip formation will make a perfect *ch* sound this way. Playing train, and saying *ch-ch-ch* like an engine may work, too.

3. Have the child prolong *sh* as though to tell someone to be quiet. When you signal by clapping or raising a finger from the table, have him quickly touch the gum of the roof of his mouth, and then go right on with *sh*. This will produce a prolonged *sh* with a *ch* in the middle.

Key Word Method.   As we have seen, one of the items in both the voice and articulation tests requires the examiner to record all words in which the usually defective sound is made correctly. Many teachers of speech correction fail to realize the value of these words in remedial work. They may be used to enable the student to make the correct sound at will and in isolation. They are also extremely valuable in getting the student to make clean-cut transitions between the isolated sound and the rest of the word. Finally, they serve as standards of correctness of sound performance. Speech defectives need some standard with which to compare their speech attempts at correct production of the usually defective sound. Although occasional cases are found who never make the sound correctly, the majority of speech defectives have a few words in which they do not make the error. The teacher should be alert enough to catch these when they do occur. Often these words are those which have the usually defective sound in an inconspicuous place—that is to say, the sound occurs in the medial or final position, or is incorporated within a blend; seldom is it found in an accented syllable. The teacher must train her ear to listen for it in the student's speech or it will escape her. At times it occurs in words in which an unusual spelling provides a different symbol for the sound. To illustrate: A child who was unable to make a good *f* in any of his words using that printed symbol, said the word *rough* with a perfect *f* sound. This was probably due to the strong stimulation given by the child's spelling teacher.

These words are worth the trouble needed to discover them, for they simplify the teacher's work tremendously, since it is possible to use that sound as a standard and guide and to work from it to other words in which error normally occurs. The experienced teacher greets these nuclei words as veritable nuggets. Similarly, even when the student is highly consistent in his errors, there comes a stage in his treatment when he is saying a few words correctly. These words may be used to serve the same ends as those mentioned in the preceding paragraph.

The procedure used in this method is roughly as follows: The teacher writes the word on one of several cards (or uses a picture representing it). Then she asks the student to go through the series one at a time, saying the word on each card ten times. Finally, the special word to be used is repeated a hundred times, accenting, and prolonging if possible, the sound which in other words is made incorrectly. Thus the lingual lisper who could say *lips* correctly repeated the word one hundred times, prolonging the *s*. He was then asked to hold it for a count of twenty, then thirty, then forty. Finally, he was required to hold it intermittently, thus; *lipssss.ssss..sss*. The purpose of such a gradual approach is that the sound must be emphasized in both its auditory and its motor characteristics to prevent its loss when the student becomes aware of it as his hard sound. For example, one baby-talker made the initial *r* in *rabbit* perfectly until told that he did. Immediately the child changed to the *w* substitution and was unable to make the initial *r* again.

After the child has emphasized the sound a large number of times, has listened to it and felt it thoroughly, and can make it intermittently and in a repetitive form, he may be asked to think the word and to speak the sound. It is often wise to underline the sound to be spoken, asking the student to whisper all but the letter underlined. Other sounds and other words may be similarly underlined if a careful approach is necessary. Through these means, the child finally can make the sound in isolation and at will.

Stabilizing the New Sound.   One of the greatest causes for discouragement in treating an articulatory case may be traced to the parent's or teacher's ignorance of a very important fact. A new sound is weak and unstable. Its mechanics are easily forgotten or lost. Its dual phases of auditory and motor sensation patterns are easily confused. Many people believe that a complicated skill (such as that involved in a speech sound) once achieved is never lost, although any musician or tennis player will tell us that a new stroke or fingering sequence must be practiced and strengthened a great deal before it can be used in competition or concert. Many speech-correction teachers become discouraged and blame the speech defective for his frequent relapse into error or his sudden loss of the sound he had been taught to make. Many children who can make the correct sound at will never learn to incorporate it within familiar words. All of these unfortunate occurrences are due to the fact that a new sound must be strengthened before it can win the competition with the error in the speaking of common words. A lisper who has said "yeth" for "yes" several thousand times cannot be expected to say the latter as soon as he has learned to make the *sss* sound in isolation. Perhaps that sound has been performed only three or four times. Yet parents and teachers constantly ruin all of their preliminary work by saying some such sentence as this: "Fine, Johnny. That was fine! You said *sss* just as plainly as anyone. Now say 'sssoup.' " And Johnny, ninety-nine times out of one hundred, will say triumphantly, "thoup." Most speech correctionists have to train themselves to resist this urge to hurry. When the child has been taught to make the new sound, the utmost patience and restraint are needed.

When a new sound has just been born, it is a tender thing and must be carefully treated. It should be repeated or prolonged as soon as possible but there should be no great hullabaloo over the achievement or it may be lost again.

During this repetition and prolongation, the student should be told to keep a poker face and to move as little as possible. A sudden shift of body position occasionally produces a change in the movements of articulation as well. As soon as the new sound tends to lose

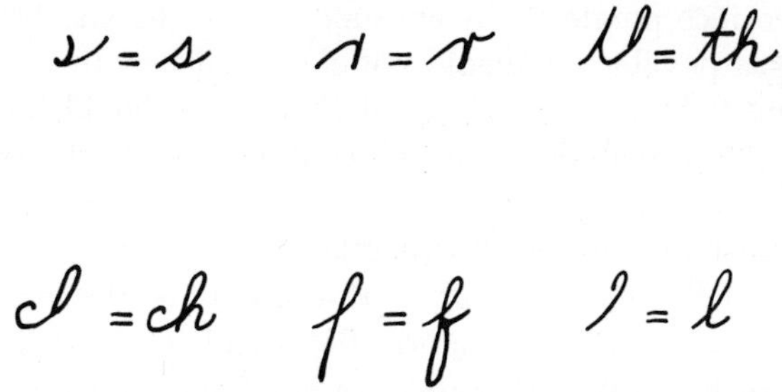

FIGURE 24. *Nonsense Symbols*

its clear characteristics, the teacher should insist upon some rest and should then review the procedure used to produce the sound. Rest should be silent in order to let maturation take place. Little intensity should be used, and when working with a pair of sounds, such as *s* and *z*, the unvoiced sound is preferable. Often sounds such as *l* and *r* should be whispered or sung.

After the speech defective is able to produce the sound readily and can repeat and prolong it consistently, the teacher can ask him to increase its intensity and exaggerate it. He should be asked to focus his attention on the "feel" of the tongue, lips, and palate. Shutting his eyes will help him to get a better awareness of the tactual and kinesthetic sensations thereby produced. Ask him to assume the position without speech attempt and, after a short period of "feeling," to try the sound. Many other supplementary devices will occur to the teacher.

After the student reaches the stage where he has little difficulty in producing the new sound, he should be encouraged to shorten the time needed to produce it. A sound which the student takes too long to produce will never become habitual. This speeding up of the time needed to initiate it may be accomplished by demanding fast repetitions, by alternating it with other isolated speech sounds, and by using signals. In this last activity, the student should keep his articulatory apparatus in a state of rest or in certain other positions, such as an open mouth, and then, at a certain sharp-sound signal, he should react by producing the new sound immediately.

One of the most effective methods for strengthening a new sound is to include it in babbling. The babbling should be initiated in the manner described in the preceding section, and the student should attempt to incorporate the new sound within the vocal flow as effortlessly as possible. It should not stand out and there should be no pausing before it. Doublings of the sound should be frequent. These babbling periods should be continued daily throughout the course of treatment.

The most important of all strengthening devices is the use of simultaneous talking-and-writing. In this procedure, the student writes the script symbol as he pronounces the sound. The sound should be timed so that it will neither precede nor follow the writing of the symbol, but will coincide exactly with the dominant stroke of the letter. Since this dominant stroke varies somewhat with different persons, some experimentation will be needed. At first the teacher should supervise this talking-and-writing very carefully to ensure clear vocalization of the new sound and proper timing. Later the student can be assigned to hand in several pages of this talking-and-writing every day. The continuant sounds should be pronounced by themselves (*sss, vvv, lll, mmm*), and the stops should use a lightly vocalized neutral vowel (*kuh, puh, duh*). Simultaneous talking-and-writing techniques not only provide an excellent vehicle for practice of the new sound, but also give a means of reinforcing it by enriching the motor aspect of the performance. They also improve the identification, and, as we shall see, make possible an effective transition to familiar words. For children who cannot write, the sound may be tied up with a movement such as a finger twitch or foot tap. In this case, as in writing, the timing is very important.

Articulation Therapy at the Syllable Level

As soon as the person has learned to produce the new sound in isolation whenever he tries to do so, we move immediately to get him to use it in syllables. You will recall that the second operational level is that of syllabic utterance in the sequence: isolated sound, syllable, word, and sentence.

Beginning with the Syllable. Some speech therapists prefer to start with this syllabic level—to teach *ree* and *ra* and *roo* rather than *rrr*, because they feel that the syllable is the basic unit of motor speech. They also point out that many sounds such as the plosives *k* and *g* can only be produced syllabically and that prolonging an isolated sound distorts its pattern in time and creates unnecessary difficulty in shifting from sounds into syllables and then into words. Why not begin immediately with the syllable and teach *la-lee-lie-lay-lo-loo* instead of the isolated *llll* sound? We will not argue the point with any real vigor for we have often begun therapy with the syllable in certain cases where the person seemed to produce the sound more easily therein than in isolation. For example, we have known several children who could produce the *l* sound more easily in a syllable such as *lee* than they could in saying the isolated *llll*.* However, since we begin with acoustic ear training rather than with the motor aspect of speech, the basic unit of auditory perception is not the syllable but the phoneme, the sound. It provides one target rather than several. It transfers easily to many syllables once it is mastered in isolation so that there is no need to teach each syllable in turn. Moreover, when we have begun with the syllable, we notice that unconsciously we kept prolonging and stressing the sound anyway. It is the sound, not the syllable, which is our first target's bull's-eye.

However, when therapy begins with the syllable, the therapist follows the same basic sequence we have outlined for the isolated sound. The standard acoustic and motor patterns of the various syllables as they occur in the speech of others are defined through ear training. Next, self-hearing of the person's own syllable production is scanned and compared with the features of the correct syllable to define the syllabic errors. Next, the same techniques of progressive

---

* These two sounds, however, are not identical. The *l* sound at the beginning of a syllable is more fricative and less vocalic than one used in isolation or at the end of a syllable such as *ol*.

approximation, auditory stimulation, and phonetic placement are used to teach the isolated syllables. The process is the same; it is the target that differs initially. Moreover, once we have trained the person to make the new sound in syllables, we usually return to the isolated sounds, pointing them out within the syllable, so that the person comes to recognize the correction he has made.

Strengthening and Stabilizing the New Sound in Nonsense Syllables. Whether we begin with the syllable or the sound, our next major step in therapy is to help our case to use the new sound in all phonetic contexts. This is very important since any sound changes slightly whenever it is preceded or followed by other sounds. The *s* in the nonsense syllable *seeb*, for example, is acoustically higher in pitch than the *s* in *soob*. Also the contour of the tongue varies a bit with differing phonetic contexts. Since we must be able to produce the new sound in all possible combinations, we must have some means of teaching these variations. The nonsense syllable provides us with such a vehicle.

Types of Nonsense Syllables.   There are three main types of nonsense syllables: CV (consonant-vowel syllables such as *la*), VC (vowel-consonant syllables such as *al*), and CVC (consonant-vowel-consonant combinations such as *kal* or *lod.*) These syllables can be readily constructed by combining the new sound with the fourteen most common vowels and diphthongs. The first nonsense syllables to be practiced are those in which the transitional movements from consonant to vowel involve the fewest and simplest coordinations. For example, *ko* involves less radical transitional movements than does *kee*. The next nonsense syllables should be those which use the new sound in the final position (*ok*), and, finally, those in which the new sound is located in the medial position (*oko*) should be practiced. Double nonsense syllables may also be used, but simple doublings are preferred (*kaka*).

These nonsense syllables should be practiced thoroughly before familiar words are attempted. The talking-and-writing technique can be used to facilitate their production if any difficulty is experienced. The student should speak the new sound as he writes the symbol until he gets to the end of the line, then should add the vowel, thus: *s s s s s s saaa*. Signal practice, such as that described later in this section, can also be used to form the nonsense syllable if it is needed. Generally, however, a simple request by the teacher to repeat the nonsense syllable he pronounces will produce the desired results. This repetition from a model is the usual way in which the syllables are used. They may also be written by the teacher and read by the student. They may be used to precede each sentence of conversation or used as substitutes for such words as *the* or *and*. Lists of them may be used for practice, and all the various vowel combinations should be employed. The student should practice them finally at high speeds.

Although most young children have no difficulty in using the standard letter symbol for the sound in these nonsense syllables or talking-and-writing, many adults and some young children who have read and written the letter while pronouncing it incorrectly will have difficulty. The letter *s*, for example, means *th* to such a lisper, and he cannot use the usual syllables in talking-and-writing. For these cases, it is wise to use a nonsense symbol in place of the standard letter. In general, the symbols should be parts of the standard symbols, though the student should not realize this fact until later. These symbols should be used for identification techniques and for all strengthening techniques. After the student has finally begun to use them in regular words, he may be shown that the nonsense symbol is really a part of the true symbol for the sound.

Nonsense Words. The big advantage of using nonsense syllables rather than words is that no unlearning is needed. Were we to use familiar words for this stabilizing, we would immediately find trouble because of the competition of the old error. A child who has said *thoup* for *soup* all his life will find it easier to say the nonsense syllable *soub* than *soup*. Moreover, by giving meanings to nonsense syllables or combining them to form nonsense words we can facilitate transfer to communication and the other functions of speech. The fingers and toes may be given nonsense names. The doorknob may be christened. The teacher can make nonsense objects out of modeling clay, giving them names which include the new sound. Nonsense pictures may be drawn and named. Card games using these nonsense pictures seem to be peculiarly fascinating to almost all cases. Through talking-and-writing techniques, repetition from a model, reading, conversation, questioning, and speech games, these nonsense names can be used repeatedly. The various sound combinations are thereby practiced, and remarkable progress will soon occur. Examples of some of the nonsense pictures are given in Figure 25.

Once we have given meanings to nonsense words, we can im-

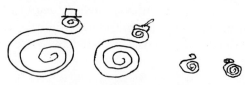

FIGURE 25. *The Sooba Family*

mediately begin to use them in the various functions of speech. The child can command us to put the *sooba* in the basket. We can ask him how many red *soobas* are in the box. He can even vent his hostility by calling us a dirty low down *poos*. Children enjoy these activities and they are much more effective than drill.

Articulation Therapy at the Word Level

We are now ready to move onward to our third operational level —the word level. The new sound has now been sufficiently strengthened so that it has a fair chance to hold its own in competition with the error if we can make sure that the odds are in its favor. We must remember that the articulation case has used his old error in meaningful words thousands of times and that it would be unreasonable to expect him suddenly to be able to speak them correctly. We therefore need new techniques to insure the successful incorporation of the newly-acquired sound into his words.

Beginning Therapy at the Word Level. There are times when we even begin our therapy at the word level. We have already discussed how we use key words to provide in-the-mouth samples of the correct sound and we have emphasized the point that inconsistency of error is much more common than we realize until we do some deep testing. These observations indicate that it might be possible to start therapy immediately by teaching correctly spoken *words* instead of isolated sounds or nonsense syllables. Indeed, most children seem to acquire correct articulation from this type of teaching. This is how parents normally teach a child to speak correctly. The fact that his method has failed with this particular person may not mean that the approach is all wrong but perhaps merely that it was not correctly administered. Although we have already stated our preference for beginning with the isolated sound for the majority of our cases, we are not prejudiced against using any approach which might be more useful with a particular case. We have taught many children to achieve correct articulation by starting at the word level.

Suitability of the Word-level Approach. Which persons seem especially suited to this approach? First, we have those who already possess many key words when they come to us; second, we have those cases who find phonetic analysis—the breaking up of word wholes into syllables and sounds—especially difficult; third, we have those children whose multiple and variable errors make their speech almost unintelligible, and lastly, we meet those who very badly need some immediate and concrete evidence that they can indeed say something right. Some children fit all four of these criteria and they certainly seem to do better when we start at the word level.

The Key Word as a Nucleus. We suspect that the failure of the traditional parental method of teaching a child words instead of sounds is due primarily to their use of too many words with too many different sounds as stimuli. When the speech therapist begins with the word level approach, she concentrates on teaching only a *few* important words, all of which contain the *same* desired sound. Parents, on the other hand, demand correction of many words containing many different errors. This confuses the child and he gives up trying to conform. The speech therapist tries to create nuclei of standard words and to insert them into the main functions of speech. We try to implant little colonies of these key words within messages, commands, emotional expressions, and even in thinking. Once planted and tended, these nuclei can attract other phonetically similar words. It is vitally important that the child *know* that these key words are ones that he can speak correctly and without error, that when he says these, he is speaking just as well as any other person, big or little. These are his yardsticks. These are his mouth models of correct utterance. He must know that when he says "Yes" he is not lisping. Only those of us who have worked long in the vineyard with discouraged children can realize how important it is that such a child can come to be completely certain that he can say at least a few words perfectly. Once he has such a nucleus, he can start a collection.

Creating Key Words. How do we get these key words? Some of them we can find, as we have said, by deep testing, by searching through the child's spoken vocabulary, by checking the lists of assimilation words we can assemble, by varying the conditions of communication. Others we must create out of the sounds and syllables which compose them, using the isolated-sound or nonsense-syllable approaches. Thus, we see that no matter where we begin, we find ourselves sooner or later at the point where we must operate on the word level, creating and collecting key words to serve as nuclei for correct utterance. With most children we find it best to begin with the isolated sound, then move into the syllable and then into key words; with some children, we start with the syllable and move into key words; with a few special children we start with the key words themselves.

Creating Key Words from Sounds and Syllables. We have two main techniques for creating key words once the child has mastered the sound in isolation and in the nonsense syllable: reconfiguration training and signaling.

Reconfiguration Techniques. Frequently the reconfiguration tech-

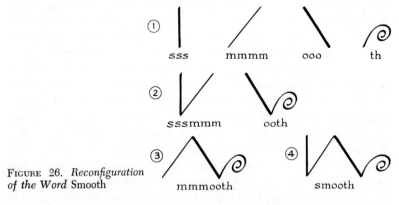

FIGURE 26. *Reconfiguration of the Word* Smooth

niques must be carried out rather gradually. Their purpose is to teach the individual that words are made up of sound sequences and that these sound sequences can be modified without losing the unity of the word. If, for convenience, we use a lingual lisper as our example, the reconfiguration techniques would follow somewhat the same sequence: (1) The student reads, narrates, and converses with the teacher, substituting the sound of *b* for that of *f* whenever the latter occurs in the initial position. He reads, for example, that "Sammy caught a bish with his hook and line." The purpose of using these non-error sounds is to make a gradual approach. (2) The student substitutes his new sound for other sounds, but not for the error. Thus: "Sammy sssaught a fish with his hook and line." (3) The student substitutes another sound for the *s* in the same material. Thus: "Bammy caught a fish with his hook and line." (4) The student omits the *s* in all words beginning with it. Thus: "—ammy caught a fish with his hook and line." (5) The student "substitutes" his new sound for the *s*. Thus: "Ssssammy caught a fish with his hook and line." Many similar techniques are easily invented. It may seem to the young speech correctionist that such techniques are far too laborious and detailed. But, after he has met with persistent error in his articulatory cases, he will appreciate the fact that careful and thorough training will produce a thoroughgoing and permanent freedom from error. Sketchy and slipshod training will enable a speech defective to make the correct sound and perhaps to use it in a few words when he watches himself carefully, but this is far from the goal that should be set. Too many speech-correction teachers have blamed the student for failure when they should have blamed themselves.

Another group of reconfiguration techniques requires the use of writing or drawing simultaneously with the utterance. For children who can read and write, these techniques are often very useful.

Simultaneous Talking-and-writing. The simultaneous talking-and-writing techniques previously described will be invaluable if used properly. The student should talk-and-write the symbol alone for one line, and then, on the next line, talk-and-write the first letter, the first syllable, and, finally, the whole word. Thus: *s s s s s s s s s; s si sick s si sick*, and so on. Later he can alternate the symbol and the word, and finally he can write only the symbol as he says the word. Assignments can be given for home practice. Frequently such a gradual approach is not necessary, and the student need write only the symbol and say any *s* word.

We also ask our cases to draw on paper or trace in the air various figures such as that shown in Figure 26. The case is trained to associate certain sounds with certain parts of the figures and then to trace continuously through the whole figure, thus producing a word.

Signaling Techniques. This group of activities uses preparatory sets to integrate the sound or syllable into the word. Signaling can generate many key words. In this, the student prolongs or repeats the new sound and then, at a given signal, instantly says the pre-arranged vowel or the rest of the word. The student should be given a preparatory set to pronounce the rest of the word by preliminary signal practice. During this practice he waits with his eyes closed until he hears the sound signal which sets off the response. Thus, during the student's prolongation of *sssssss*, the instructor suddenly raps on the table, and the syllable *oup* is automatically produced. With a preparatory set, the response is largely automatic and involuntary, and thus the new sound is integrated within the word as a whole. Often it is wise to require the student to say the word twice. Thus: *sssssss*(rap)*oupsoup*. Signal practice can also be used with repetition. Thus: *kuh-kuh-*(rap)*atkat*. After some training with this type of signal practice, the student may use other signals, such as those provided by the timing of a rhythm. Thus: *s-s, s-s-soup* or *s-s-soup, s-s-soup*. The student may also be required to repeat over and over some nonsense syllable which he can make well, suddenly saying the new word when the signal is given. Thus: *ssi-ssi-ssi-ssi*(tap)*ssip*. The nonsense syllable and the new word may also be used alternately. The isolated sound may be used in the above exercises in place of the nonsense syllable. Various other combinations may easily be invented.

Difficulties in Forming Key Words from Isolated Sounds or Syllables. At times difficulty will be experienced in making the transitions into the words. The student will say *rwabbit* and be confident that he has pronounced the word correctly. The error must be brought to his attention by the teacher's imitation and by the student's voluntary production of the error. Signal practice will help a great deal to eliminate this error.

Another invaluable technique is provided by a signal used in a slightly different way. The student is asked to form his mouth for the vowel which begins the rest of the word; i.e., for the vowel *a* in *rabbit*. He may whisper a prolongation of this vowel. Then, at a given signal, he is to say *rabbit* as swiftly as possible. This preformation of the vowel will often solve the problem. Similarly, the practice of pairs of words, the first ending in the vowel of the second, will be effective. Using pairs of words in which the first word ends with the new sound and the second begins with the same sound is occasionally useful, although the student should be cautioned to keep out all breaks in continuity.

Still another method of eliminating this error is to use some nonsense symbol to represent the part of the word which follows the new sound. Thus, one individual was asked to say *oup* every time he wrote a question mark (?), and after ten minutes of this, he was told to read the following symbols, *t?*, *kr?*, and *s?*. The last symbol was pronounced *soup* rather than *sthoup*, and no further difficulty was experienced.

Creating Key Words Directly. When we decide to forego the isolated sound or syllable approaches and to begin immediately by teaching key words, we use the same basic methods described for the other approaches. We must make sure through ear training that the person comes to realize how the *word* sounds when uttered by the therapist. He must also be made to *scan* his own utterance of the word and to *compare* it with that of the therapist. Finally he must be taught to *vary* his attempts until the correct word is uttered. All the methods used for teaching the isolated sound or syllable can be used also for the word as a whole. Here is an excerpt from an ear-training session in which the therapist is operating at the word level:

> *The child and therapist are seated at a table. There are a number of little plastic objects on the table and two glass jars, one full of water and one empty.*
> Child: Put the kitty in the water. (*Therapist does so.*)
> Child: Put the baby in the water.
> Therapist: OK. Baby have bath.
> Child: No, baby drown. All dead.
> Therapist: OK. Baby dead now.
> Child: Take baby out the water. (*Therapist does so.*)
> Child: Baby OK now. You thpank baby bottom. Baby naughty.
> Therapist: If you ask me to ssspank her I will, but you didn't. You asked me to thpank her. What's that? (*She holds baby up high.*)
> Child (*reaching*): Thpank her! Thpank her! Thpank her! (*Slaps hand hard on table.*)
> Therapist: Thpank her? . . . Oh, you mean . . . sspank her? (*Child nods.*) OK. Here goes. (*Therapist spanks baby.*)

Now let us see how we would continue, but using the word level for the therapeutic process of establishing the standard pattern for two key words.

> Therapist: No, that's no penthil.
> Child: It ith too a penthil.
> Therapist: Nope, you said it wrong. You said "penthil" . . . th . . . penth . . . penthil. That's not the same as sss, pensss, pencil. Look, here's a penthil. (*Therapist takes out of the desk a pipe cleaner with two knots and a bolt on it.*)
> OK, this is your "penthil." Look, it sssinks. The pencil swims.
> Child: Oh.
> Therapist: Shut your eyes again. I'm going to put the penthil (listen now, I said *penthil*, not *pencil*) I'm going to put the penthil in the water. Can you tell me if it swims?
> Child: No. It thinks.
> Therapist: You're right. It isn't swimming. But you didn't say sssssssinks right. It's *sss, sssih, sssinksss*, not *thinks*, but *sssinkss*. You can't peek until you can guess whether I'm saying it right or wrong. OK. Here we go: Which is right, the first or second: The *penthil thinks,* or the *penthil sinks.*
> Child: The penthil sssssssinks. . . .
> Therapist: And the pencil . . .
> Child: Sssssswims.

Not all children make such rapid progress.

We have already indicated in our play-by-play description of this interchange between therapist and child that it is possible to use several operational levels in the same activity. In these stimulation, identification, and discrimination activities, the focus of therapy has been at one time on the sentence, at another on the word, on the syllable, and even on the isolated sound. Sometimes, as our illustration suggests, the child needs little help in producing the correct sound or in incorporating it into words, sentences, and functional speech. A child who gets the words *pencil, swim,* and *sink* in this five-minute period can be taught to use them immediately in commentary, communication, and control, and he should be given opportunity to do so in the interests of stabilization. Here is how it was done in the situation described above.

> Therapist: OK. I'll close my eyes, and see if I can guess which one you'll pick up and play with.
> Child: I'll pick one up.
> Therapist: I bet it's a penthil.

Child: No, it a pensssssil.
Therapist: Is it the yellow one?
Child: Yeth.
Therapist: What are you going to do with it?
Child: I going put it in water.
Therapist: What's it doing now?
Child: It thwims.
Therapist: Thwims? What's that?
Child: It sssssssswims. You want to look?
Therapist: Good for you. That's right. It's the pencil, not the penthil

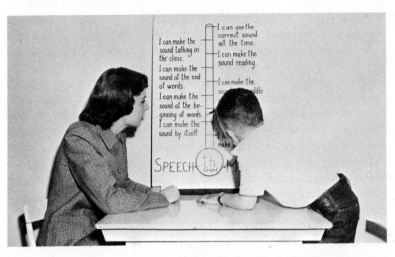

FIGURE 27. *Checking Progress*

and it's swimming all right. Now you be the teacher and boss me
around with the pencil and the penthil. Tell me what to do.
Child: Put penthil in mouth. (*Therapist does so with pipe-cleaner.*)
Child: Put pencil in water. (*Therapist does so.*)
Child: Give penthil a bath. (*Therapist puts pipe-cleaner in water.*)
Therapist: Which one do you think will get dry the faster?
Child: The pencil.
Therapist: How many penthils have I in my desk drawer here? (*Child
looks.*)
Child: *FF* . . . no, no. You got none. But four pensssils. I almost for-
got. SSS. Pencil!
Therapist: Finish this sentence: I can write with a . . .
Child: Write with a pencil.
Therapist: The only one that sinks is the . . .
Child: It's the penthil.

Therapist: The penthil is heavier than the . . .
Child: Pencil.

Articulation Therapy at the Sentence Level

Once we have taught our case a group of key words which contain the new sound in the initial, medial, and final positions, and he can now correct his misarticulations when he is being careful, we move on to the next operational level: the sentence. Again, we find here some new techniques, but before we describe them, let us tell how sometimes we begin our therapy, not at the sound, syllable, or word levels, but immediately at the sentence level.

Beginning at the Sentence Level. When we *begin* therapy at the sentence level we do so primarily to provide motivation and hope for those who have never felt they could talk normally. Usually, this sentence-level therapy is carried out only after the child has mastered the new sound in isolation, nonsense syllables, and key words. However, careful exploration sometimes reveals not only key words but key sentences, or rather key utterances, in which the usually defective sound is always spoken correctly. A child with whom we worked recently and who could not make a *th* sound in isolation, syllable, or word, was able immediately to say "Shut *the* door!" as a command. He could not say the word "the" or the sound of *th* or the nonsense syllable *shuthoo*. We found that by using other commands of a similar nature: "Shut the window," "Shut that box," in slow motion and echoed speech we could procure a nucleus of correct utterance from which we could isolate the words, sounds, and syllables and still have them articulated correctly. Most speech therapists, if they *begin* treatment at the sentence level, do so for two reasons: to convince the child immediately that the correct production of the target sound is not as difficult as he had believed, and secondly, to help him analyze the correctly spoken sentences to locate the target sounds, syllables, or words which he must use in the rest of his speech.

Thus with the lisper who can say "Oh, you're nuts!" perfectly, we want him to scrutinize this sentence-level expression of emotion to know that the final *s* sound of the last word was said as well as any other person on earth could say it; that he has said the syllable *uts* and the word *nuts* perfectly, and most important of all, that the whole insulting utterance was spoken without error. We pair these key sentences with other sentences in which errors exist and ask the case to scan them when we say them right or when we say them wrong, and to scan them again when he speaks them. Thus we locate the error and target the correct standard pattern.

Creating Key Sentences. As we have said, some of these correctly spoken sentences can be discovered by careful exploration and deep testing. It is also possible to create them, not only synthetically by incorporating sounds into syllables and syllables into words and words into key sentences, but as sentence wholes. We have several techniques for doing this: slow motion speech, echo speech or shadowing, unison speaking, cumulative speaking, and the corrective set. Each of these attempts to teach sentences as wholes.

Slow Motion Speech. In this technique the therapist and child say the error sentences in unison, but in extreme slow motion. For example: "Iiiiiz-thththththe-pennnnnsssssilll-wwwet?" The therapist should precede this with other slow-motion behavior such as walking, arm lifting, head scratching. She sets the tempo and the child follows her slowly shifting model. Often it is important that the therapist sit behind the child with her mouth slightly above his head so as to make the two sound fields similar, and so, by putting her mouth close to the child's ear for the difficult sounds or words, he can be stimulated more vividly.

Echo Speech. There are two forms of this. In the first, *shadowing,* the child tries to repeat instantly and automatically what the therapist is saying, word by word. The child's utterance should follow immediately on the heels of the therapist. For example:

Therapist: Let's play an echo game today. Try to say what I say just as soon as I say it. Don't wait. Say each word just as soon as it comes out of my mouth. Ready?
Child: OK.
Therapist: One.
Child: One.
Therapist: Two . . . seven . . .
Child: . . . Two . . . seven . . .
Therapist: Quicker, say it quicker.
Child: Quicker . . . Oh, I thee. You mean right away.
Therapist: Yes.
Child: Yes.
Therapist: I'm . . . going . . . to show . . . you . . . a picture.
Child: . . . I'm . . . going . . . to show . . . you . . . a picture.

Therapist: Good!
Child: Good!
Therapist: The dog is chasing . . . the cat.
Child: . . . The dog is chasing . . . the cat.
Therapist: Good! You said chasing, not chathing.
Child: Good! You said chasing, not chathing.

This shadowing, or echo speech, seems to be more easily learned by children than adults and it is curious to find how faithfully they can do it. Once he has learned how to shadow automatically (almost as in echolalia) the child's voice follows not only the words but also the inflections with surprising fidelity.

In the second form of echo speaking, which they have called "long-echo talk," the child repeats not single words but a *series* of words or phrases or sentences after the therapist when she pauses and signals for him to catch up and give back the echo. This should be done with a gestural or postural or behavioral accompaniment which the child must also duplicate as closely as possible. For example:

Therapist: All right, now we're going to play follow the leader, and I'll be the leader this time. You do what I do and say what I say, but wait till I stop before following me. Do and say just exactly what I do and say. If I sing, you sing. If I stand up while talking, that's what you have to do. If I scratch my nose, you've got to do so too. Ready?
Child: OK.
Therapist (*begins to shiver*): On a coooold winter night . . . (*signals*)
Child (*shivering*): On a cooooold winter night . . .
Therapist: a little boy (*therapist huddles in a crouch and signals*)
Child (*squats*): a little boy . . .
Therapist (*puts hands over face*): had a bad dream. . . .
Child (*covering face*): had a bad deem. . . .
Therapist: He thought he was out in the sssssssssssssssnow. (*Therapist claps hands on each word of this except for* snow. *On the prolonged* s *she pretends to pull a string of sound out from between her closed teeth and winds it around her ear.*)
Child (*does the same action*): He thought he was out in the ssssssssnow.
Therapist (*sings*): And he sssssssaid, "I'm cooooooooooooooold as aissssssssss." (*ice*)
Child (*sings*): And he sssaid, "I'm coooold as ice."
Therapist (*laughs*): He didn't have any covers on his bed.
Child (*laughs*): An' he waked up.

In both types of echo speech it is important that the child try to follow the therapist as automatically as possible. Children who have never produced standard sounds or who cannot seem able to do so under direct stimulation in their speech seem able to make them easily when doing this automatic kind of echo speaking. We also teach them to echo themselves.

Unison Speech. In this the child and therapist speak some previously formulated utterances together. It is important that again the child follow the therapist's movements, speech tempo, pitch, and intensity patterns. For this purpose, each utterance is spoken several times. Often the therapist cups her hands and directs her voice into one of the child's ears while the child listens with the other ear to his mouth with cupped hands, a speech shoe, or auditory training unit. This binaural listening permits a simultaneous comparison of correct and incorrect forms. Hand tapping signals are used to time the moment of attempt and to insure unison speaking. Often, as the same utterance is spoken each time, it is wise to have the child accompany it with a certain head or body movement, so that it can be stabilized thereby when the child must speak it alone. We also tape-record some of the child's own speech which is spoken without error and ask him to say it again in unison with himself. Here is an example of such unison speech, this time based upon self-expression or egocentric speech. (You will have to remember that the child's utterance will be spoken in unison with that of the therapist.)

Therapist: Now we're going to play a game in which we can grow up and be awfully big. You've got to say what I say at the same time I say it. And do what I do. We'll do and say everything at least twice, before we change. Ready?

Child: Uh-huh.

Therapist (*puts her head down by her knees*): Oh, I'm ssso ssssmall. (*Then whispers*) OK, when I touch you, say it with me, just like I do.

Child: OK.

Therapist (*in a tiny voice*): I'm ssso ssssmall. (*Touches child.*)

Child (*very softly*): I'm so ssmall.

Therapist: I'm so small, so ssmall.

Child: I'm so ssmall, so small.

Therapist (*rising up and stretching out arms*): I'm getting bigger. I'm getting bigger. (*She speaks in a low voice.*)

Child (*duplicates behavior*): I'm getting bigger, bigger too.

Therapist (*climbs up on chair and shouts*): I'm the king of the cassstle! I'm the king of the castle.

Child (*climbs up on his chair and yells*): I'm the king of the cassstle!

Therapist: No, *I'm* the king of the castle; *I'm* the king of the castle!

Child (*in unison*): *I'm* the king of the castle.

Therapist: And you're a dirty rassscal; and you're a dirty rascal; and you're a dirty . . .

Child (*chiming in*):   . . . rascal; and you're a dirty rassscal.

In this illustration, the first two sentences had previously been practiced in unison with the therapist, using a binaural auditory training unit. However, if error had occurred in the acting out, the sentences could have been then worked upon as unit utterances until they were spoken in standard fashion.

Cumulative Sentences. In this technique, the therapist has an opportunity to work on the sound or syllable or word within the sentence without losing the sentence-wholeness or gestalt. Essentially, it consists of having the child and therapist, working in unison or alternately in echo speech, build sentences and utterances word by word cumulatively. An example follows which is based on emotional expression.

Therapist: See these blocks. We're going to block-talk. I bet you never heard of that game, did you? Well, you and I must pile one block on top of another and say something at the same time, until it all falls down. I'll show you. We're going to talk about things we don't like.

Child: OK.

Therapist: You see, you have to say one word for each block, and start over again with each new block. OK. I'll start with *I* (*puts out a block*). . . . I don't (*puts another block on first one*) . . . I don't like . . . (*piles on third block*) . . . I don't like . . .

Child: Baby thithterth. I don't like baby thithterth.

Therapist: You mean baby sssssisterssss. OK, now you do it with me, and say it with me every time we put on a new block. You put on the blocks.

Both: I . . . (*one block*)

Both: I don't . . . (*two blocks*)

Both: I don't like . . . (*three blocks*)

Therapist: Now, let's just say "baby" this time.

Both: Baby . . . (*fourth block wobbles*) I don't like baby . . .

Therapist: Now remember, it's I don't like baby sssisssstersss, not I don't like baby thithterth.

(*Therapist says it very loudly in the child's left ear as they speak in unison.*)

Both: I don't like baby sisters. (*Fifth block teeters but holds precariously.*)

Therapist: Now let's say, "I don't like baby sisters very much."

Child: I don't like baby sssisters at all. (*Blocks come tumbling down as he smashes them.*)

The Corrective Set. We have also found that often a child with an articulation problem can be able to produce his usually defective sound correctly in a whole sentence when he is given a corrective set. The way we usually do this is by saying or doing many things in which our error is obvious and asking the child to correct us and to set us straight. We begin with mistakes which are so apparent that any person would be likely to recognize them. Once the child is thoroughly enjoying our stupidity and mistakes, we slip in some utterance containing his own common errors. Over and over again we have been surprised to find how easily he can show us how to say the sentence without error. Here is an example:

(*The teacher and child are seated at a table. The child lisps and has other defective sounds. The teacher has a bag with various articles in it.*)

Therapist: I'm going to say and do some things all wrong and I want you to show me and tell me how to do or say them right. Understand?

Child: Uh huh.

Therapist: See, here's a comb. I brush my teeth with a comb. (*Pretends to do so.*)

Child (*laughing*): No, No. You comb you heh.

Therapist: Show me. (*Child does so.*) Oh, I see, I comb my hair. (*Reaches into bag and pulls out a plastic spoon.*) See, here's a thpoon.

Child: Yeth.

Therapist: Oh ho! I fooled you that time. I said something wrong and you didn't catch me. I said *thpoon*, not sssspoon. O.K. Watch me fool you again.

Child: No, you can't.

Therapist (*points to her mouth*): I open my mouf.

Child (*scornfully*): You open your mouth, MOU*TH*! not mouf.

Therapist (*pretends to cry*): OK, you caught me that time. Oh look, here's a picture of a horth. See the big horth.

Child: No, no. Horsssssssssss! Not horth. Horssssssssey, and it is a little horse not a big one.

Role Playing. A most curious discovery to many speech therapists is that some children, when completely immersed in some other person's role, can speak almost perfectly the same sentences that they cannot possibly say without error in any other situation. We use fantasy, children's theater, and creative dramatics to establish these roles and much suggestion and coaching to make them vivid enough so that the child can throw himself completely into them. Identification must be very thorough. Here is a short illustration:

Therapist: All right, let's play bank robbers. Who am I?
Child: You the man at the bank. Thit there at the table. with the money.
Therapist: Where's the money?
Child: Here! (*Tears up some paper and gives it to the therapist.*) I'm going out and come in with gun.
Therapist: Don't shoot me when you come in.
Child: Oh hoh. I'll thcare you. You be thcared now when I come in.
Therapist: OK.
Child (*goes out, then enters with handkerchief over mouth and pencil in hand. Points it at therapist who pretends to be afraid*): Stick em up!
Therapist (*lifts two fingers*): Like this?
Child (*returning to his own role*): Naw. Look, when I thay "Stick em up" you've got to thtick em up like thith. (*Demonstrates.*)
Therapist: Oh I understand. Let's start again.
Child: Stick em up now!

Scanning, Comparing, Correcting at the Sentence Level. It is one thing to acquire the ability to use a new sound correctly in isolation, syllable, word, or sentence; it is another to be able to use it habitually and automatically. A person who has thought, commanded, sent messages, expressed himself in lisping speech for years needs special help in making the new unlisped speech habitual. Somehow we must build in this person a control system which will continuously scan the utterance, notice, and correct the errors automatically. No one can continually listen to the output of sound from his mouth. We need our ears to hear our thoughts and the thoughts of others. How can we automatize this corrective process? We have three main methods for doing so: (1) enlarging the therapy situation, (2) using the new sound in all types of speaking, (3) emphasizing proprioceptive feedback.

Enlarging the Therapy Situation. First of all, we must expand the therapy room to include the person's whole living space. He must be given experiences in scanning, comparing, and correcting in school, on the playground, on the job, and at home. Here are some of the ways we do this:

Speech Assignments. Some typical speech assignments to illustrate methods for getting the child to work on his errors in outside situations are:

(1) Go downstairs and ask the janitor for a dust rag. Be sure to say *rag* with a good long *rrr*. (2) Say the word *rabbit* to three other children without letting them know that you are working on your speech. (3) Ask your father if you said any word wrongly after you tell him what you did in school today.

The teacher should always make these assignments very definite and appropriate to the child's ability and environment. He should always ask for a report the next day. Such assignments frequently are the solution to any lack of motivation the child may have.

Checking Devices and Penalties. Checking devices and penalties are of great value when properly used. Typical checking devices are:

(1) Having child carry card and crayon during geography recitation, making a mark or writing the word whenever he makes an error. (2) Having some other child check errors in a similar fashion. (3) Having child transfer marbles from one pocket to another, one for each error. Many other devices may be invented, and they will bring the error to consciousness very rapidly.

Similarly, penalties are of great service, when used properly. It should be realized, however, that painful and highly emotional penalties should not be used, for they merely make the bad habit more pronounced and cause the child to hate his speech work. Penalties used in speech correction should be vivid and good natured. Typical penalties used with a ten-year-old lisper were: put pencil behind ear; step in wastebasket; pound pan; look between legs; close one eye; say *whoopee*. Let the child set his own penalties before he makes the speech attempt.

Nucleus Situations. Many parents and teachers make the mistake of correcting the child whenever he makes speech errors. It is unwise to set the speech standards too high. No one can watch himself all the time, and we all hate to be nagged. As a matter of fact, too much vigilance by the speech defective can produce such speech inhibitions that the speech work becomes thoroughly distasteful. Fluency disappears and the speech becomes very halting and unpleasant. Then, too, the very anxiety lest error occur, when carried to the extreme, seems to be able to increase the number of slips and mistakes themselves. Other errors sometimes appear.

Therefore, we recommend that the parents and teachers of the speech defective concentrate their reminding and correcting upon a few common words and upon certain nuclei speech situations. Use a certain chair as a good-speech chair. Whenever the child sits in it, he must watch himself. Have a certain person picked out who is to serve as the speech situation in which the child must use very careful speech. Use a certain speech situation, such as the dinner table, to serve as a nucleus of good speech, and, when errors occur in these nuclei situations, penalize them good naturedly but vividly. You will find that the speech vigilance and freedom from errors will spread rapidly to all other situations.

Finally, we recommend that, after a child has mastered a new sound and several words in which it occurs, he be required to say it occasionally in the wrong way. This is called negative practice, and it has no harmful effect. Indeed, it merely emphasizes the distinction between the correct and incorrect sounds.

Negative Practice. By negative practice we mean the deliberate and voluntary use of the incorrect sound or speech error. It may seem somewhat odd to advise speech defectives to practice their errors, for we have always assumed that practice makes perfection, and certainly we do not want the student to become more perfect in the use of his errors. Nevertheless, modern experimental psychology had demonstrated that when one seeks to break a habit that is rather unconscious (such as fingernail-biting or the substitution of *sh* for *s*), much more rapid progress is made if the possessor of the habit will occasionally (and at appropriate times) use the error deliberately. The reasons for this method are: (1) The greatest strength of such a habit lies in the fact that the possessor is not aware of it every time it occurs. All habit reactions tend to become more or less unconscious, and certainly those involved in speech are of this type; consciousness of the reaction must come before it can be eliminated. (2) Voluntary practice of the reaction makes it very vivid, thus increasing vigilance and contributing to the awareness of the cues that signal the approach of the reaction. (3) The voluntary practice of the error acts as a penalty.

The use of negative practice is so varied that it would be impossible to describe all the applications which can be made of it. Variations must be made to fit each type of disorder and each individual case. There are, however, certain general principles which may be said to govern all disorders and cases. Make the individual aware of the reasons for his use of the incorrect sound, for unintelligent use of the error is worthless. Never ask the student to use the error until he can produce the correct sound whenever asked to do so. Negative practice is a technique for getting the correct sound into the student's speech; it is used to make the correct sound habitual.

Set up the exact reproduction of the incorrect sound as a goal. The use of mirror observation, teacher imitation, and phonograph recording is invaluable. This is a learning process and does not come all at once. The teacher should confine all negative practice to the speech lesson until the student is able to duplicate the error consistently and fairly accurately. One should begin the use of this technique by asking the student to duplicate the error immediately after it has occurred. That is to say, the student should stop immediately after lisping on the word *soup* and attempt voluntarily to duplicate his performance.

Work constantly to make the negative practice serve the purpose of comparing the right and wrong sounds. It is often well to provide lists of words for the students to work with, speaking each of them in this sequence: correctly, incorrectly, correctly, correctly. Work first on individual sounds, then on words, then on certain words in sentences containing two words which begin with the difficult sound, one of which is to be said correctly and the other incorrectly. Have the student read material in which certain words are underlined for negative practice.

Make speech assignments for the student's use in outside situations. Examples are:

(1) Collect (write down on cards) ten words on which you have used negative practice. (2) Write down on a card two words on which you have used negative practice during each hour of the morning. (3) Write the first sentences of five phone calls, underlining the words on which you are going to use negative practice. (4) Collect,

during the day, twenty words which you have said wrongly and in which you have become aware of your error, have made a retrial and said them correctly, and then have made a second retrial using negative practice.

The preceding list of examples is merely indicatory of the type of assignments that may be used. It is vitally important that no assignment be made that does not call for an objective record of some kind. The teacher must ask for the card and discuss the fulfillment or nonfulfillment of the assignment. Assignment plus checkup will work wonders in the treatment of any speech defective. Vary the assignments to fit the case, and always make them purposeful, never a matter of routine or drill.

In concluding this section on articulatory disorders we wish to point out that in very few instances will it be necessary to spend more than five or ten minutes of individual work each day on any speech defective. Most of the work can be carried on in connection with the regular school activities, and so it should be, if the new habits are to be made permanent. Any teacher can see the possibilities for combining speech work with the language activities. In the names of the numbers themselves, arithmetic presents almost all of the speech sounds. Geography and science activities may be arranged so as to give the lisper recitations in which he is responsible for all new *s* words. Questions may be phrased so as to demand responses which involve the sound upon which error occurs. The teacher and student may have a secret signal for correction. The student should check all errors in a notebook. At times it is wise to post on the board a list of five words with which the student has trouble unless he watches himself. Occasionally, some other student may be asked to check on the speech defective's errors. Class recitations should be used not for teaching a new sound but for building up the strength of the new sound after the student can make it correctly.

Using the New Sound in All the Various Types of Speaking. In stabilizing and automatizing the new sound, we find it wise to provide systematic training which incorporates the new sound into real live message-sending, social control, thinking, emotional, and self-expressive types of speaking. Again we must make deliberate nucleic implants of good speech in all these various functions. First in the therapy room, and then in all the person's living space, we must

make sure that our case can use his new standard sounds in all the
kinds of talking he must do. When the lisper commands his dog, he
must say "Sit down!" When he responds affirmatively to a question
he must say "Yes!" When he must mentally add four and three, he
must think "seven," not "theven." In expressing his fear, he must say
"I'm scared" not "thcared." He must be able to use good sibilants
in his speech of self-display. Until certain correctly spoken sentences
are used automatically in each of these forms of speaking, we cannot
feel our task as a therapist is over.

   Emphasizing Proprioceptive Feedback. Proprioceptive feedback is
a term which refers to the perception of contacts and movements
and postures. If we place a finger on our lower lip, the felt contact
is proprioceptive; if we cock our head to the left or move a foot,
the sensations of posture and movement are proprioceptive. We
know what has happened without seeing or hearing. In much the
same way, we can know what is happening in our own speech even
when we cannot hear ourselves speaking. It is quite possible to talk
correctly in a boiler factory. We do not need self-hearing if our
proprioceptive senses are operating well.

   We believe that once a person has left babyhood, the most important automatic controls for monitoring articulation are proprioceptive. These controls see to it that we use the right movements,
the right postures, the correct contacts. We feel that when the baby
first learned to talk, self-hearing was most important. That was why
he babbled so much and did so much vocal play. But after he began
to use language and to understand the meanings of others, self-
hearing was given a less important role. Proprioception thus became
much more important, so important, indeed, that obvious errors
could persist for years without the person recognizing them audi-
torally. In articulation therapy, we must first reopen the self-hearing
circuits and put more energy into them so that these errors can be
distinguished. But we must not stop here. We must return to
proprioceptive controls if the child is to use the new sound automatically. No one can listen to himself constantly. The burden is too
great. Too many other functions interfere.

   Accordingly, in terminal therapy with the articulation case, we
teach him to use the new sound correctly by feel and touch alone.
We put masking noise in his ears so he cannot rely on self-hearing.
We ask him to speak correctly with his ears plugged. We ask him

to speak in a soft whisper and in pantomime. All these activities decrease the monitoring of speech by self-hearing and emphasize its proprioceptive control. We have found these techniques invaluable in automatizing the new sound.

Summary

In this chapter we have outlined various methods for helping a person to articulate correctly. Once we have eliminated or minimized whatever causes of the misarticulation still persist, we move immediately into a retraining program. This program consists essentially of a series of therapeutic experiences which help the person to define the standard pattern of the sound which the case utters defectively, to learn to scan and compare his own utterance with this standard, to vary his utterance and to correct it, and finally to stabilize the new sound. Four operational levels are defined: the isolated sound, the syllable, the word, and the sentence. Therapy may begin at any of these levels, but the entire sequence must be mastered. Different types of therapy are used at each level. The new sound must be incorporated into thinking, social control, message-sending, and emotional and self-expressive types of speaking in all situations. Proprioceptive monitoring and other procedures are used to make the newly acquired standard speech automatic.

PROJECTS

1. A child with a very protruding lower jaw and underbite substitutes the *p* for the *f* and the *b* for the *v* sounds. He can make the correct *f* and *v* sounds only with a very conspicuous and abnormal contortion of lips and jaw. Moreover this takes so much effort and time that the child will not even try. How can we teach him compensatory ways of producing these sounds?
2. Devise four activities which would help to improve auditory memory span.
3. A child who lalls can move the tonguetip easily in licking and sucking or chewing but seems to find it almost impossible to lift it in speech. Devise three activities which would help solve this problem.
4. A child with almost unintelligible speech due to the fact that he substitutes the *t* and the *w* for almost all other consonants has a history of prolonged and severe illness during his first two years of

life. His mother says that he still talks almost in the same fashion that he began at the age of two. She says that he showed almost no babbling or vocal play but only cried before this time. What causal (etiological) therapy would you use?

5. Put on a debate with some other member of the class in which you support the Backus-Beasley point of view as expressed in their book *Speech Therapy with Children* and your companion argues in favor of the traditional methods for teaching the isolated sound.

6. Read R. B. Irwin's criteria for selecting the first sound with which to begin therapy as explained in her book *Speech and Hearing Therapy*. Give examples.

7. Prepare a dialogue or description of interaction between therapist and case which would illustrate how to help him identify the standard pattern for the *ch* sound, using the operational level of the isolated sound.

8. Prepare a dialogue or description of interaction between therapist and case which would illustrate how to help him recognize the standard pattern of a key word in the speech of others.

9. A child can say *measure* correctly and easily produces a correct *d* sound. But he cannot say words beginning with *j* such as jump. How can you combine the *zh* sound in measure with the *d* to produce a correct *j*? Invent a dialogue to illustrate how you would do it.

10. Give three ways of helping an interdental lisper to hear and recognize his errors, using the syllable level of operations.

11. Invent three new ways of strongly stimulating a child with the isolated *r* sound.

12. Prepare a dialogue illustrating discrimination ear training at the isolated sound level.

13. Prepare a tape loop which, when run continuously through a tape recorder, would provide vivid stimulation for a child who cannot make a standard *l* sound.

14. Invent three binaural (two-ear) discrimination exercises for a child who uses the *uh* sound instead of the vowel *r* in such words as *girl* or *bird*.

15. Make (and demonstrate to the class) a speech shoe out of a quart milk carton.

16. Summarize to the class the information on ways to correct defective *l* sounds as outlined in Nemoy and Davis' *The Correction of Defective Consonant Sounds*.

17. Demonstrate to the class a series of five transitional sounds between the unvoiced *l* sound used by certain lateral lispers and the correct sound and describe how you would use them in the progressive approximation type of therapy.

18. Demonstrate a series of transitional sounds between a distorted vowel *r* sound and the standard vowel (ɝ) as you would use them in progressive approximation.

19. Make up a group of five speech assignments in terminal therapy for a child who has finally mastered his *th* sounds.

20. Prepare a tape of different types of masking noise which might be useful in helping a case to monitor his speech by proprioception.

21. Summarize to the class the information you can procure concerning creative dramatics.

22. How could you use a toy space helmet in speech therapy with articulation cases?

23. Make some nonsense objects out of clay and give them nonsense names suitable for use with a child who is mastering his *z* sounds.

24. Invent some nonsense words for common parts of the body. Call them the words which the Scamboolians use in their language. Use the *r* sound in CV, VC, and CVC syllables.

25. Practice with a companion until you can do echo talk or shadowing very well and put on a demonstration before the class. Have them attempt to shadow you.

26. Put on a demonstration of a series of activities when accompanied by a running commentary of self-talk which would provide opportunities for a lisper to use many sibilants: "I take this pencil and place it between these two fingers and . . . " Continue until you have used twenty words with sibilants in them.

27. Have another member of the class do echo speech after you and resist the occasional lisping you put into your speech.

28. Lisp and then cancel with a correct sibilant five times in speaking to a stranger. Report your reactions and those of your listener.

29. Invent three activities involving signaling. Demonstrate and explain how they would be used.

30. How could you use the isolated *rrr, sss,* and *l* sounds in thinking?

31. Read a passage before the class, lisping on every sibilant except those in two words. Do so very naturally after sufficient practice. Ask the class to try to discover these two key words. Then tell how you would use these in therapy.

32. How could you use the isolated *rrr, sss,* and *th* sounds in the expression of emotion?

33. Design two speech assignments to incorporate a newly mastered sibilant into cock-a-doodle-doo speech.

34. Invent two ways of sending messages using nonsense syllables.

35. Tell the class how you would solve this problem: A child has learned his new *l* sound in isolation and in nonsense syllables, but in words,

he inserts the old *w* error between the initial *l* and the rest of the word: "lwetter."

36. A child can use the *r* sound correctly in blends such as *tr* and *dr* but cannot use it in syllables beginning with that sound nor can he seem to master it in isolation. How would you solve this problem?

37. How could you use whispering in articulation therapy? Find five ways.

38. A child sometimes substitutes the *w* for the *l* and sometimes he uses the *y*. Invent some identification ear training exercises which will help him to identify these errors.

39. How could you use calisthenics in speech therapy with articulation cases?

40. How can we get a newly acquired *s* sound into the "body English" of a lisping child?

PERIODICAL REFERENCES

41. Altshuler, A. W. "A Therapeutic Oral Device for Lateral Emission," *Journal Speech and Hearing Disorders,* Volume 26, 1961, pages 179-182.

42. Backus, O. L., and H. M. Dunn. "Use of Conversation Patterns to Promote Speech and Retention of Learning," *Journal of Speech Disorders,* Volume 12, 1947, pages 135-142.

43. Black, M., and R. A. S. Ludwig. "Analysis of the Games Technic," *Journal Speech and Hearing Disorders,* Volume 21, 1956, pages 183-187.

44. Cable, W. A. "Dynamic Factors in the Moto-kinesthetic Method of Speech Correction," *Quarterly Journal of Speech,* Volume 31, 1943, pages 350-357.

45. Enquist, L. E., and C. F. Wagner. "Flannel Chart Technique for Rehabilitation of Speech and Hearing Disorders," *Journal Speech and Hearing Disorders,* Volume 15, 1950, pages 338-340.

46. Goda, S. "Spontaneous Speech, a Primary Source of Therapy Material," *Journal Speech and Hearing Disorders,* Volume 27, 1962, pages 190-192.

47. Hahn, E. "Indications for Direct, Nondirect and Indirect Methods in Speech Correction," *Journal Speech and Hearing Disorders,* Volume 26, 1961, pages 230-236.

48. Hawk, S. S. "Moto-kinaesthetic Training for Children with Speech Handicaps," *Journal Speech Disorders,* Volume 7, 1942, pages 357-360.

49. Hull, M. E. "Anticipatory Speech Response in Children with Articulatory Defects," *Journal Speech and Hearing Disorders,* Volume 13, 1948, pages 268-272.

50. Marquardt, E. "Carry-over with 'Speech Pals,' " *Journal Speech and Hearing Disorders,* Volume 24, 1959, pages 154-156.

51. Milisen, R. "A Rationale for Articulation Disorders," *Journal Speech and Hearing Disorders,* Monograph Supplement 4, 1954, pages 6-17.

52. Obermann, C. E. "Improving Pupils' Speech: A Practical Program of Correction," *Nation's Schools,* Volume 28, 1941, pages 51-53.

53. Porter, F. "Speech Correction in an Orphanage," *Journal Speech Disorders,* Volume 10, 1945, pages 241-249.

54. Pronovost, W. "Visual Aids to Speech Improvement," *Journal Speech Disorders,* Volume 12, 1947, pages 388-391.

55. Reid, G. "The Efficacy of Speech Re-education of Functional Articulatory Defects in Elementary School Children," *Journal Speech Disorders,* Volume 12, 1947, pages 363-368.

56. Roe, V. "Follow-up in the Correction of Functional Articulatory Disorders," *Journal Speech and Hearing Disorders,* Volume 13, 1948, pages 332-336.

57. Shames, G. H. "Use of the Nonsense Syllable in Articulation Therapy," *Journal Speech and Hearing Disorders,* Volume 22, 1957, pages 261-264.

58. Shelton, R. L., W. B. Arndt, and J. Miller. "Learning Principles and Teaching of Speech and Language," *Journal Speech and Hearing Disorders,* Volume 26, 1961, pages 360-376.

59. Smathers, S. "Speech-Play Therapy," *Journal Speech and Hearing Disorders,* Volume 24, 1959, pages 59-61.

60. Smith, M. E. "A Clinician's Story," *Quarterly Journal of Speech,* Volume 13, 1948, pages 268-272.

61. Tufts, L. C., and A. R. Holiday. "Effectiveness of Trained Parents as Speech Therapists," *Journal Speech and Hearing Disorders,* Volume 24, 1959, pages 395-401.

62. Van Riper, C. "Binaural Speech Therapy," *Journal Speech and Hearing Disorders,* Volume 24, 1959, pages 62-63.

63. Webb, C. E., and B. M. Siegenthaler. "Comparison of Aural Stimulation Methods for Teaching Speech Sounds," *Journal Speech and Hearing Disorders,* Volume 22, 1957, pages 264-270.

64. Winitz, H., and M. Lawrence. "Children's Articulation and Sound Learning Ability," *Journal Speech and Hearing Research,* Volume 4, 1961, pages 259-268.

65. Wood, K. S. "Measurement of Progress in the Correction of Articulatory Speech Defects," *Journal Speech Disorders,* Volume 11, 1946, pages 171-174.

BOOKS

66. Backus, O. L., and J. Beasley. *Speech Therapy with Children.* Boston: Houghton-Mifflin Company, 1951.
67. Berry, M. F., and J. Eisenson. *Speech Disorders.* New York: Appleton-Century-Crofts, 1956, Chapters 7 and 8.
68. Johnson, W., *et al. Speech Handicapped School Children.* New York: Harper & Row, Publishers, 1948, Chapter 3.
69. Jones, M. V. *Baby Talk.* Springfield, Ill.: Charles C. Thomas, Publisher, 1960.
70. Nemoy, E. M. *Speech Correction through Story-telling Units.* Magnolia, Mass.: Expression Company, 1954.
71. ———, and S. Davis. *The Correction of Defective Consonant Sounds,* Magnolia, Mass.: Expression Company, 1954.
72. Palmer, C. E. *Speech and Hearing Problems.* Springfield, Ill.: Charles C. Thomas, Publisher, 1961.
73. Van Riper, C. *Casebook in Speech Therapy.* Englewood Cliffs, N.J.: Prentice-Hall, Inc., 1953.
74. ———, and J. V. Irwin. *Voice and Articulation.* Englewood Cliffs, N.J.: Prentice-Hall, Inc., 1958.
75. ———. *Your Child's Speech Problems.* New York: Harper & Row, Publishers, 1961.
76. Young, E. H., and S. S. Hawk. *Moto-kinesthetic Speech Training.* Stanford, Calif.: Stanford University Press, 1955.
77. Zedler, E. Y. *Listening for Speech Sounds.* Garden City, N.Y.: Doubleday & Company, Inc., 1955.

CHAPTER ELEVEN

Stuttering: Its Nature and Causes

"O God! Cut through the backbone of my stuttering. I desire that thou shalt remove the spring of
the impediment." These are the words inscribed on a clay tablet
found by Dr. Albright, an archeologist of Haverford College, in the
ruins of the Biblical town of Beth Shemish. That lone, lorn cry of a
soul lost in antiquity has been echoed by millions of stutterers every
year ever since. Even today in this country alone there are more
than a million stutterers. Seven in a thousand, or almost one per
cent of us stutter. It is a distressing affliction and a dramatic one. It
plays no favorites. King and peasant, wise man, poor man, beggar
man, thief, all have been affected by speech that sticks and stumbles.
King Charles I of England stopped stuttering when his head was cut
off. Charles Darwin stuttered too badly to become a preacher so he
turned scientist instead. But you don't have to be royal or bright to
stutter. Although college stutterers as a group are higher in intelligence than their fellow students, there are more stutterers among
the mentally retarded than among the normal population.[1] There
are many more males than females who stutter.

Stuttering also cuts across cultures, though a few cultures seem
to have more of the disorder than others. The Germans call it
stottern; the English call it *stammering* (note: in this country the
terms "stammering" and "stuttering" are equivalent and synonymous,
but the latter has been preferred); the Fiji Islanders call it "Ka-ka";
in Japan stutterers are known as "do'mo'ri"; the Eskimo stutterer is

[1] George W. Gens in "The Speech Pathologist Looks at the Mentally Deficient Child," *Training School Bulletin,* XLVIII, 1951, pages 19-27, reports a
figure of 20 per cent.

"Iptogetok"; those of the Zulu race in South Africa are called "Amalimi"; the Salish, a tribe of American Indians, use the term "sutsuts." The only reason for giving these names is to make the point that stuttering is a common disorder, one of those universal afflictions which plague the human race.

Stuttering is also a disorder which can be worsened by ill treatment. Many well-meaning but ignorant individuals, by their suggestions and reactions, have made the stuttering not only more difficult to bear but also more severe and frequent. As in all the speech disorders, this one needs special understanding. Basic information is essential not only to enable you to help the stutterer but to keep from hurting him further.

Characteristics. There are many definitions of the disorder because it is hard to define. One reason for this is that the behavior varies widely from stutterer to stutterer. Stuttering wears many faces, none of them pretty. In the early stages of the disorder, as we shall see, the most frequently observed characteristics are excessive repetitions and prolongations of a sound, syllable, or articulatory posture, and Sheehan (55) has shown that these repetitions and prolongations are the only two behaviors common to adult stutterers who look different and sound different, one from another. Most of the variation consists of different habitual reactions of avoidance, struggle, or escape. Since different individuals avoid in different ways, struggle differently and use different methods for escaping from their sound fixations and syllabic oscillations, it is not surprising that we find such a variety of stuttering pictures. But the lowest common denominators seem to be these moments when the flow of speech is interrupted by a fixation (prolongation) or oscillation (repetition) in some of the structures used in speech. If at the very moment you read this, your right arm would begin to jerk up and down uncontrollably for a few seconds, or if you would close your left eye and then find that for an instant you couldn't open it you would come pretty close to knowing what it feels like to stutter.

Stuttering is intermittent. Even severe stutterers often speak more words normally than in a stuttered fashion. Only one of our cases, a neurotic, hysterical girl whose disorder had its onset in an emotional upheaval at nineteen, stuttered consistently on every word, big or little, and even she would occasionally forget and speak very fluently. This intermittency, however, makes the experience more distressful, since it is difficult to adapt to unpleasantness which comes and goes. In the very young stutterer, relatively long periods of fluency are followed by days when much stuttering is present. In the older severe stutterer only occasionally will an utterance have no stuttered word within it, and the only way he can have an entire day free from stuttering is to remain mute. At times volleys of stuttering occur, each consecutive word presenting new abnormality, but more commonly it is the first words and the most meaningful which present the most difficulty.

Frequency and Severity. The frequency and severity of stuttering usually vary with the amount of communicative stress. Most stutterers speak fluently when alone or in talking to pets or when reading in unison. A few do not. A few even stutter when they sing.

Why do we have such variations in the frequency and severity of stuttering? What causes it to appear and disappear? Why are some stutterings worse than others? We have tried to answer all these difficult questions by formulating one mathematical equation which we hope will not cause the student to bury his head beneath the covers but instead to recognize that it will help him assemble and remember a mass of information which might otherwise be a bit indigestible. What this equation tells us is that stuttering becomes more frequent and gets more severe

WHEN:

P Penalties are placed upon it, or past penalties are remembered
F Frustrations of any type are experienced or remembered
A Anxiety is present
G Guilt is felt
H Hostility needs to be expressed

WHEN:

Sf There are situation fears due to old memories of past unpleasantness in the situation
Wf Certain sounds and words are feared due to old unpleasant memories

WHEN:

Cs The speaking situation is full of communicative stress (listener loss, interruptions, etc.) or there are very important things to say (propositionality.)

These are the factors which make stuttering worse. They form the items on the upper line of the equation: the dividend part.

But there are other factors which *decrease* stuttering: the morale factor and the amount of fluency the stutterer also experiences along with his stuttering. Some stutterers have a lot of fluent speech; others have little. The more they have, the less likely they are to have frequent and severe stuttering. We can represent these two factors in the divisor part of our equation thus:

M   Morale or ego strength or self confidence.
Fl   The amount of felt fluency

Here then is our equation:

$$S = \frac{(PFAGH) + (Sf\,Wf) + Cs}{M + Fl}$$

This is an important equation. It explains many things about stuttering. It says that when the stutterer's morale or ego strength is high because of achievements, success, and social acceptance, he will tend to stutter less. If in any given communicative situation he expects or feels communicative stress, penalties, and frustration he will stutter more. He will stutter more if he is experiencing or anticipating anxiety, guilt, and hostility. He will also stutter more if in scanning ahead he sees words or situations coming which have been associated with past experiences of stuttering. Stutterers have more trouble talking to authority figures, to people who become impatient or mock or suffer when listening to stuttering. Most stutterers are very vulnerable to listener loss, to interruptions, to rejections, penalty, frustration, anxiety, and hostility. The pressures, then, which create more stuttering can come from without or within, from the pressures of the present, the expected agonies of the future, or the miseries of the past.

In any given speaking situation the amount of communicative stress varies. Some listeners are good listeners; others are bad ones. Some heckle us with constant interruptions. Some say the unfinished words for the stutterer. Some look away. Again, the message to be spoken may be difficult to express. Thinking may be confused and so the formulation may falter. The urgency to speak very swiftly may be present. All these factors and many others put the pressure on fluency and tend to disrupt it. We include all of them under the category of communicative stress.

Our *C* factor also includes, as we have said, the communicative importance of the utterance. This is termed "propositionality." Stutterers often can read in unison with others without stuttering. They can blurt out whole sentences as "asides" without a bit of trouble. But when they have something important to say, something urgent which must be said quickly, they have a tough time. Even little children in the first stage of stuttering often tend to have more difficulty on certain words than others (Bloodstein's so-called "consistency effect") because these words carry most of the utterance's meaning. These words therefore carry more communicative stress. When the primary stutterer comes running home from school full of important information to communicate to his parents, his stuttering comes tumbling out in volleys; when he talks to himself or his dog, he is very fluent. There's not much propositionality in what he has to say.

As part of our general equation, we referred to morale or ego strength as a favorable factor. When stutterers are feeling confident, they don't stutter as much. The better they feel about themselves, the less they stutter. This is what one of our high-school cases wrote in his autobiography:

> All I need is self-confidence. The trouble is I haven't got much, and every time I block, I lose most of what I have. I notice that when I bring home a report card full of A's, I can talk better. For a time, a little time. When I manage to get a date with a good looking girl and have fun, my speech almost becomes free. If I ask for a date and get turned down, I block all over the place. I finally got up nerve enough to ask for a job at a grocery after school, and got it! I felt so good from becoming partly independent and earning my own money that for two or three days I had more free speech than I've ever had. So what I need is for you to give me more self-confidence.

Unfortunately, morale is not a gift. It cannot be injected by any therapist. It is earned by acquiring more personality assets and by learning to cope with one's liabilities. Confidence comes when we do battle and succeed. It comes when we accept a challenge instead of running away from it. It gains strength when we lick our wounds after a defeat and return to the fray. It goes down when we grow morbid and bathe in self-pity. It rises when we confront ourselves, accept our limitations, and start working to fulfill our potentials despite those limitations. One of the tasks of the therapist, if he is to help the stutterer to talk more freely, is to assist him in understanding these things.

The other major favorable factor is the fluency factor (Fl). By this we mean the over-all amount of real fluency the person has been having in similar speaking situations. Some stutterers seldom speak a sentence without some blocking. Others can be very fluent at times. Their sentences flow smoothly, not jerkily, when they are not stuttering. We are always alert, when examining a new stutterer, to listen not only to the stuttering but also to the smoothness of his nonstuttered speech. Those who falter, pause, hem and haw, speak by spurts, can be said to have a low amount of Fl and their clinical problems are going to be more difficult. They will need to be taught how to make their normal as well as their abnormal speech fluent. When the morale is high and the person can be very fluent, it will take a lot of *PFAGH* and fear and communicative stress to make him stutter.

Definition. We have been describing stuttering. It is time to define it. Any definition is a net. It manages to hold the major features of the thing defined, but some of the lesser features, like smaller fish, escape through the meshes. Let us try to hold as many as possible. *Stuttering occurs when the flow of speech is interrupted abnormally by repetitions or prolongations of a sound or syllable or posture, or by avoidance and struggle reactions.*

Let us examine some of the items in this definition. They may help us understand what stuttering is. First of all we speak of the flow of speech. Speech consists of a sequence of sounds and movements. It is time-patterned. Each sound and each movement, within limits, must occur at a precise moment in the time sequence. A certain margin of leeway in this timing is acceptable, depending upon the cultural standards, the age of the person, and the communicative situation in which the speaking takes place. According to Lemert[2] the Polynesian cultures of the South Sea appear more tolerant of broken, nonfluent speech in their children than does the culture of Japan. Some American Indian tribes appear less tolerant than others. We do not expect little children to have as smoothly flowing speech as we expect adults to possess. We would not expect

[2] Edwin M. Lemert. "Stuttering and Social Structures in Two Pacific Societies," *Journal Speech and Hearing Disorders*, Volume 27, 1962, pages 3-10.

a person who is confessing his sins to be as fluent as one who is asking for the salt and pepper. But there are still standards of fluent utterance. When the breaks in speech occur too frequently or are accompanied by other peculiar behaviors which call attention to themselves and interfere with communication and are viewed as abnormal by the listener, we call it stuttering.

What takes place at the moment the speech flow is broken? We have used the words "repetition and prolongation of a sound, syllable, or posture." All of us repeat and hesitate and filibuster at times as we utter our thoughts. None of us is completely fluent in every communicative situation. Knowing this, we do not consider the repetition of a word or phrase or the use of pauses, um's and er's, or reformulations as abnormal. We even accept a few repetitions of a syllable. But when a sound or syllable is repeated not once or twice but many times, and when this behavior occurs too frequently, then we prick up our ears and say to ourselves that the speaker stutters. We tend to say the same thing when a sound is prolonged, as in this example: "I think what mmmmmmmmmmmy mmmmmmmmmmmother wwwwwon't let me go." The tolerance for such prolongations of a sound seems to be much less than for repetitions of a sound or syllable. We have also used the word *posture*. Not all these repetitions and prolongations are vocalized. The stutterer often makes several silent mouth postures before the word is spoken, or he may assume a fixed position and struggle silently with it before blurting out what he wants to say. These fixed postures may be located anywhere in the speech structures. One stutterer may hold his breath with both true and false vocal cords closed tightly. Another may protrude his tongue or twist his lips to one side. Since these silent postures take time, they break up the normal time sequence of speech. Finally, we have included in our definition the terms "avoidance" and "struggle." Although most beginning stutterers show little struggle or avoidance, in the advanced stages of the disorder these reactions may constitute the major part of the problem. Let us view two of these behaviors.

Uh, I, uh, well, I'm nnot (*easy prolongation, eyes turned to the right*) too sure what you, what you, what you mean by, what you mean by that. Well, well, well, uh well, d . . . do (*complete stoppage with lip, tongue and jaw tremors; eyes shut; head jerks backward*) I get sssssore (*easy prolongation*) or something, or something like that? [3]

The interiorized stutterer is characterized by constant awareness of his speech difficulty and of stuttering threats contained in speaking situations. Constant preparedness, constant vigilance to guard against revelation of his stutter, complete avoidance of all possible situations anticipated as threatening, all are evidenced. Every eventuality must be anticipated so that he can either avoid the danger entirely or meet it fully prepared. To be caught unprepared would be a tragedy. When stuttering cannot be warded off entirely, he then utilizes rather specific devices like coughing, blowing his nose, hand gestures, standing up and sitting down just at the "right" moment.[4] Most of the incredible variety in the behavior shown by adult stutterers is due to the specific ways each has learned to avoid or to escape from his unpleasant and frustrating oscillations and fixations.

Covert Features. Our definition's net has caught most of the *overt* behaviors shown by the stutterer, but the hidden or covert features have been included only by implication. Just as the outward signs of stuttering change and grow worse as the person grows older, so too do the inner experiences. Most young children appear quite unaware of their repetitions and prolongations, or at worst speech occasionally seems "hard." As the stutterer becomes aware of his broken communication, of his inability to get others to understand his message, he experiences feelings of frustration. Also, in the later stages of stuttering, social penalties cause the stutterer to experience word fears and situational anxieties. Again we find the family of Pfagh; penalties and frustration beget anxiety, guilt, and hostility.

These covert features of stuttering vary not only with age and the development of stuttering; they vary with the individual stutterer. We have known very severe stutterers who had plenty of anxiety but no specific phonetic fears. We have known others who showed the converse. Some are consumed with guilt; others feel only angry

---

[3] Charles Van Riper and Leslie Gruber. *A Casebook in Stuttering.* New York: Harper & Row, Publishers, 1957, page 11.
[4] Ernest Douglass and Bruce Quarrington. "The Differentiation of Interiorized and Exteriorized Secondary Stuttering," *Journal Speech and Hearing Disorders,* Volume 17, 1952, page 379.

frustration. One stutterer will punish himself masochistically; another, with equal feelings of hostility, will spend his life attacking other people. The particular patterns of emotional reaction shown by different stutterers are due to the particular history each has had. We know some stutterers who, because of good environments and other personality assets, have suffered very little social rejection or penality, and who seem to have learned to tolerate their communicative frustrations with equanimity. They had very little anxiety, guilt, or hostility and their stuttering was relatively mild. Others, less fortunate, live out their days in an almost constant storm of emotion. The problem of stuttering cannot be defined entirely by what emerges from the mouth.

Physiological Reactions. Certain important features of stuttering are difficult to see with the naked eye, and yet they can be revealed by instrumentation. Severe stutterers in the advanced stages of the disorder show abnormalities in heart and pulse rate, in breathing. Investigations have revealed changes in blood composition and distribution, states of general or localized tension, tremors, odd brain waves, dilatation of the pupils, and many other abnormal reactions. However, these do not seem to form the core of the disorder. All severe stutterers do not show all of them. These reactions occur during the moment of stuttering or during its anticipation. They are especially vivid during the stutterer's efforts to escape from the fixations or oscillations. They are probably no more than the reflection of the stress he feels. They are the physiological correlates of his struggle or fear. They do not occur on the shorter unforced stutterings. They do not appear in the young stutterer whose automatic repetitions and unforced prolongations do not seem to bother him. But for the older, more severe stutterer they form a major part of his internal distress. They contribute much to his feeling that something terrible is happening to him. The brain that controls the mouth is flooded with static from the viscera. The normal automaticity and monitoring of utterance is thus doubly beset. It is more difficult to talk.

The Origins of Stuttering

It is difficult to find the true source of a river; too many streams flow into it. Many explorers have attempted to trace the course of the river of stuttering to what they thought were the lakes of its origin. It should not surprise us to learn that different explorers found different lakes.

At one time, the poor student of speech therapy had to be able to describe fifteen different theories concerning the nature and treatment of secondary stuttering, and there were others they might have included in their study. While there is still disagreement and confusion among therapists with respect to their explanations of this disorder, the arguments are not so strident, and large areas of mutual thinking prevail. Formerly there tended to be various schools, each holding a definite and rigid theoretical dogma. Modern research has made available new sources of information. Cooler heads have examined the evidence again and have been able to reconcile opposing points of view. Probably the most important factor was the giving up of the belief in a *single cause* for stuttering. The fallacy of the *single cause* has been responsible for confusion in many fields, and it certainly caused plenty of difficulty in speech correction.

Nevertheless, there are still explorers who insist that the lake they have found is the only true source of the river of stuttering. Let us not argue with them; they may all be correct; let us look at their lakes. There seem to be three of them since the many different points of view concerning the origin of stuttering can be grouped into three major theories: the *learning* theories; the *neurotic* theories, and the theories of *constitutional difference*. Each has its advocates.

How shall we understand this mysterious disorder? Where shall we find the "impediment"?

Many people have tried to find the answers to these questions. Many have been sure that they knew the answer to the stuttering problem, but the honest speech therapist knows that he is still confronted with a disorder which retains much of its age-old mystery. Most of the past and present explanations contain some truth; none of them is entirely satisfactory. Many beginning students are so disturbed when they discover such a state of affairs that they tend to lose interest in the subject. But there is a similar mystery in many of the other disorders that afflict mankind—heart disease, tooth decay, asthma, and cancer, to name only a few. If there are conflicting theories concerning the nature of stuttering, there is also the ever-present fact that stutterers are with us, needing help. And we can do much to help them.

So far as stuttering is concerned, speech correction is at present in the era of "authorities" just as medicine was before Pasteur's discovery of bacterial agents in disease. Some of those early medical authorities were able and wise physicians. They had made some very keen and valid observations concerning disease. In some instances they discovered the cure for the disease long before they knew its nature. For example, the witch doctors of native tribes on the Malay Peninsula diagnosed diabetes by putting specimens of urine near ant hills, and, when the ants were attracted, prescribed certain food taboos which helped their patients cut down on sugar intake. The results were excellent, but the theories which they used to justify their diagnosis and prescription were, to say the least, confused and inaccurate. Stutterers have been helped by many different methods of treatment based on many conflicting theories. In this text we shall endeavor to present the nature and treatment of stuttering in the light of our present knowledge. There is much that we do not know about stuttering, yet we know enough to help the majority of our cases.

Stuttering as a Neurosis.   This point of view is held by many psychiatrists and some psychologists, perhaps because their clinical practice brings them, not the garden variety of stutterers, but those with deep-seated emotional problems. If you stuttered but were also deeply disturbed by emotional conflicts, to whom would you go for help—to a speech therapist or to a psychiatrist? In exploring *their* cases of stuttering, these workers therefore come to have a firm belief in the neurotic origin and character of the disorder. Stuttering behavior is viewed as the outward symptom of a basic inner conflict. Some statements of this position should be provided:

> Psychoanalysis regards stuttering broadly as a neurotic disorder in which personality disturbance is in part reflected in disturbance in speech. (Glauber[5])

[5] Peter Glauber. "The Psychoanalysis of Stuttering" in Jon Eisenson (ed.) *Stuttering: A Symposium.* New York: Harper & Row, Publishers, 1958, page 73.

> . . . stuttering is a defense created with extraordinary skill and designed to prevent anxiety from developing when certain impulses of which the stutterer dares not become aware, threaten to expose themselves. (Travis[6])

[6] Lee Edward Travis. "The Need for Stuttering," *Journal of Speech Disorders,* Volume 5, 1940, pages 193-202.

When a stammerer attempts to talk, the mouth movements are the persistence into maturity of the original sucking and biting lip-nipple activities of infancy . . . (Coriat[7])

Sometimes he is in constant fear lest he inadvertently reveal something he would his elders did not hear, (Dunlap[8])

Stuttering is by far the most important of all neurotic speech disturbances. (Freund [9])

These are but a few of the formulations of the neurotic theory. In essence, the professional workers who hold these beliefs feel that stuttering is the outward manifestation of repressed desires to satisfy such inner needs as these: to satisfy anal or oral eroticism or to express hostility by attacking and smearing the listener or to remain infantile.

As Bloodstein (25) summarizes the matter:

Such conflicts are generally considered to grow out of disturbed parent-child relationships, and to be related to abnormal feeding or nursing behavior of the mother, excessively harsh or early weaning or toilet training, parental domination, overprotection or overanxiety, or other traumatic features of the family environment which frequently go back to the parents' own neurotic conflicts.

We are pretty sure that some stutterers have this type of causation; some of our cases cannot be reasonably understood in any other way. These are in the marked minority, however. In them the stuttering is symptomatic of a primary neurosis. But there are many more stutterers in whom the neurosis, if any, is secondary. The stutterer develops the stuttering he has acquired from other sources into a defense mechanism. As one of our cases said, "Sure, I get some good out of it. If I have to stutter, I might as well use it to dodge some of the pain of living. It's not good for anything else." Most normal people are neurotic some of the time, and so are most stutterers, in this sense. A few, however, have compulsive symptoms which can only be understood in terms of psychopathology. In them, the stuttering starts in a neurosis and remains in one.

Learning Theories. Other explorers of stuttering have traced its main flow to another source. Perhaps they worked the other side of

---

[7] I. H. Coriat. "The Psychoanalytic Conception of Stuttering," *The Nervous Child*, Volume 2, 1943, pages 167-171.

[8] K. Dunlap. "Stammering: Its Nature, Etiology and Therapy," *Journal Comparative Psychology*, Volume 37, 1944, pages 187-202.

[9] H. Freund. "Psychopathological Aspects of Stuttering," *American Journal of Psychotherapy*, Volume 7, 1953, pages 689-705.

the river, i.e., the stutterers who came to them were not those who went to the psychiatrist. At any rate, according to these theories— and there are several which may be included in the category— stuttering is learned behavior. The child is so conditioned that he learns a truly broken English—or Swahili or Japanese. Beginning, as most stuttering does, in the very early years of life, it often seems to coincide with the period of speech learning and development. According to this theory, stuttering has its origin in the early fumblings and hesitancies and interruptions which seem to be a natural and common phase of the speech learning process. We have already seen what a complicated business is this speaking we take so much for granted. We must master complicated muscular co-ordinations, use the right sounds, formulate our thoughts aloud, express the glandular squirting of our emotions, control others, and use it for the communication of messages. Any of these may present many difficulties.

Rigmor Knutsen, a Danish speech therapist, said to us, "In Denmark we find a great many children who begin to stutter after the speech therapist has treated them for their delayed speech. Do you not also find this true?" We answered that we had known several cases who bore out her observation and told her about Carlene.

> Carlene, at four, had no intelligible speech. She used a few vowels and grunts with her gestures to make her wants known. She was referred to us by the psychological clinic who had found her IQ on the performance tests to be so low that they were considering suggesting commitment to a state school for the feeble-minded. By imitating her behavior until she imitated us we were able to go about getting her to produce almost all of the isolated speech sounds. By avoiding all requests to name objects, and through the use of self-talk and parallel talking, we evoked enough vocalized and whispered words to accept her for therapy. At the end of three months of daily work, she was speaking in short phrases, and retests in the psychological clinic showed her to be of normal intelligence. Her parents were very proud of her achievement, but during the summer vacation, they worked too hard upon her speech production and she began to stutter very markedly. Advised to give up all therapy, the parents cooperated willingly and within two more months the symptoms disappeared completely. The burden of trying to master her articulation and fluency skills had been too great. It was interesting that she regressed to simpler phrases and sentences as the stuttering disappeared, and for a time her articulation became worse.

Many children who do not have delayed speech go through a similar period of non-fluency when, urged by parental approvals, they try to master the adult patterns of speech too quickly. It is a long step from the single word utterance of the one-year-old to the multiple-word phrases and sentences of adult speech. Children who try to dance before they have learned to walk trip themselves, and the same thing occurs in speech. We tend to think of penalties as being provocative of stuttering but excessive approvals at the wrong times can create such a demand as to produce speech hesitation as well. Many children from happy homes can start to stutter in this way.

As we have seen in our section on how children learn to talk, some parents fail to make speech learning easy for their children. They do not listen. They demand answers which the child may not be ready to give. They may command verbal confession. They set standards of fluency and articulation which may be far beyond the capabilities of the child. Siblings may interrupt excessively. When the communicative interchange is broken either at the sending or receiving end, or when speaking becomes disrupted by emotion, there are only three things a person can do. He can repeat; he can fixate; or he can give up the attempt to speak. Some children choose the latter course and develop voluntary mutism. Others deny the parental demands to conform and talk a gibberish of fluent but distorted sounds. The stutterer keeps on talking but he falters. Driven by his urge to talk, all he can do is to repeat or prolong, to oscillate or fixate when these disrupting influences are present.

However, we have not explained why in stuttering the stoppages occur on the sound or its silent posture nor why the repetition is of the syllable and sound rather than of the whole word or phrase. Wingate's (68) critical review of the research seems to show fairly conclusively that the child who is called a stutterer shows different *kinds* of hesitancies than the one who is presumed to speak normally. The one child mainly responds to these communicative pressures by behavior our culture calls stuttering; the other primarily by hesitating or filibustering. They all show both types of non-fluencies, but the child who becomes a stutterer has many more difficulties with the sound and syllable rather than with the word or phrase. Why do some of these hesitaters become stutterers? We do not know the answer to our question. Perhaps the difference lies in the amount and intensity of the communicative stress. With minor stress, repetitions of sentences or phrases occurs; with more stress, words are repeated; with even more pressure, the oscillating occurs on syllables. When complete disruption occurs but the urge to speak still remains, first prolongations of an audible sound (mmmmmother) are shown and finally even this breaks down to a silent posture. The syllable and sound are the smallest motoric and acoustic elements into which speech can be broken.

Perhaps the normally speaking child has, for one reason or another, developed his formulative and fluency skills in speaking to such a degree of stability that only occasionally will he show the small percentage of syllabic and sound repetitions and prolongations. The stuttering child, perhaps because of constitutional difference, interpersonal relationship problems, or other reasons, may be more vulnerable to the same stress which normal speaking children handle with word and phrase repetitions. We do not know. Wyatt[10] has suggested that when breakdown occurs, a child regresses to an earlier stage. She points out the resemblance of early stuttering to the reiterative babbling of the infant. We do not know the answer to our question.

The Semantic Theory. According to Wendell Johnson, its chief exponent, stuttering begins, not in the child's mouth, but in the parent's ear. He lumps all types of repetitions and prolongations into the category of non-fluencies which he feels are quite normal reactions, common to all children. The difficulty, Johnson believes, arises when a parent hears these normal non-fluencies and reacts to them by anxiety or penalty. Johnson feels that even when the repetitions and prolongations are excessive, they are merely normal reactions to the abnormal conditions of communicative stress operating at the moment. He insists therefore, that the source of the real problem lies in parental misdiagnosis and misinterpretation. He points out that when parents become anxious or punitive about these normal hesitancies, the child, reflecting their attitudes, will begin to fear, avoid, or struggle to inhibit them.

Ricky, aged five, illustrates a source of stuttering which Johnson has vivified by his statement that "Stuttering begins, not in the child's mouth but in the parent's ear." We first met the child at the

[10] G. Wyatt. "A Developmental Crisis Theory of Stuttering," *Language and Speech,* Volume 1, 1958, pages 250-264.

age of three. He was brought to us by his mother, a former college speech teacher. She was tense and anxious about the boy, claiming that he was beginning to stutter. In three hours of observation, play, and parent conversation, we were unable to find anything but an occasional repetition of a phrase or whole word, usually under conditions of word choice which would have made any adult hesitate. Each time one of these occurred, she would roll her eyes or tug at our sleeves to point out the stuttering. Knowing that stuttering is intermittent, we even introduced some experimental stress, hurrying the child, interrupting, rejecting his statements, and averting our attention. He was remarkably fluent, much more so than most children of his age.

Recognizing the mother's anxiety, and being as careful as possible, we tried to reassure and educate her concerning the prevalence of repetition and hesitation in most children's speech. We made available some parental counseling to help her face her own problems, but she refused to participate. Said she, "You're just like everyone else. Every doctor and speech therapist I've taken Ricky to has said the same thing. You can't fool a child's own mother. He's stuttering and you know it."

A year later she brought the child back to the clinic, and sure enough, he was stuttering with all the abnormality of an adult. "See!" she said triumphantly, "I told you he was a stutterer all the time."

Frustration Theory. But stuttering need not necessarily begin in the *parent's* ear; it may also begin in the ear of the *child.* The need to communicate a message, to verbalize one's thoughts, to control another person, to express an emotion—these can be powerful drives. Besides, there are children whose appetites for speech for one reason or another are almost monstrous. They must be heard! When such speech-hungry children find these drives blocked by the repetitions and prolongations produced by listener loss or other fluency disruptors, they experience much frustration. If you have had to use a typewriter or piano on which the keys stick occasionally, you will understand. The urge to consummate the response is blocked and impeded by the delay occasioned by the repetitions and prolongations. Interruptions frustrate, whether they come from others or from one's own mouth. Too many of the young stutterers we have studied do not appear to have the origin of their difficulty in parental mislabeling of normal nonfluencies for us to accept blindly Johnson's thesis. Some parents actually deny the existence of any problem. Usually, stuttering has had a gradual history of growth in frequency and severity before it ever gets labeled. We feel that the role of frustration in the development of stuttering must receive the attention it deserves. Not only can frustration account for the initial breaks in the flow of speech; it also can help us understand why children eventually begin to struggle and avoid. Frustration is unpleasant; we avoid unpleasantness and we fear it. Frustration also leads to aggression, and so we struggle.

Jimmy, aged four, was in most respects a rather ordinary normal child. But he differed markedly from other children his age in his outstanding inability to tolerate frustration. This was not inborn, but the result of poor handling by his parents, his uncle, and his older sister. The whole family loved to tease each other, to play practical jokes, to upset apple carts and egos. Even as a baby, Jimmy was teased with the bottle being held tantalizingly to the lips, or withdrawn, or waved from side to side. The adults liked to pretend to drop him; they put obstacles in the way of his crawling; they greatly enjoyed seeing him become purple with rage. At the age of two he was holding his breath until his face became blue. Toilet training was slow and his family interpreted his occasional urinary lapses upon those who held him as a sign of his family-belongingness. As is obvious from the foregoing description, a good amount of hidden hostility permeated the entire family living, but it appeared only in joking and teasing forms. The approved culture pattern was to be a good sport, to be able to take it and dish it out.

Jimmy, however, never quite managed to adopt these values. He fought back; he threw temper tantrums; he kicked and bit and howled. They called him a poor sport and, since they despised poor sports, they worked hard to toughen him to their teasing. He had spoken well and without any nonfluency until his fourth birthday when his sister began to kid him about his pronunciation of words beginning with the *s* blends which he had not mastered.

At this point they gave him, for the first time, a nickname "Twaberry Bwonde" since his hair was that color and he pronounced the words in that way. He reacted by going berserk, and so more teasing occurred, this time focused primarily on speech. The sister learned that he would tend to make more articulatory errors if she interrupted him, finished his sentences, or hurried him, and she went to work. Within one week he was stuttering severely, though in a repetitive fashion. Two weeks later, he was showing facial contortions and severe struggling in breathing. At this point the parents became alarmed and brought the child to the speech therapist.

Although the parents and family changed their policies and all teasing was eliminated, the stuttering persisted. It was not until a lot of release therapy through play was administered and a course of training in frustration tolerance was instituted that first the struggle, and later the repetitions, subsided and disappeared.

Approach-avoidance Conflicts. This position, which has been most clearly expressed by Sheehan (55), is also one of the learning theories. It can be called the "conflict reinforcement" theory of stuttering. It treats the disorder from the viewpoint of modern learning theory. The primary symptoms are seen as the result of competitive and opposing urges to speak and not to speak. When these tendencies are approximately equal, oscillations and fixations in behavior occur. These are the repetitions and prolongations of the primary symptoms. The conflicting urges may come from many sources. The child may want to speak but may not know what to say or how to say it. He may need to speak at a time when he thinks his listener is not listening or does not want to hear him. He may have the urge to say something "evil" which may receive penalty. He may want to speak like big people, yet not have the fluency or articulatory skills to keep the flow going. He may have an urge to express himself at a time when he feels ambivalent. The lag of a clumsy tongue may oppose a strong need to talk quickly. Any of these and many other situations could produce the opposing forces. All this theory considers is what results when the urge to speak meets a contrary urge not to do so. In essence, this theoretical formulation holds that stuttering occurs when, in Sheehan's words, "there are conflicting urges to speak and to hold back from speaking." Here is a case study illustrating an approach-avoidance conflict.

One of our cases began to stutter severely on Christmas morning, repeating sounds and syllables, hesitating, and prolonging vowel sounds so markedly that he was referred to us that very afternoon. We had seen the child the week before and had noticed no speech abnormality, nor had his parents, according to their report. He spoke normally that morning until he asked the question "Dih-dih-dih-dih-dih-didn't I g . . . ggg . . . ge . . . get a-a-a-anything fr . . . om mmmmmmy Da . . . da . . . daddy?" The father was not present, having been on a business trip, and he had expected to return that afternoon, bringing his presents with him. However, he was delayed for three more days, and his return did not allay the problem. Subsequent exploration revealed that the child felt profoundly rejected by his busy father.

These three variants of the learning theory seem to complement one another. Together they provide a description of how stuttering starts and develops. We are certain that each of them explains how certain children began to stutter. We are not sure that all of them explain how all stuttering starts.

The Constitutional Theories. The final explanation of stuttering states that the child who stutters has a constitutional difference or predisposition to stuttering. This theory has been slain many times but refuses to die. Such vital tenacity itself deserves some recognition. One of the early formulations of this theory was couched in terms of *cerebral dominance.* Stutterers were said to have a constitutional difference called "dysphemia." This word refers to an underlying neuromuscular condition which reflects itself peripherally in nervous impulses which are poorly timed in their arrival in the paired speech musculatures. It was felt to be an inherited problem or one due to a shift of handedness. At the present time few subscribe to the cerebral dominance theory in its original form but the concept of dysphemia has been broadened to include what Gutzmann called "a weakness in the central coordinating system."

The importance of the concept of dysphemia is that it explains the stutterer's speech interruptions in terms of a nervous system which breaks down *relatively easily* in its integration of the flow of nervous impulses to the paired peripheral muscles. In order to lift the jaw, for instance, nervous impulses must arrive simultaneously in the paired muscles of each side. In some stutterers these arrival times are disrupted; they are not synchronized. It is very difficult to lift a jaw or a wheelbarrow by one handle. The dysphemic individual is able to time his speech coordinations pretty well as long as the coordinating centers in the brain are not being bedeviled by emotional reactions and their backflow of visceral sensations. He can talk pretty well when calm and unexcited. But his thresholds of resistance to emotional disturbance are low. His coordinations break down under relatively little stress. We have all known pianists and golfers who could play excellently by themselves but whose coordinations were pitifully inadequate to the demands of concert or tournament pressures.

It may well be true that the term *dysphemia* is merely a cloak for our ignorance, yet there are many evidences that such a condition exists in certain individuals. Chief among these are research findings which indicate that (1) the tendency to stutter seems to be inherited; (2) the stutterer is often more poorly coordinated in swift or rhythmic movements of the speech musculatures during silence; (3) the stutterer exhibits metabolic and biochemical differences; (4) the stutterer frequently shows confusion in handedness and other peripheral signs of central laterality; (5) the brain waves of stutterers differ from those of nonstutterers. These research findings are not entirely conclusive, since other investigations have challenged their accuracy; yet when we consider that among the groups of stutterers tested there must have been many whose stuttering was of neurotic or developmental origin, the positive findings seem to have increased significance.

Many expressions other than dysphemia have been used to indicate that stutterers are neurologically differentiated from nonstutterers. Some of these are: "neuropathic diathesis," "lack of a sufficient margin of cerebral dominance," "constitutional incoordination," and "nervous instability." Greene[11], for instance, says:

> The stutterer is psychobiologically a variant. Whatever the exact nature of the underlying inferiority—and as yet we do not know—it appears to be an hereditary factor that predisposes the individual to emotional instability and disorganization in general, and to stuttering speech in particular.

Hahn (41), whose text summarizes the current views concerning the theories and therapies of stuttering, declares:

> Most authorities view stuttering as the result of a malfunctioning nervous system, and contend that in the early or primary periods of onset the central nervous system has not reached a maturation point sufficient to withstand certain shocks, childhood diseases, ego competitiveness or malnutrition. These and other "trigger" causes affect the nervous system, and speech, dependent so much on finely adjusted muscle groups under brain leadership, naturally is affected.

A more recent statement of the constitutional theory is that by West (66). He believes, as do all who advocate a constitutional theory, that an underlying condition is activated by communicative and emotional pressures, and hence there is no need to wonder why the stutterer does not always stutter. (Allergies also run in families

[11] J. S. Greene. "Stuttering: What About It?" *Proceedings American Speech Correction Association,* Volume 1, 1931, pages 165-176.

and seem to have a background in the biochemistry of the individual, but they are often precipitated by psychological pressures.) West's idea is that the stutterer has a convulsive disorder akin to epilepsy or rather to its milder childhood form called "pyknolepsy" and has its basis in an imbalance of blood chemistry. The moments of stuttering are triggered by stress and resemble tiny seizures which interrupt the flow of speech and come to be feared by their victim.

Cluttering Origin. Another statement of the constitutional theory, which finally is arousing real interest in speech pathology in this country although it has had a long history elsewhere, is the concept that stuttering is rooted in cluttering, which itself is viewed as the reflection of a constitutional difference. Weiss (64) has called this difference "central language imbalance" and others have used the term "specific language disability." The clutterer is usually late in speaking, has a family history of cluttering and stuttering and retarded speech development, speaks very swiftly and in a disordered manner. Speech is poorly organized, both linguistically, motorically, and perceptually. Reading, writing, and other language difficulties are often present. The articulation is slurred. The onset of speech is delayed. All these features, it is said, point to a basic constitutional difference. Weiss believes that most stuttering begins in the disorganized repetitions of cluttering. Freund (33) does not agree with this sweeping statement but has reported that of those children whose stuttering first appeared at puberty, about 50 per cent had a history of former cluttering. It is our clinical impression that some of our cases did show this origin. There are clutterers who do not stutter, stutterers who do not clutter, some stutterers who have cluttered, and some who still do. But when we find this pattern of cluttering coexisting with the stuttering either in the present symptomatology or in the past histories of these individuals, we tend to suspect the presence of an original constitutional difference or predisposition. Stuttering has more than one source.

Two other final forms of the constitutional theory may be mentioned. Karlin (45) attributes stuttering to delayed myelination of those nerve tracts in the brain which coordinate the muscles used in speech. He explains the fact that there are four times as many males as females who stutter by pointing to the research which shows that myelination in girls is always advanced over that of the boys during the critical age from two to four years, when most stuttering begins.

We also have the formulation of Eisenson,[12] who feels that stutterers possess a constitutional difference which shows itself in a tendency to perseverate in motor activity. Again, some research supports this point of view even as some research seems to support all other theories.

Summing Up. What is a student to believe when so many different explanations exist? Our own resolution of this problem is an eclectic one. We feel that stuttering has many origins, many sources, and that the original causes are not nearly so important as the maintaining causes, once stuttering has started. We can find stutterers who partly fit any one of these various statements of theory and some stutterers who fit several. All stutterers are not cut from the same original cloth. It is important that we know these various explanations because the problems of some of the stutterers we meet can thereby be best understood. The river of stuttering does not flow out of only one lake.

The Development of Stuttering

One of the key characteristics of stuttering is that it changes its form as it develops. This is important because the way we treat any given individual stutterer depends upon the stage of development shown by that stutterer. By treating the beginning stutterer in the same way we would treat an adult, we would almost surely make his stuttering worse. The beginning and the terminal stages of the disorder differ greatly in terms of both the overt and the covert symptoms. The stages in between are less clearly definitive and all stutterers do not seem to follow the same pathway. However, there seems to be a general growth in abnormality, and in frequency. The form of stuttering changes as the years go by. The development of stuttering seems to pass through four main stages, each of which is characterized by different types of outward behaviors and by different kinds of inner feelings. We will describe each a bit later in this chapter. It should be understood, however, that this development is not directly in a straight line. Its path is an oscillating one, but one which usually moves forward in the direction of increasing severity. We

---

[12] J. Eisenson. "A Perseverative Theory of Stuttering," in Eisenson, J. *Stuttering: A Symposium.* New York: Harper & Row, Publishers, 1958, pages 225-271.

have studied the growth of stuttering in hundreds of individual children and we have watched many of them leave the first stage, move into the second, return to the first, move again to the second, and then into the third and fourth stages. Rarely, without help, do we see the person return to earlier stages once he has entered the fourth stage of secondary stuttering, but up to this point reversal and regressions are not unusual.* Let us attempt to trace this growth.

First Stage.   Shortly after its onset, most stuttering seems to consist of short, effortless repetitions and prolongations of the syllable or sound. The general tempo of speech is not disturbed. The child seems quite unaware of his interrupted speech. He bubbles and bounces his way along. He shows no fear of talking, little frustration, and only rarely is there any evidence of momentary struggle. There are periods at times for weeks and months when the speech is normally fluent, only to be followed by another period of frequent stuttering. More trouble seems to occur in states of excitement, ambivalence, or strong communicative need. More difficulty is experienced at the beginning of utterance. For many years this first stage of stuttering has been called *"primary stuttering"* to distinguish it from the chronic, complex adult form, which has been termed "secondary stuttering." Stage one, the primary stage, roughly corresponds to what Bloodstein (27) terms the "first phase" in stuttering development.

Some workers in the field, especially Johnson (42) and others who hold to the semantic theory, do not like the term "primary stuttering" since they feel that the only behavior shown is normal nonfluency. They prefer to reserve the word stuttering for the advanced stages of the disorder. They claim that all nonfluency is normal until the person begins to fear it or struggle with it. Only then does it become abnormal and deserve the term "stuttering." They argue that if all the conditions surrounding the moment of hesitation or repetition were known, it would be a perfectly natural response of a normally functioning human being. Unfortunately our culture does not agree. Unlike the Indians (see Johnson) *we* have a word for excessive repe-

---

* Although we are also sketching the development of stuttering in four stages, we wish to make clear that these are not the same as those described by Bloodstein (Reference 12). His study was based on cross sections of children at certain age levels, which probably accounts for many of the inconsistencies of his findings. Only by studying the growth of stuttering in the individual child sequentially can we hope to understand what takes place.

titions, prolongations, or breaks in the fluency of speech and we call it "stuttering." Perhaps we shouldn't use it, but we do. To try to tell a culture it is thinking or talking incorrectly is to try to sweep back the ocean with a broom. If a boy is saying "Mmmummy, ca . . . ca . . . ca . . . ca . . . can I-I-I-I- I gggggo tuh-to th---e st-st-stu-store wwwwith y-you?" it is terribly difficult to convince his mother that she and her husband and their friends and his teacher are all wrong, and that he is not stuttering at all but merely nonfluent. We in this book prefer to achieve a reduction in their anxiety and puni-tiveness by using the term "primary stuttering."

We have said that *most* stutterers begin by showing the behavior of stage one. Not all of them do. Those whose stuttering stems from a primary neurosis often show facial contortions, hypertension, and struggle from the first beginnings of the disorder. Those in which the stuttering seems to stem from constitutional factors often have more prolongations than repetitions and more quick but transitory struggling is shown. They also tend to show cluttering, delay in language development generally, and few periods of normal fluency are evidenced. The stuttering dates from the beginnings of speech.

Second Stage. Tracing the growth of stuttering in individual stut-terers, we find that certain changes appear in the repetitions and prolongations of sounds. They become faster and more irregular. No longer do they fit smoothly into the normal tempo of syllabic utterance. Instead of saying: "Da. .da. .da. .daddy" he now says "Da. . . .da.da.da. . . . .dadadadaddy." The prolongations become longer, and many of the repetitions end in prolongations, either of the sound or of the posture required by that sound. These are def-initely danger signs and all parents and speech therapists should recognize them. The horse is beginning to run away. Most of the time the child still seems to be unaware of his broken speech but occasionally the discerning parent will report looks of surprise on the child's face, or occasionally he may cry and say, "I can't talk!" But again, the stuttering seems to come in waves and periods of good speech still appear.

Third Stage. After surprise, comes frustration! As the frequency of the moments of stuttering increases, as the repetitions of a sound double and triple, as the prolongations become longer, the child becomes not only aware of his difficulty but profoundly frustrated by it. Now he begins to struggle. The repetitions become forced and often they increase in pitch and irregularity. At times a sirenlike shift upward in pitch is heard on both repetitions or prolongations. Tiny little vibrations called tremors appear on the tensed silent postures of certain sounds. Breathing abnormalities appear as the child attempts to blow open the closed doors of tongues and lips. Facial contortions show themselves as the child struggles to escape from his oscillations and fixations. These are the *overt* symptoms of stage three. The basic covert symptom, as we have said, is the feeling of frustration.

The Stuttering Tremor. We feel we must expand a bit on the subject of tremors for they play a part of supreme importance and are often overlooked or disregarded by those who could seek to understand the nature of stuttering. Their appearance at this stage in the development of the disorder constitutes a danger signal of the greatest significance. The stuttering tremor appears when a fixed articulatory posture is suddenly invested with a surge of tension. In this third stage the repetitions tend to terminate in fixed postures or prolongations. Tight closures of the lips, the tongue, or the vocal cords occur and tiny but very swift vibrations appear in these structures as a result of the tension. These are called tremors.

The lips, for example, in uttering the word *paper*, are pressed tightly together when a series of repetitive syllables fails to result in communication or brings a parental scowl. The child says, "puh-puh-puhpuhpuh-ppppppp . . . aper." In the struggling which takes place the lips are highly tensed. This of course prevents the breath from getting past this articulatory dam. The more tense the stutterer becomes, the tighter the lips are pressed, until finally a sudden localized burst of tension sets into motion a vibrating tremor. Like the "intention tremor" or the "athetoid tremor" of brain-injured individuals, the stuttering tremor creates in its possessor a vivid feeling of inability and frustration. He feels blocked. His lips seem locked by some mysterious force over which he has no control. His response to the awareness of tremor is to increase the tension, which only speeds up the tremor, or to make a sudden jerky movement of the structures involved. If this movement is out of phase with the tremor, he often finds release and the word is uttered. If it is in phase, then he bounces right back into his tremor and the same impasse of self-defeating struggle. These tremors are devastating experiences for most stutterers. To them, they seem as threatening as a sudden inability to move an arm would seem to us. The loss of one's power to control one's limbs or mouth can produce anxiety very quickly, and it does so in the stutterer. Some stutterers begin to avoid feared words because of the penalties society inflicts upon abnormality, as we shall see in the next section. But many others develop their first fears and withdrawals as a result of experiencing tremors.

During this transitional period the stutterer begins to spend his energies, not only in trying to utter the word but also in escaping from the tremors. He begins to battle himself. Many of the spasmodic, bizarre contortions that mark the adult stutterer were originally movements that in the random struggle by chance happened to precede release from tremor. Whatever is done just before an escape from punishment becomes strongly reinforced.

At this time the child often regresses to earlier infantile behavior. He may show temper tantrums, enuresis. He may begin to suck his thumb again. He is under stress now. He knows that he has trouble talking, and the behavior is so obvious that others react to it unfavorably and give it a name. Perhaps he does not think of himself as a "stutterer" but he knows that he "stutters." He feels angered and upset by the breaks in his communication.

It is in this third stage that the temporary remissions from stuttering tend to disappear. Seldom are there long periods of fluent speech. Most days will show some speech difficulty, although it increases in frequency and severity with communicative pressures or emotional upheaval. He still does not avoid speaking and has not analyzed his difficulty enough to locate feared sounds or words. All he knows is that he has trouble talking, that he stutters. He knows that it is unpleasant and frustrating to himself and he is just beginning to realize that it is also unpleasant to others. This is the frustration stage of stuttering.

Some children with low frustration tolerance, due to parental pampering or other factors, enter this third stage very quickly. Also, as we have said, the stutterers whose difficulty is of emotional origin, although they usually begin to stutter later than the others, jump almost immediately into the behavior described. Those whose stuttering stems from the larger reservoir, that of learning to be fluent under conditions which tend to disrupt speech, often linger in the first and second stages for several years. Many of them feel their first frustrations and begin their struggling when they enter school and have to compete with other more fluent children. It is our impression that the stutterer of constitutional origin lingers longest in the first two stages. Perhaps he is accustomed to inadequacy.

Fourth Stage. In this stage, which has usually been termed "secondary stuttering," we find *fear* as the major covert symptom and *avoidance* as the overt one. The stutterer, as a result of the penalties and frustrations he has experienced, not only has fears of specific words, communicative situations, and certain listeners; he also tends to develop general anxiety states. He becomes worried and a worrier. It is also at this stage that shame and guilt appear as covert symptoms of the disorder. He feels guilty for having smeared the conversation, for having appeared so communicatively impotent, for making his listeners wait or suffer. He feels socially objectionable, a verbal leper in a world of words. Also, he often feels hostile toward himself or his listener. These are the extreme reactions shown by the more severely handicapped stutterers. All sorts of gradations of fear, anxiety, guilt, and hostility may be found in specific stutterers in this stage, but each of these emotional reactions is usually found in some degree. They also seem to increase as the stuttering persists. It is in this fourth stage of secondary stuttering that marked personality changes tend to occur.

As in each of the preceding stages, those behaviors which characterized earlier phases can still be seen in stage four. The secondary stutterer still has a few repetitions and prolongations of the types characteristic of stages one and two, though their proportion has decreased. He also shows the struggling behavior of stage three, the frustration period. But in stage four, something new has been added: *fear* and *avoidance*. Stuttering is cumulative in its development. It grows by addition.

In the early days of the airplane, we heard much of the "point of no return." This phrase referred to that point on a transoceanic flight where the supply of gas was no longer sufficient to enable the pilot to fly back to his starting base. In the development of stuttering there is a crudely similar point of no return. It comes with the fixing of situation and word fears. When a case shows marked fears of speaking situations, when he fears certain speech sounds or avoids certain words, the disorder has taken a definite turn for the worse. Many children with marked primary stuttering symptoms, and even quite a few who are struggling in the transitional stage, seem to be able to unravel their speech problems and find perfectly normal speech. They respond readily to indirect therapy of the type we have described. Some of these children show a spontaneous recovery without specific speech therapy even of the indirect kind, as their environments become more favorable or their ego status improves. But once a stutterer begins to objectify his difficulty, to scrutinize approaching situations and words with anxiety, this favorable prognosis is no longer present. The disorder becomes self-perpetuating.

How does this happen? What is the method by which the disorder becomes self-reinforcing? These are tough questions and there are many possible answers. Some authorities insist that a neurotic *need for stuttering* is created once the case becomes aware that his symptoms can help him as well as hurt him. They say that often the stuttering serves as an acceptable excuse, as a defense against the exorbitant demands of conscience or culture. Most stutterers reject this explanation, but some secondary gain from stuttering is often to be found, in the adult case at least.

How Situation and Word Fears Precipitate Stuttering. More immediate and probably more important is the fact that the fear of stuttering, like most fears, creates its own hesitancy and tension and ambivalence. These factors are the very ones which create nonfluency in the normal speaker, and they have a more potent effect on the stutterer's speech. Very often, too, feelings of guilt may create the disturbed emotions so disruptive of fluency.

> The fact that I am Chinese is very important in my stuttering. We are trained from infancy never to do anything which would cause our families to lose face. I cannot tell you how strong this need is, but maybe you can understand by my telling you how I cut off part of my tongue when I stuttered in front of my father when I was only five. I almost bled to death. I don't think at all about my own trouble, only about what a disgrace I am to my family. I fear stuttering more than anyone I have ever known. I am even afraid to talk to myself sometimes. I sleep on my face so I will not speak in my sleep. And the more I think about it, the more I stutter. The more I try to hide it or avoid it, the worse it gets. . . .

The emotions generated during the approach to a feared situation or word are far more powerful than most nonstutterers would be likely to suspect. One of our cases with a normal pulse rate of 74 beats per minute found an increase to 87 as he dialed a phone number, a rate of 114 at the moment his listener said "hello," and a final peak of 123 as he attempted his first speech. Intense feelings of panic, frustration, and self-disgust become clustered about the act of talking, and they are bound to interfere with the smoothness of the functioning. Thus, the fear of stuttering produces more stuttering.

Approach-avoidance Conflicts. Another way of explaining how nonfluency can be increased by word fear is that based on the concept of the approach-avoidance conflict. Suppose the stutterer wants to order a cup of coffee. He starts out: "I would like a cup of. . . ." At this moment, he suddenly becomes highly aware that on the next word his face may become repulsively contorted, that he may find himself frustrated in a long, tremorous prolongation of a tightly pressed-back tongue posture, that his listener may be startled or irritated. Instantly, he feels pulled forward by the need to complete his communication and he feels a strong urge to utter the word "coffee" as quickly as possible. But at the same time, the expected unpleasantness pulls him backward. A tug of war ensues. Sometimes, when neither force is strong enough to win, oscillation occurs and repetitions, hesitations, retrials, and half-hearted speech attempts reflect the equality of the two competing urges.

To speak or not to speak, that is the stutterer's vital question. At times the struggle shows itself in a complete impasse. The urge to attempt the word "coffee," and the fear of the subsequent abnormality counteract each other to such an extent that the person's mouth is immobilized, frozen in a fixed grimace. Thus, either repetitive (clonic) or prolonged (tonic) symptoms may be created by adding fear to the forward flowing process of communication. Fear is the refrigerant that always congeals action. It inhibits. And when one's fluent utterance is suddenly frozen by fear, hesitancies are bound to occur. It is for this reason that we speak of secondary stuttering as being a disorder infinitely more dangerous and difficult than either primary or transitional stuttering.

How the Stuttering Symptoms are Reinforced. There is another basic concept which must be understood by those who wish to help the secondary stutterer. It is this very significant fact: the contortions, tremors, and other unpleasant abnormalities which cause the stutterer so much distress are terminated by the utterance of the word. No matter what silly gyrations his mouth goes through, finally the word comes out. When it does, the panicky fear belonging to that word subsides. In essence, what the stutterer does then is to make a very serious error of judgment. He attributes his release to the struggle and the abnormality. He says, "I squeezed my eyes and then the word came out. If I want to have any future word come out, I'll have to squeeze my eyes."

When any bit of behavior in a punishment situation is followed by release from punishment, it gets powerful reinforcement and strengthening. The stutterer is like the cat in a puzzle-box who happens to look under its left leg at the moment its tail hits the lever that opens the cage. The cat will tend to assume the same head position when it is put back in the cage.

In most cases, the actual release from blocking is due to the fact that the stutterer has had sufficient abnormality to satisfy his morbid expectation. Once the fear is satisfied, the tension subsides, and with it, the tremor. The word can now be uttered. If, at this instant, the stutterer by chance happens to gasp for breath, he will tend to feel he must gasp henceforth. The release has rewarded the behavior which preceded it. Why do secondary stutterers show such an amazing variety of bizarre symptoms? The only ones they have in common are repetitions and prolongations. All others are diverse. We would account for this variety in terms of the reinforcement given certain items of struggle behavior occurring at the moment of release. Anxiety reduction is a powerful conditioner. So also is the escape from punishment. Both of these powerful reinforcers play an important part in secondary stuttering. They create new symptoms and help to perpetuate the disorder. Therapy must be so designed as to prevent them from doing their foul work. They cannot be ignored.

How the Fears of Stuttering Develop. By fear we mean the expectation or anticipation of unpleasantness. The unpleasantness in stuttering can be (1) the experience of frustration, of being unable to communicate, of being unable to move a tongue or lip out of its tremor, of being unable to inhibit facial contortions or abnormal sounds; or (2) it can be the unpleasantness of feeling rejected by one's associates, of being on the receiving end of social penalties, of finding one's speech attempts greeted with anxiety, impatience, pity, or laughter.

Most texts on stuttering stress the fears but ignore the importance of the frustrations which are equally vivid parts of the stuttering experience. The intermittent nature of stuttering makes it all the more unpleasant.

> If I were blind, I could get used to it and learn to make the best of a bad situation. If I were deaf, I could learn to read lips and face the fact that I could never hear again. If I had no arms, I could finally learn to feed myself with my toes or let others feed me. But I'm a stutterer only part-time. Sometimes I talk as well as the best speaker on earth. Then again, boom! I'm stuck, helpless, petrified in the mouth. The next moment I'm normal again. It drives you crazy and you can't ever adjust to it.

The inability to move or control a part of the body is profoundly disturbing. It has some death threat in it. If suddenly you could no longer raise your arm, you would find yourself terribly frightened. You would struggle and be afraid. You would know frustration of a peculiarly vivid kind. The stutterer feels the same way when he finds his jaws frozen in a tremor or his tongue stuck quiveringly to the roof of the mouth.

This temporary inability to move the speech muscles can be explained in many ways: as a manifestation of a latent dysphemia, as a conditioned inhibition, or as a moment of emotional blankness. It may be merely symptomatic of a chronic speech hesitancy which has been practiced so often that it has become habitual. It may be only the result of simultaneous and opposing desires to speak and to remain silent. But introspectively, the dominant feature of the stuttering experience is the feeling of being "blocked" in the forward flow of speech. As one stutterer said:

> What happens is that I can't go on. I can't complete the word I want to say. I'm stuck. I either hang there struggling on a consonant or find my mouth repeating the same syllable over and over again like a broken record. Sometimes I'm talking great guns when bang! I'm hung up higher than a kite. Something seems to freeze my tongue or throat shut or else it turns it over to an automatic repeater.

In our first chapter we described some of the ways our society reacts to the person handicapped in speech. In it we traced the historical progress from attitudes of rejection, through humor and pity to the more modern policy of retraining and reeducation. The stutterer knows all these reactions and more, too. Here are some excerpts from autobiographies:

What hit me worst of all and something I've never forgot or forgiven was how the parents of other kids would yank them away from me when they would hear me stutter. They wouldn't let me come in their yard to play. They told me to go home and stutter somewhere else. They didn't want their kid to get infected.

. . .

Elsie was the worst. She was always teasing me, calling me "stutter-cat" or "stumble-tongue" or mocking me. She was so slick at it that hardly anyone but me noticed it. She'd say it as she went by my desk, under her breath, so only I got it. I could have killed her if I hadn't been so hurt and helpless. And I couldn't hit her, because boys can't hit girls, not even out on the playground.

. . .

Whenever I'd stutter, Dad would slump down behind his paper, or if he didn't have any, he'd just look away and pretend to think. Some-times, he'd just drum on the table with his fingers or hum an absent-minded little tune, as though to say, "I'm not listening so it doesn't count." He never teased me or said anything about my stuttering. No one did. It was as unmentionable as Sex. My father, as a small town minister, believed in letting sleeping dogs lie. I grew up feeling that stuttering was somehow pretty sinful.

. . .

My nickname was "Spit-it-out-Joe" or "Spitty" for short. I got it from my third-grade teacher, an impatient, aggressive old dame who couldn't bear to hear me block. Every time I did, she'd yelp, "Spit it out, Joe!" and the kids picked it up and I've carried the tag for years. I still have dreams of killing the old hag.

. . .

My mother only did one thing when I stuttered. She held her breath. She never teased me, punished me or seemed embarrassed. Her lovely face was always serene. But she held her breath. She was entirely pa-tient, sweet and understanding. She gave me the feeling that she was proud of me and was completely confident that everything would turn out all right. But she held her breath every time I stuttered. That breath-holding sometimes sounded louder than thunder to me.

It is from experiences such as these that most young stutterers begin to expect unpleasantness in the act of speaking. This expec-tation may at first be specifically focused on a single word, the one on which the unpleasantness occurred. Or it may start with a more general fear of a certain situation, such as talking over the telephone, or speaking to a hard-of-hearing grandmother. Stuttering fears are of two main types: situation fears and word fears.

Word Fears. The first word fears arise from two main sources: (1) from words which are remembered because of the severe frustration or vivid penalties experienced when uttering them, and (2) from words which because of their frequent use under stress accumulate more stuttering memories upon them.

> The question words have always been hard for me to say, ever since I can remember. What? Where? When? Why? How? My folks were always so busy. I always had to interrupt something important they were doing. They either answered without paying any real attention so I had to say it again, or else they told me not to bother them, or they told me to stop asking so many questions.

> My own name is my hardest word. Too many big people have asked me, "What is your name, sonny?" I've had to say it too many times when I got into trouble. I've said it so often and stuttered on it so often that I almost think it should be spelled with more than one *t*, like T-T-T-Tommy.

> I believe I remember the very first time I stuttered or at least it was the first time I ever noticed it. I was in the second grade, in the third row, last seat. The teacher asked me several simple *times* problems in multiplication, and I stuttered and she got irritated and asked me something simpler until finally she said, "Okay, dummy, how much is two and two?" and I couldn't say, "Four." I've been afraid of that number and of all *f* words ever since.

These fears, starting from such simple instances, grow swiftly. Often their growth almost seems malignant, constantly invading new areas of one's mental life. A child begins by first fearing the word *paper*. He has had an unpleasant experience in uttering it. He sees it approaching and expects some more unpleasantness, either frustration or penalty. He finds more difficulty. Soon he is fearing many *p* words besides *paper*. He recognizes *pay* and *penny* as hard words to say. Then the fear generalizes or becomes fastened to other features of the stuttering experience. It spreads to other words having similar visual, acoustic, kinesthetic, tactual, or semantic features.

The visual transfer, for example, may be in terms of spelling cues. Because of his fear of *p* words, he may see the word *pneumonia* as dreaded, even though the actual utterance begins with a nasal sound. Or, to illustrate the acoustic transfer, he may come to fear the *k*, *ch*, and *t* sounds because they, like the *p*, are ejected with a puff of air. Or tactually and kinesthetically, he may soon be fearing all the other lip sounds, starting with the *b,* then spreading to the *w, m,* and even the *f* and *v* sounds. The spread of fear can take several directions. The following example illustrates how the cues precipitating fear of stuttering can spread semantically.

I had never, so far as I remember, had any real trouble on words beginning with a *w.* Oh, I might have had some, I suppose, but generally I considered them easy sounds to say. And I had very frequently used the word, "well," as a sort of handle, saying it as a kind of way to get started. Sometimes, of course, I might have to say it three or four times before the next word came out, but, anyway, I could always say "well." It was a handy trick to cover up and postpone. Then one day I had an experience which ruined that word for me forever. To this day, "well" is a very hard word for me to speak without stuttering, and it all happened because of that one experience. It happened like this. I was in a grocery store, asking for five pork chops, and I got blocked in saying the name of the meat. It was a long one with hard sticking in my throat and I kept trying to break it by saying "well." I must have used too many of them because a man behind me impatiently shouted, "Well, well? You aren't well, young lady. Get out of here and go home to bed. You're sick. Not well, sick! Do you hear, sick!" I fled without the pork chops, but I can never use the word in the sense of healthy without blocking completely. I sometimes can use it as a starter, but if I happen to think of it as the antonym of "sick," I block on it immediately.

Situation Fears. We have been describing the stutterer's conflicting urges to utter and to avoid the utterance of a given word. Shall he or shan't he attempt it? He scrutinizes the word for cues which might indicate danger, for resemblances to other words formerly provocative of great unpleasantness. The same sort of process occurs on the situation level. Sheehan (55) puts the matter as follows:

At the *situation* level there is a parallel conflict between entering and not entering a feared situation. The stutterer's behavior toward using the telephone, reciting in class, or introducing himself to strangers illustrates this conflict. Many situations which demand speech hold enough threat to produce a competing desire to hold back.

Often in word fears there occurs an actual rehearsal of some of the expected abnormality. Breathing records show that even prior to speech attempt the stutterer's silent breathing often goes through the same peculiar pattern that he shows when actually stuttering. In situation fears this is not the case. Situation fears are more vague, more generalized, more focused on the *attitudes* of the listener and the stutterer than upon the *behavior.* Situation fears can range in intensity all the way from uncertainty to complete panic. We have known stutterers to faint and fall to the floor in their anticipation of a speaking situation. The fear fluctuates in intensity from moment to moment. It is often set off by the stutterer's recognition of certain features of an approaching speech situation as similar to those of earlier situations in which he met great penalty or frustration. Stutterers learn to scan an approaching speaking situation with all the concentration of a burglar looking over a prospective bank. Like word fears, situation fears generalize. They may begin from a simple recognition on the part of the child that he was having much difficulty in talking to a certain storekeeper. Remembering this, he may begin to fear speaking in any store; or to take another tack, he might begin to fear talking to all strange men, or to mention still another, he might fear having to relay any message given him by his mother. Situation fears are like word fears in another way, too. Avoidance increases them greatly. The more the stutterer runs away from a given speaking situation, the more terrifying it becomes.

Both situation and word fears can serve as *maintaining* causes of the disorder. By constantly reinforcing them by avoidance, the stutterer keeps his stuttering "hot." Any therapy worthy of the name must have as one of its basic aims the elimination of this avoidance. Stuttering begins to break down and disappear as soon as the stutterer ceases his constant reinforcing.

Avoidance Behavior. The stuttering picture shown by those who have progressed to this fourth stage in the development of stuttering can best be understood in terms of avoidance and escape. Let us be very clear about what is being avoided and escaped. It is the experience of finding a part of the body mysteriously oscillating or fixating; it is the experience of having communication blocked and retarded; it is the experience of behaving in a way which other people penalize.

No one likes to have feelings of frustration, anxiety, guilt, or hostility. When these feelings appear in conjunction with repetitive or prolonged interruptions in the flow of speech, those interruptions will be viewed as highly unpleasant. The stutterer will seek to prevent, avoid, or escape from repetitions which keep repeating, from prolongations of a sound or posture which persist. It is very important that we understand that to the secondary stutterer, this repeating and prolonging appears to be involuntary, uncontrollable, mysterious. When this behavior is anticipated, the stutterer tries to avoid it; when it has occurred, the stutterer tries to escape from it.

How the Stutterer Avoids Stuttering. Since, in stage four, the secondary stutterer has learned to scan approaching speech situations for clues that indicate he will probably have difficulty, and since he has also learned to scrutinize the formulation of his sentences for "hard" words and sounds, he naturally tends to avoid these words and situations. One of our child cases just stopped talking altogether; one of our adults became a hermit in the Ozarks. But most stutterers cannot use this drastic solution to their problem. They continue to talk but they talk as little as possible in these feared situations, and avoid or alter them if possible. It is often difficult for the nonstutterer to realize that much of the abnormality he witnesses in examining a stutterer is due to the latter's efforts to avoid unpleasantness. The desire to avoid stuttering may lead to such jargon as "To what price has the price of tomatoes increased today?" when the stutterer merely wished to say "How much are your tomatoes?" Dodging difficult words and speech situations becomes almost a matter of second nature to the stutterer. He prefers to seem ignorant rather than to expose his disability when called upon in school. He develops such a facility at using synonyms that he often sounds like an excerpt from a thesaurus. He will walk a mile to avoid using a telephone. And the tragedy of this avoidance is that it increases the fear and insecurity, makes the stutterer more hesitant, and doubles his burden.

Postponement. Procrastination as a reaction to approaching unpleasantness is an ordinary human trait, and the stutterer has more than his share of the weakness. We have worked with stutterers whose entire overt abnormality consisted of the filibustering repetition of words and phrases preceding the dreaded word. They never had any difficulty on the word itself, but their efforts to postpone the speech attempt until they felt they could say the word produced an incredible amount of abnormality. One of them said, "My name is . . . my name is . . . my . . . my . . . my name is . . . my name . . . name . . . name . . . what I mean is, uh . . . uh . . . my name is Jack Olson." Others will merely pause in tense silence for what seems to them like hours before blurting out the word. Others disguise the postponement by pretending to think, by licking their lips, by saying "um" or "er." Postponement as a habitual approach to feared words creates an anxiety and a fundamental hesitancy which in themselves are precipitative of more stuttering.

Starters. Stutterers also use many tricks to start the speech attempt after postponement has grown painfully long. They time this moment of speech attempt with a sudden gesture, or eye-blink, or jaw-jerk, or other movement. They return to the beginning of the sentence and race through the words preceding the feared word in hope that their momentum will "ride them over their stoppages." They insert words, phrases, or sounds that they can say, so that the likelihood of blocking will be lessened. One of our stutterers hissed before every feared word, "because I get started with the *s* sound which I can nearly always make." Another used the phrase "Let me see" as a magic incantation. He would utter things like this: "My name is Lemesee Peter Slack." Another, whose last name was Ranney, always passed as O'Ranney, since she used the "oh" as a habitual device to get started. Starters are responsible for many of the bizarre symptoms of stuttering, since they become habituated and involuntary. Thus, the taking of a deep breath prior to speech attempt may finally become a sequence of horrible gasping.

Antiexpectancy. The antiexpectancy devices are used to prevent or minimize word fears from dominating the attention of the stutterer. Thus, one of our cases laughed constantly, even when saying the alphabet or asking central for a phone number or buying a package of cigarettes. He had found that, by assuming an attitude incompatible with fear, he was able to be more fluent. Yet he was one of the most morose individuals we have ever met. Other stutterers adopt a singsong style, or a monotone, or a very soft, whispered speech so that all words are made so much alike that no one will be dreaded. Needless to say, all these tricks fail to provide more than temporary relief, and all of them are vicious because they augment the fear in the long run.

How the Stutterer Tries to Escape. As we have said earlier, the experience of finding one's mouth repeating a syllable uncontrollably or discovering one's tongue or lips frozen in a fixed posture is not only unpleasant but almost terrifying. There is an overwhelming desire to escape from this experience, to "break the block," to "get free from it," to find release. These are the stutterer's own words. Williams (67) has clearly expressed this common experience of the mysterious something which holds the stutterer in *its* mysterious grip. Undesired perseveration in any activity is traumatic. It makes one doubt one's will. It violates the integrity of the self.

Interrupter Devices. The fast little vibrations called tremors which first appear during the third stage are very prevalent in secondary stuttering. They are produced by highly tensing the muscles that form a fixed posture, often an abnormal one. When triggered by a sudden ballistic movement or surge of tension, the tremors come into being. The stutterer doesn't know what they are, or how he sets them off. All he knows is that some part of him is vibrating and it scares him as it would you. In some stutterers several structures will be vibrating at the same time—the lips, the jaw, and the diaphragm, and often at different rates. The case attempts to free himself from the tremor by increasing the tension or by using some interrupter device similar to the starter tricks he has used to initiate speech attempt after prolonged postponement. He tries to wrench himself out of the frozen vibration of the tremor by sheer force. Even as he closes the articulatory door of the tongue or lips and holds it tightly shut, he strives to blow it open with a blast of air from below. When the opposing forces are equal, nothing happens except the quivering of the muscles. Oddly enough no stutterer tries to open the speech doors voluntarily; he must break them down with a surge of power. As in transitional stuttering, the random struggling often results in out-of-phase movements of the vibrating structures which cause a release from tremor and make possible the utterance of the word. One stutterer may squeeze his eyes shut; another will jerk his whole trunk; another may suck air in through his nostrils. These peculiar reactions have become habituated through their chance presence at the moment of tremor release. The anxiety reduction, the freedom from punishment, give them their compulsive strength. The stutterer comes to feel that only through using them can he ever escape from the dreadful feeling of inability which the tremor creates in him. Even when they do not give release, he will try them over again, sniffing, not once, but twenty and thirty times in his desperate effort to free himself from the mysterious closure that his opposing efforts have produced. There are easier ways to terminate tremors than these, but few stutterers ever find them without the aid of a therapist.

Other Reactions of Escape.   It is obvious that the same devices used to interrupt tremors can also be used to interrupt repetitions or prolongations of sounds, syllables, or postures. A few stutterers split their words, giving up the attempt to produce an integrated word and finishing it after a gap. They would say "MMMMMM. . . .other." More frequently the stutterer responds to the experience by ceasing the speech attempt and making a retrial, often only to find himself again in the same predicament. He may stop upon feeling an interruption in speech flow and try the entire word again, to stop and use some starting device on the retrial, to stop and use a distraction, to stop and assume a confident behavior, to stop and postpone the new attempt for a time, to stop and avoid the word, and to stop and wait until almost all breath is gone, subsequently saying the word on residual air.*

Stuttering as a Self-reinforcing Disorder.   We have said that usually when stuttering develops into its fourth stage, little hope can be held that it will be "outgrown" or disappear. Even when the environment is changed so that it is permissive and free from fluency disruptors, the person continues to stutter. A few individuals are able to escape even after they enter this stage only because their morale factor in the stuttering equation is powerfully strengthened through other achievements. But usually, once fear and frustration, avoidance and escape have shown themselves, the disorder becomes self-perpetuating. As a response, it becomes the stimulus to other stuttering responses. It is necessary to understand how this comes about.

The Vicious Circle.   Not only is word fear able to beget stuttering symptoms; it almost seems to be able to reproduce itself. When words or situations are perceived as being full of unpleasantness, the stutterer tends to avoid them. He not only becomes more hesitant in his speech, but also in his general behavior. He escapes from the approach-avoidance misery by refusing to talk, or by using a synonym instead of the word that scares him, or by putting off the speech attempt as long as possible. But the future fear is increased

---

* A detailed description of the procedures used in examining a stutterer is provided in the Appendix. See pages 485-490.

by each successful avoidance. Here is an excerpt from a stutterer's autobiography:

> For years I ducked *k* and *g* words. They were my "Jonah" sounds. They always made me stutter. So I just wouldn't use them. There are lots of ways a stutterer has of hiding his running away from the words he can't say and I knew all of them and used them. But then, when I was fifteen, my folks moved to Kenmore Street in Greenwood and I had to give my address using the feared sounds. I would avoid all I could but there are some times when you can't and you just have to say it. Well, I stuttered harder and longer and more awful on that Kenmore word than any other I've ever said. And even now I'm more afraid of *k* words than of any other. I think it's because I backed away from them so long.

What happens is this: The successful avoidance causes some anxiety reduction. Then, when a similar situation presents itself, the need to avoid is even stronger due to the preceding reinforcement. But now, no avoidance is possible. The conflict becomes even greater. And so several vicious circles (or rather spirals) are set into motion. The more one stutters, the more he fears certain words and situations. The more he fears, the more he stutters. The more he stutters, the harder he struggles. The more he struggles, the more penalties he receives, and the greater becomes his fear. The more he fears, the more he avoids; and the more he avoids speech, the more he fears speaking. And so the stutterer becomes caught in the tangled ropes of his own knotting. Once stuttering creates fear, and this fear, more fear and more stuttering, the disorder can exist on a self-sustaining basis. It can maintain and perpetuate itself even though the original causes may long since have lost all effectiveness and importance. Predisposing or precipitating causes have little importance, once the chain reaction gets going. Perhaps it is for this reason that deep psychotherapy has had but meager success with stuttering. Once stuttering becomes not only a response but also a stimulus, it must be attacked directly.

Personality Changes. In our own clinical studies of stuttering development over the years, it seems that many stutterers begin to show marked changes in personality after they enter the fourth stage of secondary stuttering. Many of them respond to their unpleasant experiences, by becoming shy, withdrawn, and aloof. This is supported by Goodstein's (39) review of the research. He concludes that when a group of adult stutterers is compared with a comparable group of normal speakers, the stutterers "do appear different, usually more anxious, tense and socially withdrawn." However, he also concludes that adult stutterers *as a group* are not primarily neurotic or severely maladjusted. Perhaps the wisest course is to assess the degree of maladjustment in any one case. Some stutterers have more traumatic experiences than others. Some are more vulnerable. Some show marked personality changes; others do not. As Murphy and Fitz-Simons[13] write: "A reasonably broad interpretation of the greater number of research findings on the stuttering personality may be that the personalities of stuttering persons can be distributed along a very broad adjustment *continuum* extending from psychotic to normal adjustment."

In our clinical work with severe adult stutterers we find this range described by Murphy. Some of them show obsessive, compulsive behavior and general anxieties, guilts, and hostilities which are far from normal. They show the pattern characteristic of what Freund (33) calls an "expectancy neurosis." This is how Freund describes it:

> The expectancy neuroses represent neurotic disturbances of learned but automatized skills, and also of simple motor or vegetative functions. They are all based on actual traumatic ("primary") experiences of helplessness and failure in the performance of these activities. The activities therefore become dreaded and the anticipation of their recurrence leads, via inhibition, etc., to a repetition of the failure, thus establishing a vicious spiral.[14]

What we are saying is that the experiences of a stutterer in the final stage of stuttering are such that the *possibility* of a marked change in personality can be expected—the possibility, not the certainty. Indeed, in working with these people, we are constantly surprised that so many of them appear pretty normal except in communication. We find the odd ones, but we also find others who seem to have made the best of a bad situation. It is our impression that those whose stuttering seems to stem from constitutional factors make the best adjustment; those of developmental origin, the next

---

[13] Murphy, A. T., and Fitz-Simons, R. M. *Stuttering and Personality Dynamics.* New York: Ronald Press, 1960, page 153.

[14] H. Freund. "Psychopathological Aspects of Stuttering," *American Journal of Psychotherapy,* Volume 7, 1953, 689-705; p. 679.

best, and those whose stuttering comes from basic emotional conflicts, the worst.

Summary

Perhaps the best way we can summarize this material is to use the picture or map in Figure 28. Stuttering has three sources; the major one represented by the largest, Lake Learning, into which the stream from Constitutional Reservoir flows. Neurosis Pond is

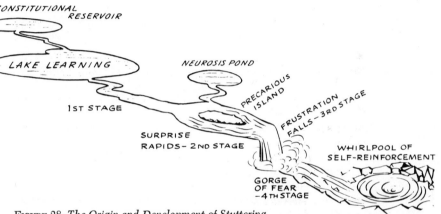

FIGURE 28. *The Origin and Development of Stuttering*

also one of the sources of stuttering but it is smaller. Its contribution to the flow also occurs further down the river's course. Stuttering can come from any of these three sources.

As the stream leaves Lake Learning it flows slowly and many a child caught in its current may make it to shore by himself or with a bit of parental or therapeutic help. Some of them are cast up on Precarious Island and become fluent for a time, only to be swept away again by the swift moving emotional currents from Neurosis Pond. The second stage in the development of stuttering is represented by Surprise Rapids, and the stutterer begins to know that he is in trouble. It isn't hard to rescue him, however, if you know how to do it.

Once he is swept over Frustration Falls, however, he takes a beating from the many rocks that churn the stream. Despite their random struggling, a few make it to shore even at this stage, the third stage, but they usually need an understanding therapist and cooperative parents to help them. The river flows even faster here and soon it enters the Gorge of Fear. This is the worst stretch of the whole stream of stuttering for below it lies the Whirlpool of Self-reinforcement. Once the child is caught in its constant circling, there is little hope that he will ever make it to shore by himself. Only an able and stout swimmer who knows not only this part, but all of the river of stuttering, can hope to save him. Where does the river end? King Charles the First knows.

PROJECTS

1. Demonstrate to the class all the various types of postponement devices. Insert them before all words beginning with *l*.
2. Present a stutterer before the class and describe in your commentary afterward his avoidance and release reactions.
3. Stutter severely to three strangers and report your feelings and the audience reactions.
4. Pretend that all words beginning with *s* are feared and use synonyms or circumlocutions to avoid using them in telling of an experience before the class.
5. Interview a stutterer concerning his feelings of fear and frustration.
6. Go with a stutterer into a feared speaking situation and with his help try to assign numerical values to each of the factors in his stuttering equation so that they reflect the items which are more potent.
7. Interview some stutterer to find the history of his feared situations.
8. Analyze some stutterer's tremors to ascertain their location, how they are set off, and how they are terminated.
9. With some other member of the class, present a debate on the nature of stuttering in terms of its causes. One of you should take the neurotic and the other the semantic point of view.
10. Demonstrate to the class the overt behaviors shown in each of the four stages of the development of stuttering. Also comment on the covert features of each stage.
11. Have a tape-recorded conversation with a friend in which both of you tell anecdotes about similar experiences. Listen to the tape and analyze and list all of your nonfluencies. Then compare them with those of a stutterer.

12. Make a polygraphic recording of the breathing of a stutterer in silence, when speaking alone, and when speaking to an audience. What differences do you find?

13. Have a stutterer read and reread a paragraph four times. Count the number of stutterings on each reading and prepare a graph showing what changes occur. Explain the results in terms of the stuttering equation.

14. Make a list of items under each of the three main theories concerning the nature of stuttering which will show contrasts between them.

15. Make a large wall chart of the figure given in the chapter showing the development of stuttering.

REFERENCES

16. Abbott, J. A. "Repressed Hostility as a Factor in Adult Stuttering," *Journal of Speech Disorders,* Volume 12, 1947, pages 428-430.

17. Ainsworth, S. "Integrating Theories of Stuttering," *Journal of Speech Disorders,* Volume 10, 1945, pages 205-210.

18. ———. "Method for Integrating Theories of Stuttering," in L. E. Travis (ed.) *Handbook of Speech Pathology.* New York: Appleton-Century-Crofts, 1957, pages 947-964.

19. Arnold, G. E. "Studies in Tachyphemia: I. Present Concepts of Etiological Factors," *Logos,* Volume 3, 1960, pages 25-45.

20. Aron, M. L. "The Nature and Incidence of Stuttering among a Bantu Group of School-Going Children," *Journal Speech and Hearing Disorders,* Volume 27, 1962, pages 116-128.

21. Barbara, D. A. *Stuttering: A Psychodynamic Approach to Its Understanding.* New York: Julian Press, Inc., 1954.

22. Bleumel, C. S. "Concepts of Stammering: A Century in Review," *Journal Speech and Hearing Disorders,* Volume 25, 1960, pages 24-32.

23. ———. "Primary and Secondary Stammering," *Quarterly Journal of Speech,* Volume 18, 1932, pages 187-200.

24. ———. "Stuttering: A Psychiatric Point of View," *Journal Speech and Hearing Disorders,* Volume 23, 1958, pages 263-267.

25. Bloodstein, O. "Stuttering as an Anticipatory Struggle Reaction," in J. Eisenson (ed.). *Stuttering: A Symposium.* New York: Harper & Row, Publishers, 1958, pages 1-70.

26. ———. "The Development of Stuttering: I. Changes in Nine Basic Features," *Journal Speech and Hearing Disorders,* Volume 25, 1960, pages 219-237.

27. ———. "The Development of Stuttering: II. Developmental Phases," *Journal Speech and Hearing Disorders,* Volume 25, 1960, pages 366-376.

28. ———. "The Development of Stuttering: III. Theoretical and Clinical Implications," *Journal Speech and Hearing Disorders,* Volume 26, 1961, pages 67-82.

29. Coriat, I. H. "The Psychoanalytic Conception of Stuttering," *The Nervous Child,* Volume 2, 1943, pages 167-171.

30. Davis, D. M. "The Relation of Repetitions in the Speech of Young Children to Certain Measures of Language Maturity and Situational Factors," *Journal of Speech Disorders,* Volume 5, 1940, pages 235-246.

31. Douglass, E., and B. Quarrington. "The Differentiation of Interiorized and Exteriorized Stuttering," *Journal Speech and Hearing Disorders,* Volume 17, 1952, pages 377-385.

32. Dunlap, K. "Stammering: Its Nature, Etiology and Therapy," *Journal of Comparative Psychology,* Volume 37, 1944, pages 187-202.

33. Freund, H. "Psychopathological Aspects of Stuttering," *American Journal of Psychotherapy,* Volume 7, 1953, pages 689-705.

34. ———. "Psychosis and Stuttering," *Folia Phoniatrica,* Volume 7, 1955, pages 133-152.

35. Glasner, P. J., and F. D. Vermilyea. "An Investigation of the Definition and Use of the Diagnosis, 'Primary Stuttering,'" *Journal Speech and Hearing Disorders,* Volume 18, 1953, pages 161-167.

36. ———. "Personality Characteristics and Emotional Problems in Stutterers under the Age of Five," *Journal Speech and Hearing Disorders,* Volume 14, 1949, pages 135-138.

37. ——— and D. Rosenthal. "Parental Diagnosis of Stuttering in Young Children," *Journal Speech and Hearing Disorders,* Volume 22, 1957, pages 288-295.

38. Goda, S. "Stuttering Manifestations Following Spinal Meningitis," *Journal Speech and Hearing Disorders,* Volume 26, 1961, pages 392-393.

39. Goodstein, L. D. "Functional Speech Disorders and Personality: A Survey of the Research," *Journal Speech and Hearing Research,* Volume 1, 1958, pages 359-376.

40. Gray, M. "The X Family: A Clinical and Laboratory Study of a 'Stuttering' Family," *Journal of Speech Disorders,* Volume 5, 1940, pages 343-348.

41. Hahn, E. F. *Stuttering: Significant Theories and Therapies.* Stanford, Calif.: Stanford University Press, 1943.

42. Johnson, W. (ed.). *Stuttering in Children and Adults.* Minneapolis: University of Minnesota Press, 1955.

43. ———. "The Indians Have No World for It: I. Stuttering in Children," *Quarterly Journal of Speech,* Volume 30, 1944, pages 330-337.

44. ———. "The Indians Have No Word for It: II. Stuttering in Adults," *Quarterly Journal of Speech,* Volume 30, 1944, pages 456-465.

45. Karlin, I. N. "A Psychosomatic Theory of Stuttering," *Journal of Speech Disorders,* Volume 12, 1947, pages 319-322.

46. King, P. T. "Perseveration in Stutterers and Nonstutterers," *Journal Speech and Hearing Research,* Volume 4, 1961, pages 346-357.

47. LaFollette, A. C. "Parental Environment of Stuttering Children," *Journal Speech and Hearing Disorders,* Volume 21, 1956, pages 202-207.

48. Lemert, E. M. "Some Indians Who Stutter," *Journal Speech and Hearing Disorders,* Volume 18, 1953, pages 168-174.

49. ———. "Stuttering and Social Structure in Two Pacific Societies," *Journal Speech and Hearing Disorders,* Volume 27, 1962, pages 3-10.

50. Milisen, R., and C. Van Riper. "A Study of the Predicted Duration of the Stutterer's Blocks as Related to Their Actual Duration," *Journal of Speech Disorders,* Volume 4, 1939, pages 339-345.

51. Moncour, J. P. "Parental Domination in Stuttering," *Journal Speech and Hearing Disorders,* Volume 17, 1952, pages 155-165.

52. Selson, S. E. "Personal Contact as a Factor in the Transfer of Stuttering," *Human Biology,* Volume 11, 1939, pages 393-418.

53. Nelson, S. E. "The Role of Heredity in Stuttering," *Journal of Pediatrics,* Volume 14, 1939, pages 642-654.

54. Robinson, F. "Nature and Treatment of Stuttering in Children," in N. M. Levin (ed.). *Voice and Speech Disorders.* Springfield, Ill.: Charles C. Thomas, Publisher, 1962, pages 698-728.

55. Sheehan, J. H. "Conflict Theory of Stuttering," in J. Eisenson (ed.) *Stuttering: A Symposium,* pages 121-166.

56. ——— P. A. Cortese, and R. G. Hadley. "Guilt, Shame and Tension in Graphic Projections of Stuttering," *Journal Speech and Hearing Disorders,* Volume 27, 1962, pages 129-139.

57. Snyder, M. A. "Stuttering and Coordination," *Logos,* Volume 1, 1958, pages 36-44.

58. Travis, L. E. "The Need for Stuttering," *Journal of Speech Disorders,* Volume 5, 1940, pages 193-202.

59. ———. "The Unspeakable Feelings of People with Special Reference to Stuttering," in L. E. Travis (ed.) *Handbook of Speech Pathology.* New York: Appleton-Century-Crofts, 1957, pages 916-946.

60. Van Riper, C., and L. Gruber. *A Case Book in Stuttering*. New York: Harper & Row, Publishers, 1957.

61. ———. *Stuttering*. Chicago: National Society for Crippled Children and Adults, 1948.

62. ———. "The Effect of Penalty upon the Frequency of Stuttering Spasms," *Journal of Genetic Psychology*, Volume 50, 1937, pages 193-195.

63. ———. "The Growth of the Stuttering Spasm," *Quarterly Journal of Speech*, Volume 23, 1937, pages 70-73.

64. Weiss, D. A. "Therapy of Cluttering," *Folia Phoniatrica*, Volume 12, 1960, pages 216-228.

65. West, R. "A Neurological Test for Stutterers," *Journal of Neurology and Psychopathology*, Volume 10, 1929, pages 114-118.

66. ———. "An Agnostic's Speculations About Stuttering," in J. Eisenson (ed.) *Stuttering: A Symposium*. New York: Harper & Row, Publishers, 1958, pages 167-222.

67. Williams, D. E., "A Point of View about Stuttering," *Journal Speech and Hearing Disorders*, Volume 22, 1957, pages 300-397.

68. Wingate, M. E. "Evaluation and Stuttering, Part I.: Speech Characteristics of Young Children," *Journal Speech and Hearing Disorders*, Volume 27, 1962, pages 106-115.

69. ———. "Evaluation and Stuttering: II. Environmental Stress and Critical Appraisal of Speech," *Journal Speech and Hearing Disorders*, Volume 27, 1962, pages 244-257.

70. Wischner, G. J. "Stuttering Behavior and Learning: A Preliminary Theoretical Formulation," *Journal of Speech and Hearing Disorders*, Volume 15, 1950, pages 324-335.

CHAPTER TWELVE

Stuttering: Its Treatment

Here is an excerpt from a recent letter written us by a public-school speech therapist.

The one arena in which I still feel incompetent after eleven years of practicing my profession is that of stuttering. I've had more failures with my stuttering cases than with any of the others. Perhaps I haven't had time enough to give them the intensive treatment they seem to need but it isn't only that. It's that I'm not sure what I'm trying to do. I try lots of things, and some of them seem to work for a time, but the improvement doesn't last. Oh a few of them do get better but I don't see what I've done when they do. The worst of it is that you are often judged by what you do with the stutterer. He stands out in any school-room. I can help a hundred children with articulation problems to get good speech and no one seems to notice. All they can see is that one stutterer I don't seem to be able to help.

And here is an account of something that happened forty years ago, when speech pathology as a profession was in its infancy.

In 1920 at an evening session Erastus Palmer, City College of New York, was called up by the president (McKean) to fulfill his promise to "start something." He did so by issuing a blanket challenge to any-one to cite a single instance of a stammerer who had been corrected and had stayed corrected for more than six months when not under the direct influence of his teacher. . . . In the end no one was able to take up the challenge and no instance of a permanent cure was cited.[1]

Are we to conclude from these two accounts that the stutterer presents an insoluble problem? Not at all. He usually presents a

---

[1] Anon., "Notes," Quarterly Journal of Speech, Volume 6, 1920, page 87.

difficult one, and one which requires more than token treatment. We have learned much about the successful treatment of stuttering in the last forty years. We even know some ways of preventing it,[2] and its incidence in the general population seems to be decreasing. However, if we are to help the stutterer, we must know what we are doing and why we are doing it.

A Design for Stuttering Therapy.   Two very important facts serve as the foundation of our therapy for stuttering: (1) stuttering is intermittent, and (2) its specific occurrence, frequency, and severity vary systematically with the strength of certain factors which can be defined and manipulated. If we can focus our therapy on these factors so that those which make stuttering worse are weakened sufficiently and those which make for less stuttering are strengthened, the frequency and severity of stuttering will decrease and ultimately stuttering will disappear. Therapy then is viewed as selective reinforcement and extinction. Stuttering is no mysterious curse to be eliminated by incantation or voodoo practices. Like all human behavior it obeys certain laws. It may be awful but it's also lawful.

The Focus of Theory.   In our general stuttering equation (see page 309 for an explanation) we said that these were the things which made stuttering worse: (1) penalty, frustration, anxiety, guilt, and hostility, (2) situation fears based on memories of past stuttering unpleasantness in similar situations, (3) word and phonetic fears based on memories of past stuttering unpleasantness on similar words and sounds. There is also a fourth factor, C, representing the communicative importance of that which is being said. Stutterers stutter more on messages and words which are especially important in communication. Stuttering, as numerous researches have shown,[3] increases with the propositionality (communicative meaningfulness) of the material read or the thing said. There are also many things which seemed to make stuttering better but all of them appeared to be able to fit into the category of morale or ego strength. Our equation then is as follows:

$$\frac{(PFAGH) + (Sf\,Wf) + Cs}{M + Fl} = \text{Stuttering frequency and severity.}$$

[2] See the booklet "Stuttering: Its Prevention," Speech Foundation of America, Memphis, Tennessee, 1962.

[3] Jon Eisenson (ed.). *Stuttering: A Symposium.* New York: Harper & Row, Publishers, 1958, pages 235-244.

The task of therapy is to weaken each of the factors in the numerator and to strengthen the denominator. The smaller the resulting fraction, the more the fluency.

Therapeutic Methods. One of the fascinating things about this disorder is that literally hundreds of methods for successfully helping stutterers have been reported. Many of these are mutually contradictory; some of them, on first glance, make no sense whatever. Yet we do not doubt the honesty of these reports. Some stutterers have been helped and even cured by each of these many diverse procedures; the same procedures applied to other stutterers have failed.

> We know an elocutionist who cures stutterers by drill in mental multiplication. We have seen a few of them before treatment and afterward. There is no doubt that they were helped. We have also seen some of her cases who showed no improvement and who actually got worse. We would explain her successes as the result of the increased M factor. The children who improved were deprived, young, rather dull children. They had few personality assets and their initial morale was low. They were not severe stutterers. Their situation and word fears were mild and infrequent. Most of the penalty they had received was for their poverty and poor grades in school. They had not reacted very much to their stuttering by frustration, anxiety, guilt, or hostility. No one had expected much of them, nor had they expected much of themselves. In terms of our stuttering equation, then, the numerator above the line was rather small. The elocutionist is an older woman, child-hungry, unmarried, and she gave these children her love and time and faith without measure. She was very patient with them. She believed that they would be cured if they could only learn how to multiply in their heads; and they also came to believe it. She did not penalize their stuttering. She ignored it. As a result of her drilling, they became able to astound and astonish their schoolmates, their parents and teachers with their often-paraded ability to solve these problems. Their stuttering decreased and finally disappeared. The elocutionist believed it was the mental multiplication that was the healing agent. Our own belief is that it was the Mm factor, the morale and motivation and self-confidence they had attained.

It is important that we understand that any individual stutterer may present different values for each of the factors above and below the line of our equation. Two stutterers with about the same amount of stuttering may have completely different problems so far as therapy is concerned. One may have very little *PFAGH* but, be-

cause of his habitual avoidance of speaking, his situation and word
fears can be very intense; another stutterer may show the reverse, or
his morale and motivation may be so much lower that the stuttering
quotient (frequency and severity) may be equal to that of the first
stutterer. It is the therapist's task to study each individual stutterer
until she knows which *factors* are especially important in the picture
he presents and then to work especially hard to weaken or strengthen
these, while not forgetting the others.

We especially wish to emphasize the plural of the word *factors*.
The weakness of most therapy with stutterers is that it has con-
centrated on only one or two of these. The psychiatrist who works
to relieve anxiety, guilt, and hostility may do his job well, but the
person will still stutter if his stuttering still brings penalty or frustration or if his situation and phonetic fears have not been decreased
by speech therapy. And morale alone, like love, is not enough for
many stutterers. It may be for a few special ones, such as the
occasional television or movie star who says he formerly stuttered—
but not for most stutterers. We need a many-pronged therapy if we
are to help most of our stutterers. A one-pronged therapy will help
the special few who present unusual equations in which the factor
hit by the prong is of major importance. It will fail with the others.
There are too many factors operating in stuttering.

In the light of what we have just said, let us look at some of the
ways stuttering has been treated. One of the earliest accounts goes
back to ancient Greek literature and it tells of one Battos who went
to the Oracle of Delphi to find out how he could be freed of his stuttering. The Oracle gave him this prescription: "Exile yourself forever
to a foreign land and never come back." We have had a few ornery
cases to whom we were tempted to offer the same advice. But there
is a fighting chance that Battos was helped by the Oracle's prescription. A change of environment often decreases situation fears and
also permits an escape from some of the sources of *PFAGH* in the
original life situation. Or perhaps he found a Parthian maiden who
loved him completely even unto the elbows and so his self-esteem
soared. Let us hope that Battos was cured, but if he was, let us
understand why.

During the Middle Ages, the tongues of stutterers were burned
and even as recently as fifty years ago they were sliced surgically.

Cures were reported. Once, long ago, the French government paid several hundred thousand francs for the secret stuttering cure of a Madame Leigh who was said to have phenomenal success in treating stammerers. Her secret, when finally exposed, consisted of a small pad of cotton rolled up and held under the tongue during speech. Bizarre? Of course, but even apart from the faith healing and confidences which might have been engendered, we can see why a few stutterers might have been helped at least for a time. If your mouth and tongue were hurting or if you had to hold a pad under it, you'd have a hard time pressing that tongue hard enough to precipitate a tremor. You'd find yourself not struggling so hard. You'd find yourself expecting to have some long hard blocks and then having little ones or not having any. And so the frustration would go down and so would the fears of words and sounds. And so would the stuttering.

About 150 years ago, a man called Columbat treated stutterers by having them say each syllable of their speech as they waved their arm or tapped on a table. This method is still in use today even though it has had a long history of failure. But doubtless, like every other method, it has had a few successes, because, for the moment, it can reduce or eliminate most of the stuttering in most stutterers. In terms of our equation, what it does is to make all words very much alike. It reduces phonetic fears by distraction. It reduces the C factor, the communicative meaningfulness of speech. It is an anti-expectancy device. Like most distractions, however, as soon as it becomes habituated, it loses its power to distract and often becomes a part of the compulsive symptomatology. There are better ways to reduce the fears of sounds and words.

Treatment of Early Stuttering. In our discussion of the development of stuttering we have seen that most children show their first marked stuttering behavior during the ages from two to six. There are a few who begin later. Usually the latter are individuals whose stuttering originates in a primary neurosis or follows a severe illness such as encephalitis. They begin to struggle, fear, and avoid almost from the first. Most stutterers whose disorders seem to originate in the communicative pressures of speech learning or whose histories indicate a possible constitutional etiology tend to show the excessive repetitions and prolongations of syllables and sounds and postures characteristic of stages one and two. And they appear to have very little

situation or word fear. Accordingly, they present a different therapeutic problem than those of the more advanced stages. Their
problem, expressed in terms of our equation is this:

$$\frac{(PFAGH) + Cs}{M + F} = S$$

Penalty Reduction.   Our task, then, is to reduce the penalties they
are experiencing, not only those which parents are placing on the
speech interruptions but all penalties. They need more permissiveness and less punishment.

> One of our primary stutterers, showing the behavior of the first stage,
> was having a very bad time with his speech. The first word of almost
> every utterance was spoken with repetitions or prolongations. Often
> the repetitions would continue for several seconds. He would say, "Ca-
> ca-ca-ca-ca-ca-ca-ca-can I go now? His frantic parents who had been
> asking him to "Stop that!" or to "Stop and begin over again!" followed
> our advice and ceased these admonitions. The reduction of this pen-
> alty reduced the stuttering but too much still remained. We then dis-
> covered that they were also "breaking him of the habit of sucking his
> thumb." As soon as we persuaded them to stop their efforts in this re-
> gard, the child stopped stuttering completely. We had reduced the *P*
> factor in his equation.

Reducing Frustration.   Children in the first stage usually experience
little frustration so far as their stuttering is concerned. A bit of it
comes in during the second stage when the major reaction is the
occasional expression of surprise and bewilderment, and the repetitions become faster, irregular, and end in prolongations of a sound
or posture. The child, without knowing why, is beginning at this
stage to sense that speaking is hard work at times, that it isn't easy.
But the major frustrations come from other sources, from the daily
business of living in a world geared to the needs of others as well as
to one's own needs. One of the sad things about our culture is that
the age of speech learning is made to coincide with the application
of so many taboos. During the preschool years, there are so many
things that a little child must learn he musn't do. The frequency of
usage of the word "No!" by mothers of children of this age is probably exceeded only by that of the expression, "Oh dear!" Anyway,
all children of this age hear a hundred "No's" each day of their lives
and some children hear more, or feel the sharp slap of a heavy
hand on their bottoms. We do not wonder that the age of three is a

negativistic age; the demands for conformity are especially heavy then. All this means frustration. The child must indeed learn to behave the way our culture says he must. But he can't help feeling plenty of frustration.

In counseling our parents we must help them to understand the role of frustration in precipitating stuttering. We cannot ask them to stop being culture carriers. Their own needs for a peaceful, reasonably quiet and orderly home life would then be frustrated. They know that each of us must learn to inhibit some of our infantile urges if we are to live in a civilized society. A child must learn to respect the needs of others. A totally ungovernable and spoiled child is an excrescence in any household. Are we then caught in a dilemma? On the one hand, to reduce the stuttering, we must reduce the frustration; on the other, if we do so, we create a continuing annoyance in the home who will provoke penalty outside the home if not within it.

The solution to the dilemma is simply to help the parents do two things: (1) *reduce* the number of the child's frustrating experiences, and (2) build up his frustration tolerance. There is no need to eliminate all frustration; we merely need to decrease it. Indeed, since life is always bound to hold many frustrations in store, it is wise to help our children learn to tolerate them.

In counseling the mother of another of our primary stutterers, we first got her to express most of her own frustrations not only in child rearing but also in other areas. Then when the river ran dry we explained a bit about the role of frustration in stuttering, gave her a little hand counter and asked her to click it every time she used a forbidding "No!" to the boy. The first day's total was 186; the second day's 132; the third day's 71; and on the fourth day she brought back the counter, saying that Junior had stopped stuttering.

We need not, we cannot eliminate frustration; we always can reduce it.

Increasing Frustration Tolerance. Many an adult should learn the lesson that it is possible to increase one's tolerance for frustration. The inappropriate infantile behavior shown by our frustrated friends (never ourselves!) is evidence that somewhere along the growth line, many of us fail to learn this lesson. Perhaps it is because we have never had the teacher we needed. There are two major ways in which we can build up frustration tolerance. One is through the empathic understanding of the needs of others; the second is through desensitization or adaptation. We shall not go into the first of these save to say that children should learn that parents have rights too, and to give one illustration.

> Willy was an *enfant terrible*. He had conquered his parents. He controlled them. The mother, a frantic neurotic wisp of a woman, was very infantile herself and totally unable to cope with his nagging, his defiance, his temper tantrums. She even feared the little stuttering monster for once he had chased her up the backstairs with a butcher knife. The father was a weak, colorless individual whose response to his miserable home life was to stay away from it as much as possible. We managed to get them to send the boy away for the summer to a camp and for the rest of the year to an uncle's family where the laws of the Medes and the Persians and of the parents were clear and enforced. He had a bad time of it at first but his stuttering disappeared as he learned to curb his pampered infantile urges and become a member of society. He had learned to recognized the needs of others.

The second way to build frustration tolerance involves conditioning. It follows one method for breaking a horse. First you put a cloth on the horse's back, then later a sand bag, then a saddle, then a brave little boy, and then you can jump aboard. It takes time and patience and plenty of gentling and loving along the way, but some horses are taught to accept their riders this way. Through parental counseling and observation of the child, the major frustrating factors are defined. Then they are introduced into the child's life very gradually, but persistently, and only to the degree that he can tolerate them. The consequence is that the child will adapt and gradually be able to tolerate more and more frustration.

> Grant was almost four years old when volleys of stuttering appeared and went away in their usual fashion. For a week he would be very fluent; the next, he could hardly say a sentence without many repetitions. After several months of this, the repetitions began to come out irregularly and faster. Often they would end in a prolongation that rose in pitch. He did not seem to be aware of these interruptions, perhaps because he was so anxious to talk. He talked incessantly to anyone who would listen and to those like his elder brother and sister who often would not. The slightest loss of the listener's attention or any sign of the listener's impatience or any interruption seemed to precipitate a burst of stuttering. The periods of remission were shorter and further apart. He was in real danger. Occasionally he would stop and look bewildered. Talking was getting hard.

The parents fortunately were both understanding and cooperative. They loved the boy and there were no penalties to be decreased. There was little communicative stress in the picture. If anything, they had created conditions which made his communication too easy. If he began to talk, they stopped their own conversation. They asked few questions, talked slowly and simply, and gave him the floor whenever he wanted it. We could discern little evidence of emotional conflicts or anxiety or guilt or hostility. It was a wonderful home. Even the brother and sister seemed to understand and they made things easier for Grant than most children would. The boy had simply developed an abnormal appetite for attention and for communication. He had been a bit delayed in speech and still had some errors in articulation. Perhaps, once he learned the magical power of speech, it was too good to lose. He had logorrhea. The more that appetite for speech was fed, the bigger it grew, and the less he could bear to have it frustrated.

We asked them to institute a progressive change in policy. First they were to give them their complete attention but gradually to introduce a few mild interruptions, a consciously averted glance, a slight delay in answering his questions, or doing what he wanted. They were to do this judiciously so that the amount of his frustration would not be sufficient to precipitate stuttering. But they would put a bit of pressure on him. Then they were to return to the former policy of giving him complete attention, putting an arm around him and listening intently. Then they were to give him another dose of communicative frustration, a little larger one if possible, but again returning to the complete attention. We asked them to do this eight or nine times a day, gradually increasing the dosage of their inattention. Within a week they reported that Grant was now able to wait his turn, to accept delay in responding, to tolerate an occasional interruption. Within a month the stuttering was gone. We had reduced the large F value in his stuttering equation by increasing his ability to tolerate frustration. Frustrations other than those in speech can be handled in the same way. It is possible to build up frustration tolerance.

There is also another way of breaking a horse. You can jump on his back, drive in the spurs, and break his spirit to your will. We do not advocate this method for children, but we have known a few instances in which parents used this policy to teach their children to bear frustration. And again we have seen the stuttering disappear. But we do not advise this method. We want our children free.

Reducing Anxiety, Guilt, and Hostility.   In Chapter Three we have described in detail some of the ways we can reduce these reactions. First they can be lessened by reducing the penalties and frustrations which beget them. Secondly, outlets other than stuttering should be made available. Thirdly, the beginning stutterer needs extra reassurance that he is loved and accepted. We have already considered the first of these three sources; now let us discuss the second.

We find many homes where the need to express one's feelings of anxiety, guilt, and hostility is neither understood nor accepted. If a child reveals that he is afraid of big dogs, thunderstorms, going to bed, or anything else, he is subjected to ridicule and "shamed out of his silly fears." His confessions of guilt and shame evoke a slap or a smile or parental embarrassment. His expressions of hostility are punished. He soon learns to keep them to himself. But we repress these emotional acids at our peril. They want out! And they always find a way. With the stutterer, that way is often stuttering.

These taboos against emotional release can be changed for some children by parental counseling but some parents are themselves too inhibited or emotionally involved to make the necessary changes. As Sander[4] says, "When parents cooperate in a counseling program with insight and determination, the outlook for the young stutterer is most favorable." But there are parents who do not cooperate, who cannot accept counseling. What do we do then?

Play Therapy.   We can offer the child an opportunity through play to release his forbidden feelings. We can provide him with at least one situation in which he finds a loved and loving adult who understands and accepts his feelings, who actually rewards their expression whether the child expresses them verbally or through acting out. A quotation from the excellent book by Murphy and Fitz-Simons[5] helps us understand what takes place in play therapy.

> "One of the clinician's prime tasks is to estimate how the child is perceiving self, parents, and the world as well as how much he is distorting, misperceiving, and misinterpreting. In order to do this the clinician must provide situations and materials which will give the child the opportunities to *externalize* and project his deeper feelings. Play's therapeutic value lies in giving the child a chance to communicate some aspects of his inner world to an understanding adult, to re-evaluate his perceptions and confusions; in short, to integrate. The clinician enters the child's world by allowing him to speak his own

---

[4] E. K. Sander. "Counseling Parents of Stuttering Children," *Journal Speech and Hearing Disorders,* Volume 24, 1959, page 262.

[5] Albert T. Murphy and Ruth M. Fitz-Simons. *Stuttering and Personality Dynamics.* New York: The Ronald Press Company, 1960.

language, often a highly nonverbal, symbolic esoteric one. The child will express his needs to be aggressive; to be infantile; to suck; to mess; to do what he wants and needs to do. The child's formerly suppressed and derogated behavior will be reacted to differently by the clinician whose role is one of "new parents." The clinician submits and resubmits the child's fears, desires, hostilities, condemned wants and wishes to the child's self or conscious awareness for relearning and resocialization, for differentiation and the integration of self.

We have used play therapy with many of our young stutterers and not only with those in whom we suspect a primary neurosis. Where anxieties, guilts, and hostility play an important part in the child's stuttering problem and when their expression at home is denied or prevented by the parents, play therapy is absolutely essential. Not all young stutterers need it. There are some children who show no more than a normal amount of these feelings and in whose problems other factors are more important. With the neurotic stutterer it is the treatment of choice.

Creative Dramatics. Another method for relieving the pressures of anxiety, guilt, and hostility so that they do not contribute to the stuttering problem is that of creative dramatics. In this activity, a group of children, guided by an imaginative adult leader, improvise a play, take the various parts, and invent their own dialogue. Children frequently select and play parts which provide for the expression of their more intense feelings. Here is an account of an eight-year-old nonfluent child having this experience.

> He joined a creative dramatics group but took a relatively inactive part until one day when the children were playing the story of *King Midas and the Golden Touch*. Most of the children characterized King Midas as a grumpy man but not as a cruel one. Finally John said he wished to play King Midas. Suddenly the character of the king became completely different. Midas screamed at the servants, hit the table, ordered the impossible, ranted and raved and almost completely forgot the plot of the story. The children were impressed with the idea of the king, and a discussion followed. Several of the children thought that John had made King Midas too mean. Others thought maybe the previous attempts to play the king had been too mild. The children turned to John to get his opinion. "I think King Midas was a very cruel man. He's as mean as my teacher." [6]

---

[6] B. M. McIntyre and B. J. McWilliams. "Creative Dramatics in Speech Correction," *Journal Speech and Hearing Disorders,* Volume 24, 1959, page 277.

We have found creative dramatics especially useful when much of the emotional conflict was due to sibling rivalry, fears of the local bully, or teasing by the child's playmates. In such instances, the child needs more than a permissive parent figure; he needs a permissive group. We find it very useful when play therapy fails because this particular child cannot come to have any trust in the therapist or any other adult. There are such children. There are also some children whose contact with reality is precariously slim. We do not use creative dramatics with these latter ones. Fantasy and role playing have their dangers.

Parental Counseling. We have referred frequently to the counseling of parents in the reduction of all of the factors which increase stuttering. Parents need education and information, but this is not all that counseling provides. They also need relief from their own anxieties, guilts, and hostilities. They need the opportunity to verbalize their own feelings in the presence of a permissive, understanding listener. They need to learn to view the stuttering child with strange eyes, objectively. Jointly with the therapist, they must explore all his problems, not just his stuttering. In so doing, they often realize their own perfectionistic strivings, their own childhood conflicts, their own present acting-out of relationships they had with their own parents long ago. There are many problems in this counseling of parents which produce difficulty. Some should be referred to the psychiatrist. With some, the conferences should be confined primarily to the giving of information. The depth of the counseling relationship should depend upon the therapist's own training and competence and on the severity of the interpersonal relationships which exist. There are Pandora's boxes no speech therapist should open.

Group Counseling. Often when the therapist can get a small group of parents together in the evening over coffee to discuss their mutual problem, the stuttering child, some real advantages are to be had. First of all, we are able to meet the fathers of these children and often they play a most important role in the stuttering boy's difficulties. Secondly, through free discussion parents come to view their own children differently, more objectively. They get the opportunity to air and share their problems of parenthood. Each is a mirror for the other. Again the anxieties are verbalized, the guilt feelings explored, and the irritation exposed. Again the therapist plays the role of the catalyst. Group counseling can be very helpful.

Reducing the Communicative Stress. The final factor, C, in the dividend of our stuttering equation is communicative stress. All stutterers at any stage show more stuttering when they are bedeviled by the fluency-disrupting influences we now list. The beginning stutterer is especially vulnerable and we have been able to cure more stutterers in stages one and two by reducing the fluency disruptors in the speech environment than by any other means.

How to Prevent Hesitant Speech. Hesitant speech (pauses, accessory vocalization, filibusters, abortive speech attempts) occurs as the resultant of two opposing forces. First, there must be a strong need to communicate, and second, this urge must be blocked by some counterpressure. Some of the common counterpressures which oppose the desire for utterance are:

1. *Inability to find or remember the appropriate words.* "I'm thinking of-of-of-of-uh that fellow who-uh—oh yes, Aaronson. That's his name." This is the adult form. In a child it might occur as: "Mummy, there's a birdy out there in the . . . in the . . . uh . . . he's . . . uh . . . he . . . he . . . he wash his bottom in the dirt." Similar sources of hesitant speech are found in bilingual conflicts, where vocabulary is deficient; in aphasia; and under emotional speech exhibition, as when children forget their "pieces."

2. *Inability to pronounce or doubt of ability to articulate.* Adult form: "I can never say sus-stus-susiss-stuh-stuhstiss- oh, you know what I mean, figures, statistics." The child's form could be illustrated by "Mummy, we saw two poss-poss- uh- possumusses at the zoo. Huh? Yeah, two puh-possums." Tongue twisters, unfamiliar sounds or words, too fast a rate of utterance, and articulation disorders can produce these sources of speech hesitancy.

3. *Fear of the unpleasant consequences of the communication.* "Y-yes I-I-I- uh I t-took the money." "W-wi-will y- you marry m-me?" "Duh-don't s-s-spank me, Mum-mummy." Some of the conflict may be due to uncertainty as to whether the content of the communication is acceptable or not. Contradicting, confessing, asking favors, refusing requests, shocking, tentative vulgarity, fear of exposing social inadequacy, fear of social penalty in school recitations or recitals.

4. *The communication itself is unpleasant, in that it re-creates an unpleasant experience.* "I cu-cu-cut my f-f-f-finger . . . awful bi-big hole in it." "And then he said to me, 'You're f-f-fired.' " The narration of injuries, injustices, penalties often produces speech hesitancy. Compulsory speech can also interrupt fluency.

5. *Presence, threat, or fear of interruption.* This is one of the most common of all the sources of speech hesitancy. Incomplete utterances are always frustrating and the average speaker always tries to forestall or reject an approaching interruption. This he does by speeding up the rate, filling in the necessary pauses with repeated syllables or grunts or braying. This could be called "filibustering," since it is essentially a device to hold the floor. When speech becomes a battleground for competing egos, this desire for dominance may become tremendous. More hesitations are always shown in attempting to interrupt another's speech as well as in refusing interruption.

6. *Loss of the listener's attention.* Communication involves both speaker and listener, and when the latter's attention wanders or is shifted to other concerns, a fundamental conflict occurs. ("Should I continue talking . . . even though she isn't listening? If I do, she'll miss what I just said . . . If I don't, I won't get it said. Probably never. . . . Shall I? . . . Shan't I?") The speaker often resolves this conflict by repeating or hesitating until the speech is very productive of speech hesitancy. "Mummy, I-I-I- want a . . . Mummy, I . . . M . . . Mumm . . . Mummy, I . . . I . . . I want a cookie." Disturbing noises, the loss of the listener's eye contact, and many other similar disturbances can produce this type of fluency interrupter.

We must remember that the beginning stutterer is still learning to talk. His speech is not stabilized. But the mere fact that he has some fluency, and all stutterers do, indicates that, with a little less pressure, stabilization may occur. If, through counseling the parent and often by demonstrating better practices before her in play therapy, we can just ease his burden a little, the stuttering goes away. Often we are surprised to find how quickly these children respond to the reduction of any one of the precipitating factors. This is not so true of the children whose stuttering comes from constitutional or neurotic causes however, but it is true of the large proportion of garden variety stutterers. And even the others are helped thereby.

Lowering the Standards of Fluency.   Communicative stress can also come from the need to talk like others do. If the parents or other children set standards of fluency far beyond the child's ability to imitate, he is almost certain to falter. In our chapter on the development of speech we emphasized this, but here we wish to point it up again. Parents provide the models for all behavior whether they want to or not. It is not enough for parents to become better listeners; they must also provide models of fluency which are not too difficult for the child to follow. It is difficult for some parents to simplify their manner of talking to children, but most of them manage it once they understand why they should do so.

We observed that one of the primary stutterers with whom we were working spoke in compound, complex sentences and used vocabulary which was not only that of the adult level but almost that of an English professor. We even heard him stutter on the word "innocuous," and this at six years of age. He was the only child and his parents were in their forties. They were voluble and precise in word choice. They read him to sleep each night and the selections they chose were *good* literature. They italicized the word when they told us about it. They also played word games and lost no opportunity to teach the boy a new word.

The counseling was difficult but finally they came to see that they were setting exorbitant standards of speech and they asked us for suggestions. We told them to stop reading any stories to the child. We told them to make up some tales instead about very little boys. We asked them to speak in simple sentences to the child as often as they could, to stop the word play and teaching, and to falter a bit in their own talking. We asked them to stop talking so much. We asked them at times to play games in which they pretended that the boy was a little baby and to encourage him to talk like one. They had kept him out of school because of his stuttering and we insisted that he be placed in the kindergarten forthwith. We continued to counsel them. In two months the stuttering was gone.

Reducing the Communicative Demands. Parents frequently report that the young child has more stuttering when he first comes back from school or from playing with the other children. They think it is because of the excitement or some baleful influence of the teacher. The better explanation often is that this is the time that parents give the child a cross-examination. "What did you do at school today?" No child remembers. He did lots of things but he didn't memorize them. One question follows another when all he wants is a cookie and to go out to play.

Parents never seem to realize how much they question their children nor that questioning always puts the child under communicative stress. The mother gets lonely. She needs someone to talk with and her husband, when he does get home, hides behind the paper until after dinner. She also wants to keep her close umbilical relationship with the child. She wants to know what he's thinking and feeling and doing. We can understand and sympathize, but if her needs are making her child stutter, they've got to be satisfied in other ways.

> Peter, aged five, never stuttered in school or on the playground, but he sure did so at home. Or when he talked to his mother (who illustrated the pattern outlined above). We did no counseling. Instead, with all the force and authority at our command, and enlisting her husband's aid in the matter, we insisted that from that moment she was to ask the boy *no* questions. None! Not another one for two months! She could answer his questions but she was not to demand, or wheedle any speech from him. She could talk all she wanted but it had to be commentary, not questioning. We also got her to serve as a volunteer nurse's aid in the hospital each afternoon. The boy stopped stuttering and the father gave me a cigar. Not a very good one.

Removing the Stimulus Value of the Stuttering. A final, but very important, component of communicative stress is the unfavorable attention given to the stuttering by the parents. They call attention to the repetitive speech. They tell the child to "stop it," or to "stop stuttering." We know of no quicker way to throw a child into the third and fourth stages of stuttering than by such suggestions. They should be terminated immediately. Other parents interrupt the child when stuttering and ask him to relax or to stop and think over what he is about to say. When we tell them not to do so, they protest and say, "But it really works. If we stop him and tell him to relax or to stop stuttering he does stop stuttering. Why shouldn't we do this?" Advice again is not enough. Parents must understand how stuttering develops, how frustration and fear are born. We do point out that the child is still continuing to stutter, and is probably getting invisibly worse, that the policies they are using are frustrating in themselves, and that they are training him to fear and avoid. We help them to see that they should reduce the stimulus value of the stuttering, not make it more vivid.

Other parents do not nag their children when they hear them stuttering but they respond to it by signals of alarm and distress which are probably worse. They freeze in their conversational tracks. They hold their breath; they become jittery. Their faces suddenly become masks. Any little child will respond to such signals as though they were cannon shots. When the doe suddenly grows stiff with alarm, the fawn freezes. Quite as much as when the old buck snorts! We must reduce these signals. They add too much to communicative stress.

Usually, the only way to help parents change these attitudes is by providing counseling and information. Occasionally we actually train them out of their signaling behavior by being with them as they interact with their children and helping them to respond to what the child is saying rather than to how he is saying it. But we had one set of obstinate parents who would not accept our picture of the problem and its solution. Under their constant nagging, the boy was growing worse and worse, but they still felt they should "correct him" every time he had some repetitions. Finally, in desperation, we put them into a therapy room with a group of our very severe adult stutterers and locked the door. When we let them out they were a changed couple and from that time on followed our suggestions and the child became fluent.

Building Ego Strength. We now turn to the favorable part of our equation, to those factors which reduce stuttering. These are the factors we must do our utmost to facilitate. The first of these is the M factor representing morale, ego strength, self-confidence, security, whatever you wish to term it. It is difficult to define but we know when it's low and we know when it's high. It rises and falls in all of us depending upon our success-failure ratio but its basic ingredients are love, faith, and opportunity. Some of our stuttering children are denied all three.

One of our beginning stutterers had a father who hated him, perhaps because he wanted the babying which the mother gave only to the child. He had not desired to have children. The boy's stuttering provided the excuse he needed for the expression of his hostility. At any rate, he made no bones about his feelings. Whenever the boy tried to talk to him, the father cut him short and showed his disgust and rejection. The mother's attempt at protection only redoubled the intensity of the father's dislike. He forbade the boy to play with other children, made him stay in the house or yard "so he wouldn't get hurt," refused to let him ride a tricycle so he wouldn't get hurt, and in every way made the boy feel he was both unpleasant and inadequate. We had no success with this child despite some heroic efforts. He is now in high school, a lonely, frightened unhappy boy, barely passing in his school work despite a high IQ. His teachers say that he has no confidence in himself. In one of our recent interviews we asked him why it was so hard for him to work on his speech. He said, "I've been brainwashed all my life. Nobody thought I could do anything and I can't. Every time I make a half-hearted attempt I hear my father saying what I've heard a hundred times: "My God, I'll have to support you all my life." He said that whenever I stuttered bad. I think he's right."

This parent was the exception, fortunately. We have come to have a great respect for parents once they realize their child is in danger and know what to do. Some parents have to be taught to show their love. Some have to be shown how to put aside their own anxieties and to let the child run the risks of living in a dangerous world. Better to break a leg than break a spirit! We have found the overprotective mother to be one of our major problems in this regard. The child must have opportunity even to fail. Security does not come from success alone; it comes from the ability to take failure in one's stride, to lick one's wounds and return to the fray. It comes from the acceptance of liabilities as well as the possession of assets. These attitudes can be taught and parents can change their practices and policies.

How do we build up ego strength, morale, self-confidence? It is difficult to generalize. Often the therapist must accept much of the responsibility for doing the job. We ourselves have done many things. We have taught a boy to box, another to swim, another to read, another to ride one of our horses. We once took a child to a cowboy movie every week for a whole semester. Each child has his own needs.

> One little girl stutterer, the next to the youngest in a family of six girls, had failed to show any improvement in her stuttering for almost a year despite all our attempts to reduce the denominator of her own particular stuttering equation. Then one of our student therapists bought her a puppy and she stopped stuttering. I asked the therapist, a girl, why she had bought the puppy. "It was obvious," she answered. "I have been out to Nancy's home several times and it was clear that she had no status whatsoever. She's shy and quiet and the other girls dominate her completely. I felt that she ought to have something she could dominate or feel superior to, someone to whom she could talk and not be interrupted, something to love. I had a puppy once and I remember."

We aren't sure that her analysis was correct but we are sure that the stuttering disappeared. And we are certain that self-confidence, morale, and ego strength can be increased with love, faith, and opportunity.

The Fluency Factor. *Fl* stands for fluency in our equation, and as we have mentioned, all stutterers have a share of it, often a remarkably large share. No child stutters all the time. Under certain conditions even the secondary stutterer is very fluent. The beginning stutterer in stages one and two can be provided with much more fluency by a few simple procedures. It is the responsibility of the therapist to see that the average amount of fluency is increased.

First of all, with the beginning stutterer, we should arrange things so that during the periods of more severe stuttering, he talks less. The converse is also true. Since early stuttering comes in waves, during the periods of excellent speech, the parents should provide him with every possible opportunity to exercise it. This simple policy has eliminated the disorder in many children.

Secondly, both in the play therapy sessions and in the home, self-talk should be encouraged. Parents should do it as they go about their ordinary activities, telling aloud what they are doing, perceiving, or feeling. In the sessions with the therapist, she should provide the same models of commentary. Few children stutter in their self-talk. It should be facilitated.

We also institute games which might be called "speech play." No attention to the stuttering of course should be involved. The child should only know that he and the therapist or parent are having verbal fun. Some of these games involve speaking in unison, or echoing, or speech accompanied by rhythmic activities, or talking very slowly and lazily. Even baby-like babbling seems to help. There are hundreds of variations but the purpose of all of them is to increase the experience of fluency.

Desensitization Therapy.* Any fluency under any conditions is to be sought, but fluency under conditions of communicative stress is especially to be prized. Most beginning stutterers respond favorably to a coordinated program of the type we have described, but there are some who become worse as the environmental pressures are removed, and there are many whose parents and teachers cannot be persuaded to change their unfortunate policies. What can we do with these children? Give up the case and blame the failure on the child's peculiar constitution or the parents' guilt? No, there is an-

---

* The author owes his initial interest in this therapy and subsequent experimentation with it to George O. Egland, who first brought the concept to his attention.

other alternative, if we can toughen the child, build up his tolerance to stress, and create callouses against the hecklings, rejections, or impatience. Human beings learn to adapt to extreme noise levels, to incredible heat and cold. The housefly can even eat DDT and like it. Should we not try some desensitization, just as the physician gives the shots for hayfever? Instead of lowering the fluency disruptors at home while being unable to do anything about them on the school playground, should we not train our stuttering child to be able to tolerate them without breakdown? As we indicated earlier, some children shift downward their thresholds of speech breakdown as soon as the parents decrease their home pressures. This just makes such a child all the more helpless outside the home.

At any rate, this is what the speech therapist does. He first establishes a social relationship with the child in which the latter does not realize that he is doing any speech therapy. They may be setting up a toy railroad on the floor or participating in any other similar activity. The speech therapist then works to achieve a basal fluency level on the part of the child. This may in rare cases have to begin with grunts or interjections, but usually it consists of simple statements of fact, requests, observations, etc. The therapist, as he works, thinks aloud in snatches of self-talk, commenting on his activity. Soon the child will begin to do the same, and by appropriately altering the communicative conditions, and his own manner, the therapist gets the child to speak with complete fluency. In the primary stutterer, this is not too difficult. Then, once the basal fluency level has been *felt* by the child, the therapist begins gradually to inject into the situation increasing amounts of those factors which tend to precipitate repetitions and nonfluency in that particular child. He may, for instance, begin gradually to hurry him, faster and faster. *But*, and this is vitally important, the therapist stops putting on the pressure and returns to the basal fluency level as soon as he sees the first signs of *impending* nonfluency. How can he tell? Experience and training will help, but we have found usually, that just before the non-fluencies appear, the child's mobility begins to decrease—he freezes, or his general body movements become jerkier, or the tempo of his speech changes. There are other signs peculiar to each child, and a little experimentation will help the therapist know when to stop putting on the pressure just before the stuttering appears.

As soon as the therapist returns to the basal fluency level, he again begins slowly to turn up the heat, to hurry the child a little faster, to avert his gaze more often, or whatever he happens to be trying to toughen the child against. Then an interesting thing occurs. The child can take more pressure the second time than he could the first. The increment is very marked. But again, the first signs of approaching stuttering appear, and again the therapist goes down to the original basal fluency level. Most children do not seem to profit from more than four of these cycles per therapy session, since the tolerance gain decreases somewhat with each subsequent "push." It should be made clear that throughout this training, the child never does stutter, if the therapist has been skillful. What he feels, probably, is that he is being fluent-under-pressure. Fluency becomes associated with the feeling of being hurried. Perhaps this is why there is a remarkable transfer. The effects of this toughening to stress are not confined to the speech therapist. The child seems to be able to stay fluent even when his father keeps interrupting him. This technique, for lack of a better term, we can call "desensitization therapy." We have found it very useful.

Prognosis. If we can locate the child soon enough and initiate the type of therapy outlined above, the chances of a favorable outcome are excellent. Children in the first two stages of the disorder usually seem to present no great difficulty if systematic treatment can be administered. For these children it seems as though all that is needed is the reduction of one or two of the factors that are precipitating the speech hesitancy so that homeostasis, self-healing, can take place. Indeed many children seem to heal themselves without treatment. Glasner and Rosenthal,[7] in a questionnaire study given to parents of 996 first-grade school children, found that 15 per cent of them said that their children had stuttered at one time (a percentage which indicates both the confusion of normal nonfluency and stuttering and also the vulnerability of theories which attribute all stuttering to misdiagnosis). Half of these children had overcome the disorder without professional therapy. Moreover, when these parents were asked how they had handled the problem, 47 per cent of them testified that they had done all the wrong things, according to our

---

[7] P. J. Glasner and D. Rosenthal. "Parental Diagnosis of Stuttering in Young Children," *Journal Speech and Hearing Disorders,* Volume 22, 1957, pages 288-295.

beliefs, and yet their children had stopped stuttering. We would suspect that most of these children were not real stutterers, but even so, we are certain that many children who start stuttering are able to overcome it without professional therapy. Therefore the prognosis is favorable.

Jameson (18) found that among her cases, 80 per cent of those who were referred to her within one year after the onset of stuttering acquired "normal or near normal speech," whereas only 44 per cent did who came to her after a longer time had elapsed. Johnson[8] reports that within two and one half years after the initial counseling of parents (soon after onset), his 46 stuttering subjects acquired normal or near normal speech. So the prognosis for the stutterer in stages one and two is very good. It is our impression that those whose stuttering appears to be of constitutional origin offer a less favorable predicted outcome and need all the help we have to offer. So, certainly, do those whose stuttering seems to be a symptom of a primary neurosis.

Treatment of the Stutterer in the Third Stage. As we have seen from our discussion of the development of the disorder, once the child begins to be frustrated by the repetitions and prolongations which interrupt his communication, the picture changes. Something new has been added to the F factor above the line of his stuttering equation. He is not only frustrated by having his other needs and desires blocked; now he is also frustrated by the speech itself. This is one of the major eddies in which the stutterer finds himself swirling, helpless. It too is a vicious circle or spiral. The more he struggles to release himself from the perseverative repetitions and prolongations, the more he feels frustrated, and the more he struggles. His efforts bring tensed musculatures, hard contacts, tremors, jerks, and facial contortions, all of which make speaking more difficult and unpleasant. He does not fear speaking yet but he is having a hard time. His stuttering equation is the same except that the frustration factor has shown a drastic increase.

$$\frac{PFAGH + Cs}{M + Fl} = S$$

---

[8] W. Johnson. *Stuttering in Children and Adults.* Minneapolis: University of Minnesota Press, 1955. Chapter 3.

The treatment of children in this stage follows much the same course as that used in the treatment of primary stuttering. We must increase the essential emotional security, remove the environmental pressures that tend to disrupt speech, and increase the amount of fluent speech which he experiences. Every effort should be made to prevent traumatic experiences with other children or adults who might tend to penalize or label the disorders. By creating a permissive environment in which the nonfluency has little unpleasantness, much can be done to help the child regain his former automaticity of repetition. The wise parent will find ways of distracting the child so that the struggling will not be remembered with any vividness. Some parents have increased their own nonfluency, reacting to it with casualness and noncommittal acceptance. One of them used to pretend to stutter a little now and then, commenting, "I sure got tangled up on that, didn't I? What I meant to say was . . ." It is also wise to provide plenty of opportunity for release psychotherapy, for ventilation of the frustration. Let them show their anger. Help them discharge it.

If teasing has reared its ugly head and the child does come home crying or unpleasantly puzzled by the rejecting behavior of his playmates, the situation should be faced rather than avoided. Here is a mother's report:

Jack came home today at recess. He was crying and upset because some of the other kindergarten children had called him "stutter-box." And they had mocked him and laughed at him. He asked me what was a stutter-box and for a moment I was completely panicky though I hope I hid the feelings from him. I comforted him and then told him that everybody, including big people, sometimes got tangled up in their mouths when they tried to talk too fast or were mixed up about what they wanted to say. Stutter-box was just a way of kidding another person about getting tangled up in talking. I told him to listen for the same thing in the other kids and to tease them back. Later on that day he caught me once and called me a stutter-box. We laughed over it, and I think he's forgotten all about it today. I hope I did right. I just didn't know what to do.

The desensitization therapy used with the third stage stutterer varies in one respect from that used in the first two stages. We do not use complete fluency as our basal level from which we start and to which we return after gradually increasing the stress. Instead, it is wiser to use the first appearance of tension in the repetitions or postural fixations as the cue to return to the basal level. As in primary stuttering, we try to harden the case to the factors that precipitate his nonfluency, but in this third stage of stuttering we keep putting on the stress (the interruptions, impatience, hurry, etc.) even though the repetitions begin to appear. But we stop short, and return to our basal fluency level, just before the tension, forcing, or tremors show themselves. By this technique, it is possible to bring the child back to a condition where there may be many of the primary symptoms, but little or no struggle reactions.

Direct Therapy. Depending upon how far the child has entered this third stage of frustration and struggle, there comes a moment when direct confrontation of the stuttering is necessary. There comes a time when the child needs some adult to show him that he need not struggle, that it is better to let his speech bounce and prolong easily, that this way "the words come out faster and easier."

This new direct attack on the problem should be done by the professional therapist but we have found it wise to do it in the presence of the parents so that they can feel the objective attitude employed and observe what we do. Here is a glimpse from the transcript of one such session:

> Therapist. I understand that you've been having a lot of trouble talk-
> lately, Peter.
> Peter. Yea, I, I, I, I've been sssssss . . . . stutt . . . . stuttering." (*The
> boy squeezed his eyes shut and fast tremors appeared on his
> tightly closed lips. The word finally emerged after a surge of tension
> and a head jerk.*) "I've been stuttering bad."
> Therapist. So I see. Let's try to help you. I know what you're doing
> wrong. You're fighting yourself. You're pushing too hard. Let me
> show you how you just stuttered and then show you how to do it
> easy. (*Therapist demonstrates.*)
> Peter. Oh!
> Therapist. Now I'm going to ask you a question and if you stutter
> while answering it, I'll join you but show you how to let it come out
> easy. OK? All right, how close is the nearest drugstore to your house?
> Peter. It's over on the next b . . . b . . . bbbbbbblock. (*While the boy is
> struggling, the therapist first duplicates what he is doing, and then
> slowly slides out of the fixation without tension. The child hears him,
> opens his eyes to watch him, and an expression of surprise is seen on
> the child's face.*)

Therapist. Yea, I told you I was going to stutter right along with you but you'll have to watch me, if you're to learn how to let the words come out easy. Let's try another. If I went through the front door of your house, how would I find your room?

Peter. YYYYYYYYYYYou'd . . . (*The child joined the therapist in his grin.*) Yyyou'd have to ggggggo upstairs.

Therapist. That second time you didn't push it so hard, did you. Good. You went like this . . . (*Therapist demonstrates.*) Look, you've got to learn how to stutter my way, nice and easy, either like th-th-th-this or like th . . . is. (*Therapist prolongs the sound easily and without effort.*) Now let's play a speech game of follow the leader. You be my echo and say just what I say and stutter just like I do. Sometimes I'll stutter your way and sometimes my way, the better way, the way you've got to learn to do it.

The session continued along this line and, before the end of the half-hour, Peter was beginning to cease his struggling. It took four more meetings before he really learned how to stutter easily but the parents reported a marked reduction not only in the severity but in frequency as well. We saw him again after four months and the only stuttering behavior he showed was that of the first stage. Within a year it was gone. Children learn quickly and forget their troubles quickly.

The Conspiracy of Silence. Many parents have been told so often that they should always ignore the stuttering that they continue to do so even when it sticks out like a second nose. This is very unwise. When the child is struggling with his stuttering, when he is obviously reacting to it, no good is obtained by pretending that it doesn't exist. There is a time for ignoring it, for distracting the child's attention from it, but there also comes a time when we must confront it and share the child's problem with him. Otherwise he will feel that his behavior is shameful, unspeakably evil. He will feel that his parents cannot bear even to mention it. This is the road to fear and avoidance. It is a dangerous road to travel alone and in the dark.

Treatment of the Secondary Stutterer. The stutterer who shows the behavior characteristic of the fourth stage of stuttering presents the most difficult therapeutic problem. Something new has been added —fear. The equation is now complete:

$$S = \frac{(PFAGH) + Cs + (Sf \times Wf)}{M + Fl}$$

Situation fears times word fears (and we think they multiply rather than add) create a most potent influence in determining stuttering frequency and severity. Often this influence of fear overshadows in importance all the other factors. Certainly it makes for more penalty, creates more frustration in communication because of the avoidance, and adds a constant supply of anxiety, guilt, and hate. We now cannot content ourselves with reducing *PFAGH* and communicative stress, building morale, and providing more experiences in fluency. We must do these things but we must do more: we must now find ways of reducing the fears of speaking situations, the fears of words and sounds. Stuttering now has become its own cause. It is self-reinforcing. Somehow we must get the person out of the whirlpool.

Current Methods.   There are presently three major ways of treating the secondary stutterer being employed in this country. One is through psychotherapy alone. We are not impressed with the results of this method. A few are healed, usually those whose stuttering is fairly mild or of neurotic origin. Psychotherapy certainly can reduce anxiety, guilt, and hostility but in the stutterer who has spent some time in the fourth stage of the disorder, the situation and word fears together with the habituated struggle reactions cannot be ignored. These also need therapy.

The second major method for treating secondary stuttering does attempt to eliminate the fear and struggle components but it does so largely by suggestion and distraction. This school of speech correctionists, numbering among its adherents many of the older workers in the field, attempts to teach the stutterer methods for avoiding or preventing fear and occurrence of stuttering blocks. It aims to eliminate the emotional factors which precipitate the symptoms. The stutterer is urged to believe in the theory advanced by the clinician, and nothing is left undone to convince him he can be cured. Strong clinical suggestion and even hypnosis are used to strengthen his confidence in the remedial techniques. Routine breathing and vocalization exercises and rituals are employed. Through the use of distractions of all kinds, the fear of stuttering is kept from consciousness. Gestures, head movements, and other forms of muscular reinforcement are used as starters. Strange methods of vocalization—preceding all consonants by a vowel, singsong speech, the "octave twist," stereotyped rhythms of stress or phrasing, slurring of the consonants, and many other similar devices—are used to keep the fear from becoming potent enough to precipitate stuttering. Every effort is made to get the stutterer to forget his fears and symptoms. He is urged to consider himself a normal speaker. By the use of speech situations and types of communication arranged according to graduated levels of difficulty, his confidence is nursed along until it becomes sufficient to enable him to speak without fear or stuttering at each successive level. Group techniques help to decrease the fear and increase the suggestion.

In most cases, this type of treatment produces immediate release from fear and stuttering. The stutterer believes that at last a miracle has happened. Hesitantly he applies the formula and lo! it seems to work. His confidence grows by leaps and bounds, and, as it does, his fears decrease. He writes his clinician a glowing letter of praise and thankfulness and departs for his home. Occasionally, his new speech fluency continues for the rest of his life. Whenever fears arise, and they are inevitable, he applies the formulas given to him by the speech correctionist. If the environmental pressures are not too great, and novelty, suggestion, and faith are still effective, the formulas successfully dispel the fear. He realizes that he can still speak without stuttering.

Unfortunately, like most of the devices the stutterers themselves have invented, the formula devices soon become habitual and relatively unconscious. When this happens, they no longer are able to take the place of fear in the stutterer's mind, and relapse usually occurs. Giving the stutterer a period of free speech does not solve his problem if, and when, fear returns. Nevertheless, in the safe haven of the speech clinic, where belief and novelty are important factors and both group and clinical suggestions are everywhere, the stutterer finds great relief. Under such conditions, few stutterers experience much trouble, but unfortunately, such conditions do not exist in ordinary life. When the stutterer returns to his home or former environment, or meets situations which remind him of past failures, there is no one around to tell him that his fears and blocks are mere bugaboos which will disappear if he follows the formula. Life is not made up of easy speech situations or optimal conditions for communication. He finds that he cannot remain relaxed when he applies for a position. He finds it impossible to remain permanently unemotional. The self-confidence so carefully and painstakingly nurtured by the speech correctionist collapses like a house of cards. The formula suddenly seems to have lost its charm. Faith crumbles. The stuttering returns in all its viciousness, often with greater frequency and severity than before. The stutterer attempts to relax, but fear and panic prevent relaxation. He starts his arm swing, or "octave twist," or whatnot, and finds that suddenly it does not keep out the blocks. After repeated failure, he finally gives up and resumes his hunt for a new miracle worker to cast out his "stuttering devil." Meanwhile, the speech correctionist has new stutterers to whom the formula may be taught.

Relaxation. Another basic technique used in helping the person not to stutter is that of relaxation. For many years it served as the basis of all therapy with stutterers. They were asked to relax completely, on the cot and off. They were told to put themselves to rest, that all was well on the blue horizon, that no thunderclouds were visible. Powerful suggestion, even including hypnosis, was used. When a state of relaxation was obtained, the case was then asked to speak, quietly and serenely, the carefully graded sounds and sentences of his therapist. Usually no stuttering appeared when the person followed these directions and was safe in the harbor of his therapist's arms or voice. It was almost as easy as speaking alone. There were no tensions to form the substructure of tremors; no sudden ballistic movements were permitted. There was no stress—often no real communication. But it is hard to be a rag doll in a steel world, as Martin Palmer once said. To be serenely relaxed under a descending sword or pile driver is not a natural response. Life for the stutterer is full of threats, old and new. To ask him to be relaxed is to ask him not to fear. Sure, he can do it when he is safe, but not otherwise. Some few stutterers have been cured this way. Through relaxation many of them have had a bit of temporary relief and hope, but most of them have been left still stuttering and with added guilt feelings because they do not relax as they've been told they should. It's a nice treatment—for the therapist.

The third method is now perhaps the most widely used, although the way it is administered often differs with clinics and therapists. First of all, it is devoted to a total attack on all the factors which increase stuttering. It provides a nonpunitive situation in which stuttering is sought and encouraged. The exhibition and confrontation of stuttering are rewarded so that it can be studied and explored. When possible, other penalties being suffered by the stutterer are reduced by environmental manipulation. The P factor is therefore treated. Frustration (the F factor) is also reduced by this permissiveness about stuttering, and at the same time definite steps are taken to build up the stutterer's frustration tolerance. Anxiety, guilt, and hostility (A, G, H) are not forgotten. Through group sharing of experiences, through acting out the conflicts during the speech assignments, or by professional counseling or other forms of psychotherapy when indicated, these factors are also reduced. Communicative stress (the Cs factor) is not, as in the earlier stages, primarily treated by reducing the stress and creating especially favorable speaking situations. Instead, the stutterer is deliberately subjected to judiciously chosen speaking situations in which stress is present, and he is taught to resist this stress. The M factor (morale) is augmented in many ways: through the close support of a sharing therapist, through the creation of new assets and the elimination of old liabilities, but especially by means of the sense of achievement procured by the successful performance of speech assignments and the conquest of fears. Through various means, later to be described, the stutterer is made aware of the amount of fluency (the Fl factor) that, despite his stuttering, he always possesses, and especially of the fact that one can stutter and still be fluent. To sum it up, this total approach tackles each of the features of the disorder, not just a few of them.

In the preceding paragraph we have shown how this type of therapy treats the $PFAGH$ and Cs and M and Fl factors. But it is in the way this therapy attempts to reduce the situation and word and phonetic fears (the Sf and Wf factors) that it seems to be unique. It stresses the welcoming of stuttering as behavior to be confronted, analyzed, and manipulated or controlled. It works hard to eliminate all forms of avoidance, since avoidance increases fear. It also attempts to associate more fluent forms of stuttering with the situational and word cues which formerly produced avoidance or struggle. It teaches the stutterer that he can stutter fluently. The expected unpleasantness is reduced and with it the fears. As Bloodstein[7] phrases it, this new therapeutic approach was one which

    . . . aimed directly at a reduction in the fear and avoidance of stuttering while at the same time attempting to reduce the amount of diffi-

[7] O. Bloodstein. *A Handbook on Stuttering for Professional Workers.* Chicago: National Society for Crippled Children and Adults, 1959, page 70.

culty through gradual modification of the stuttering pattern based on study and understanding of the behavior.

It is obvious that the author of the test is an advocate of this methodology, perhaps because, as a stutterer himself and as a speech therapist, he has experienced the inadequacies and restricted scope of the other two methods. This brief summary of the purposes of this particular variety of stuttering therapy was intended to point up the contrast between it and the other two. Now let us outline the sequence of therapy and tell what we do.

The Sequence of Therapy. Let us coin another acronym to put the matter succinctly: *MIDVAS*. The separate letters of this word refer to the main phases of our therapy for the secondary stutterer and they follow the order of the letters of the word. *M* is for motivation; *I* is for identification; *D* for desensitization; *V* for variation; *A* for approximation; and *S* for stabilization. This is the sequence of our therapy. We structure our therapy plan so that each new phase has a special emphasis but all preceding goals are continued. New experiences are added but the old are reviewed. It is cumulative therapy. For convenience of exposition, we shall describe the treatment as though it were being administered to severe adult stutterers. Modifications must of course be made for young children or for the very mild stutterer, as well as for the special needs of any given individual. All stutterers present special problems. All need special treatment, but there still are general principles and practices which help all of them.

Motivation. One who has not worked much with secondary stutterers would expect to have little trouble motivating them to do the things necessary to find relief. Certainly, the interruption to communication, the social implications and deprivations, the struggling and the fear, are unpleasant. Why then do we find so much resistance? For we certainly do. We think there are two answers. First, it is always difficult to confront one's abnormality, to expose it enough to modify it, and this resistance is found in healing all emotional ills. Indeed, unless resistance occurs in psychotherapy, we can be pretty sure that any apparent insight and improvement in adjustment is superficial and temporary. Secondly, the fact of the stutterer's fluency when alone or in nonstressful situations makes him feel that no major overhaul is needed. But deep in his bones he knows he has a tough job to do, that the seizure-like behavior and the panic of his fears are not going to yield to any waving of a savior's hands, yet it is only human to hope for easy miracles. We keep in our desk a little bottle full of pink aspirin with a label reading: "One of these will cure stuttering forever." In an early session, we always hand a new stutterer the bottle. He always grins and hands it back. We have never had one as much as open it in thirty years. They know.

The Role of the Therapist in Motivation. When the secondary stutterer first comes for therapy, he speaks with great difficulty usually and we have found it wise to begin by revealing our own role and competence. We don't tell him how good we are; we let him find that out. But we do define our role, not as a teacher or preacher or medicine man, but as a guide and companion on a joint quest. We do this in the initial interview, explaining why we ask the questions we do, and sharing with him the implications of his answers. When he stutters, we provide a running commentary of our own objective evaluations of his behavior. When he avoids, or postpones a speech attempt on a feared word, or uses some trick to start his utterance or disguise the stuttering which occurs, we recognize and identify what he has done with complete acceptance. This always seems to surprise the stutterer. He always seems to feel that his little devices for avoiding or escaping from his difficulty are his own personal secret. And he is always surprised at the acceptance. The only listener responses he has remembered are those of rejection or embarrassment or pity. Suddenly he finds not only a permissive listener but one who understands. This is one of the crucial experiences in all successful therapy. Often, at this point, he will begin to stutter very severely as if to test the genuineness of the therapist's acceptance, and again he is surprised to find that the behavior is welcomed, rewarded.

Another crucial experience which the stutterer should have as soon as possible is that of observing his therapist actually *sharing* his abnormality. Here is the transcript of one such experience:

Therapist. You had a pretty long and complicated block on that word "people." Let's see if I can duplicate it. First of all you squeezed, then protruded your lips like this. Then I think you gave a quick little gasp like this . . . and then . . . No, I don't have it right. Let me have another bad one so I can learn what you do.

Subject. Pppeople. That time it came out easy.

Therapist. Yes it did but I wish you could show me a more severe one, the kind that make you panic, as you said a moment ago. I've got to feel it in my own mouth to know what you do so I can understand what the problem is. You've got to teach me.

Subject. Yyyyou mmmmean you want me, you want me, you want me to teach you to sttttt . . . sttttttttttutter like I do?

Therapist. To know how you feel, to know what you do, I've got to do it too. And not just here but in real speaking situations. As soon as I've learned how you do it, I'll make a phone call and try it out, and you can tell me how close I am, and if my feelings are similar to yours.

Subject. Holy C-C-Cow!

We do not only repeat the stutterer's behavior; we also share it as it is happening. By pantomiming what he is doing as he is doing it, we become a human mirror for him. When he first experiences this, old memories of the mockery of playmates long ago flood back and suspiciousness is aroused, then allayed as he finds that the therapist is actually trying to understand and share his burden of abnormality. This interaction not only helps to produce a close relationship of the stutterer with the therapist but it also partially extinguishes some of the persisting evil effects of old traumatic wounds.

Another important experience occurs when the therapist reveals that he is interested and desires to share not only the outward behavior of the stutterer but also to understand his inner feelings. We find it wise to begin with the feelings created by the immediate moment of stuttering. A few stutterers are able, with skillful counseling, to express these feelings, but most are not. The stuttering itself interferes with expression. As Fenichel put the matter in a nut shell, when speech, the healing tool of psychotherapy, is itself infected the task of the therapist is hard. We have therefore found it wise to verbalize his feelings for him. We do this tentatively and ask for corrections and additions. Here is a portion of the transcript of a session in which this took place:

Therapist. When you were stuck that time, what were your feelings?

Subject. I don't know. All, all mmmmmmmmmmmmixed up, I gggggguess.

Therapist. You probably felt helpless . . . sort of as though your mouth had frozen shut . . .

Subject. And, and and I cccccouldn't open it. Yeah.

Therapist. You couldn't open it. It was almost as though you had lost the ability to move a part of yourself when you wanted to . . . Sure must be frustrating . . .

Subject. Sssure is. BBBBBurns me up. I, I, I, jjjust hate mmmmm . . . Oh, skip it . . . I don't know.

Therapist. (*Acceptingly*): It almost makes you hate yourself when you get stuck like that.

Subject: Yeah, dih-dih-disgusted with mmmmmyself and everything else. . . .

Therapist. Some stutterers even find themselves hating the person they are talking to.

Subject. Yyyyeah. I, I, I, I, I wwwwwas huh-huh-huh-hating yyyyyy-yyyyyou just then.

Therapist. Uh huh. I know.

Subject. (*Blurting it out*) How, howcome you know all these th-things?

If these three crucial experiences, which will be repeated many times in many different forms, are scrutinized, it is apparent that we are already at work on the stuttering equation. The case finds for the first time that stuttering is not being penalized but encouraged. Frustration declines a bit as he discovers that his therapist is in no hurry, that his ear is always open no matter how long the blockings last. He learns that here he can pour out a bit of anxiety, guilt, and hostility with impunity. In the therapy situation, communicative stress is reduced. It is easier to talk here. Moreover, since stuttering is actually sought and encouraged, the fears are reduced. We do not fear that which is rewarded. Finally, and perhaps most important of all, there comes an increase in morale as the stutterer finds that he is not alone, that someone who seems to understand his problem has faith that he can solve it. Moreover, burdens which are shared are thereby divided. The load lightens. All of these changes reflect themselves in increased motivation. The M in the equation can also stand for motivation.

Goal Orientation. But the therapist is not only an understanding companion sharing part of the load; the stutterer soon comes to feel that this person is also a competent guide. At least he seems to know one way out of the swamp. Let us outline how we help him to come to this conclusion.

First of all we try to provide some person whom he can see or hear who has been able to learn to conquer his stuttering problem. Usually we have several around who are determined, despite our usual discouragement, to become speech therapists. We also have

the tales of many others on tape, tales that often exaggerate a bit
the difficulties encountered and we must use them with care so that
the new sprout of hope will not be withered by the frigid windiness
of their exaggerated accounts of what they had to do. We use films
for the same purpose.*

Next we try to help the stutterer to realize that he possesses in
his own present speech both a certain amount of fluency and also,
what is more important, a certain amount of stuttering which does
not interrupt communication unduly or show much abnormality.
This latter item is of utmost importance. All stutterers have some
moments of stuttering which are unforced and unaccompanied by
struggle or avoidance. We point these out when they occur and
often make a tape in which many samples of these fluent, unabnormal stutterings are combined. We ask the stutterer to listen to this
tape frequently. Also in our pantomimic sharing of his stuttering, we
often repeat again and again these fluent stutterings so that he can
see them, and we ask him to repeat them also. We point up this
easy fluent sort of stuttering as a goal object. Even a rat runs a difficult maze better when he has a taste or smell of the cheese to be
found at the end of that maze.

At this point the stutterer often objects.

Subject. Yyyyou mean, you mmmmmmmean that it's possible to stutter
   easy like that even when you're scared green?
Therapist. You feel it isn't possible. (*Nods acceptance of the feeling.*)
Subject. Oh nnnnnnot when you're really petrified, nnnot wheh, when
   you can see th . . . em c-c-c-coming and the fffffffffffffear builds up.
Therapist. Real hard fears are bound to throw you into long hard
   blocks. . . .
Subject. Yeah, but mmmmmaybe, maybe not. Maybe it is ppppposssible
   to let them kind of leak out, hey? MMMMaybe I c-c-could lllllearn.
   . . . (*He shakes his head.*)
Therapist. But you have your doubts. . . .
Subject. SSSSStill those other gggguh-guys say they can stutt . . .
   stutter . . . Hey, I'm doing it right now. I just had an easy bbbblock
   on sssss, on sssssssstut . . . Why can't I say it now? On sssssssstutter.
   I, I, I ddddddid have one, dddddidn't I?
Therapist. Sounded like it.
Subject. And, and, and mmmaybe the ffffears wwwwwwwon't al, al, al,

---

* One which we have found useful in this regard is "Great Clinicians: Stuttering," which can be procured on rental from the audio-visual department of
the University of Wisconsin.

al, always be so strong. Even already I dddddon't seem to bbbbe quite sssssssssssso sceh, scared. YYYou know it's true. I, I, I, I dddddo have dddddifffferent kkkinds of bbbbblocks.

At some such moment it is possible to help the stutterer to have another very important experience: the realization that it is possible to stutter in many different ways and that some ways may be better than others. We make it possible for him to observe and duplicate the kinds of stuttering shown by other stutterers. We also ask him to experiment a bit in modifying his own.

> Therapist. I notice that usually on a word beginning with *b* or *p* you squeeze your lips tightly and then open them and suck in a little air just before the release comes—like this. . . . (*Therapist demonstrates.*)
>
> Subject. YYYYeah, and it, it, it, it mmmmakes a sssssssssssssssssucking sound I don't like.
>
> Therapist. You hate that sucking noise.
>
> Subject. Yeah. (*It is evident that he is not going to pursue the subject further.*)
>
> Therapist. Then let's see if you stutter on words like that without sucking.
>
> Subject. Huh?
>
> Therapist. Let's see if you can say these names in the phone directory beginning with *P* and try to keep the sucking noises out.
>
> Subject. (*Doubtfully*) OK. PPPP(*suck*)Partridge; PPPPPP(*suck*)Parsons . . . I can't.
>
> Therapist. OK. (*Acceptingly*)
>
> Subject. LLLLLLet me rrrrreally try th . . . is tttttttime . . . PPPPuh-puhparparpartridge. Hey! I did it! What do you know! Yyyyou mean I, I, I, I don't have to ssssssuck?
>
> Therapist. Looks like it.

This is another of the crucial experiences which are the mile markers on the road to freedom. There are many of them.

Mapping the Route to the Goal. It is also necessary that a clear picture of the course of therapy be given to the stutterer. He needs some kind of a map before he becomes willing to undertake a journey, even though he now knows he has a guide. We have found it useful to give him some understanding of *MIDVAS* and also of the stuttering equation. This first phase of therapy requires the imparting of information. The stutterer is usually as ignorant of the nature of his disorder as he is of the behavior he uses so compulsively. He needs to know something of the causes of stuttering and the way it develops, and we also help him to find information about the way stuttering has been treated in the past as well as how it is being treated today by other therapists. We do not believe in blind therapy. We want him to know where he's going, where he is, and what he has to do. We find that we get a better motivated case this way.

The Second Phase of Therapy: Identification

As soon as possible we move directly into the second phase of our therapy, in which the basic goal is the identification and evaluation of the various factors in the case's *personal* stuttering equation. There is no emphasis on trying to speak more fluently. Just the converse. The stutterer is to seek out stuttering experiences and to analyze the behavior and identify the forces which created it. This is the period of self-study, of self-exploration. Note that this goal-structuring increases the approach and decreases the avoidance vectors in the approach-avoidance conflicts. The objective observation of the stuttering behavior gets down to what the semanticists might call "first order facts." The more the stutterer stutters, the more opportunity he has to make his observations. The therapist shares and rewards these discoveries. He also provides structured experiences which will make them possible.

Speech Assignments.   One of the unique features of this type of therapy is the use of the speech assignment. In addition to the stutterer's own attempts in self-therapy, certain required activities and experiences are devised by the therapist to provide guidelines and models for what the case should be doing himself. Some stutterers need few of these; others need many; but the emphasis is always on self-therapy. The devising of self-assignments is constantly and vividly rewarded. Usually, the therapist-formulated speech assignments are given more frequently in the early phases of therapy, and especially during the phase of identification. Reporting of the experiences *and feelings* evoked by these experiences is a very necessary part of the clinical routine. This may be done orally either in private sessions with the therapist or in group sessions with other stutterers, or the reports may be written in certain instances. Often we use both oral and written reports. The mere act of preparing and handing in reports of self- and therapist-assigned experiences gives a sense of achievement which has profound and cumulative effects upon the M factor in the equation. Moreover, these assignments often provoke the resistances and testings of the relationship between stutterer and therapist which, when worked through, create new insights and energies for healing. They make it possible for the therapist to share significant moments in the stutterer's life; they reveal the basic feelings which can then be accepted and reflected. They help the stutterer to know where he is and how much he is doing and how much he still must do. They provide an objective account of the course of therapy. We have found them very useful.

Typical Assignments in Identification. Since this is a general and introductory text in speech correction and not a manual for stuttering therapy, we can do no more than provide one or two typical assignments for each of the sub-goals involved. There are hundreds of other possible assignments which might be more appropriate for a particular case. The stutterers themselves often invent better ones than we can design. Since the basic goal of this phase of the therapy is the identification of the various factors in the stutterer's personal equation, the illustrative assignments will be organized about these factors. Often, in a single day's work, the stutterer will perform one of the therapist's assignments for each of the factors, and also a self-invented one of his own for each of them. There are also times when he may do nothing. He gets the therapist's warm approval for the first of these responses and the other is accepted as part of the difficulty. However, if the case proves entirely unwilling to work, therapy is terminated. Even a psychoanalyst has to get them on the couch now and then.

Penalties. Many secondary stutterers have become a bit paranoid about the reactions of listeners to their stuttering. Even when no overt rejection is evidenced, they think the listener is merely covering up a punitive or embarrased reaction. It is vitally necessary that they do some reality testing. Some assignments which could begin this testing might run like this:

> Keep track of the number of listeners who frown or show objective signs of impatience when you stutter. What proportion do not? Get a sample of ten strangers with whom you stuttered obviously to determine the proportion.

How many store clerks did you talk to before you found one who showed signs of mirth or mocking when you stuttered? Try a minimum of five.

If possible, ask one of your friends how he really feels when you stutter to him. Ask him to tell you the truth. Report what he said and whether you think he was honest.

Here is one stutterer's own self-assignment report:

I've been wondering maybe I've been blowing this fear business all up. Maybe most people don't really give a damn whether I stutter or not. Maybe they figure it's my problem, not theirs and they let it go like that. Then I got to thinking how many people can I remember who really did laugh in my face when I stuttered and you know I couldn't remember a single one except Wilbur Ketchum when I was a kid and he was goofy anyway and laughed all the time. So I got to thinking and thought I'd try something out. I called on the phone a whole mess of people and asked them things like "Is Wilbur home" or "May I speak to Jane, please" and I stuttered plenty but I cocked my ear to see if I could hear any laughing or giggling. I just got one who did. It was a little girl who answered the phone. All the rest just waited till I got it out. I was sure surprised. Maybe I have been exaggerating.

And here is another:

Had a lulu of a penalty today. It threw me. Was talking to a stranger. Man about sixty and asked him how to get to the bank. He got mad when I stuttered. He said, "If you can't talk any better than that don't ask questions." And turned away. Felt like quitting right there. Made me feel dirty mouth. But I said to myself why does he act like this? What kind of a guy is this? So I follow him around and listen. He gets some tobacco in a store and he raises hell with the clerk for not having his kind. Then he goes to another place and gets his tobacco but growls at that clerk. I tailed him into Gilmores and there he was giving some other clerk hell for something. So I guess I got a bad one and it wasn't just my stuttering. Felt pretty good after.

These assignments happen to revolve about the speech disorder itself but we wish to make clear that we explore all penalties, not just those evoked by stuttering. Punishment of any kind seems to add an increment of stuttering. During this phase of treatment the case tries to locate and assess the importance of all penalties, present and past. He becomes aware of sources of rejection other than his stuttering. One girl changed her hairdo and bought new clothes and a red hat instead of the mousy-looking apparel she had been wearing. A boy learned how to dance when he found he could get dates easier for such affairs than for the movies. As a result of some vivid experiences, one man began to see that he was getting more rejection for his aggressive sarcastic reactions to other speakers than for the fairly mild stuttering which he exhibited. And he also found that his stuttering began to decrease. One of our college students wrote an essay on "My History of Penalty" and won a prize for the composition. Often, in group sessions, the memories of past penalties are ventilated, and again not just those concerning stuttering. In this phase of therapy, we make no attempts to eliminate the behavior which provokes the penalty but merely to explore and to define it, but often the stutterer starts making some changes anyway. The emphasis at this phase of therapy is merely to *identify* those penalties which contribute to stuttering.

Frustration. In exploring this factor the stutterer compiles an account of the frustrations characteristic of his present situation and also a history of those of the past. He also thereby becomes aware of basic drives and needs other than to speak fluently. Many stutterers become so focused on stuttering that other major problems are completely disregarded even though they contribute to the disorder and may be more easily rectified. In the identification phase of therapy, the whole target, not just the bull's-eye of stuttering, comes into view. Here are a few typical assignments:

Keep a pad and pencil with you all morning and write down *every* time you feel frustrated, not just those times when you stutter. Try to report why you felt this way and what the frustrating situation was.

Frustrate your roommate three times and report how you did it. Then ask him to frustrate you as often as he can for an entire day and report how he did it.

In speaking to some friend, keep on stuttering on a word until he says it for you or finishes your sentence. Do this a minimum of three times. Report your feelings.

In what ways were you especially frustrated as a child? What were your parents' major frustrations? Prepare a written and comprehensive answer to these questions.

Here is the report of a self-initiated assignment in exploring the frustration factor.

My roommate in our girls' dormitory has a nasty little habit that's been driving me to distraction. She sniffs. She sniffs when she's studying. When it's quiet all I can hear is that sniff sniff and I almost go wild. It's a tic or something. I used the radio for a while to cover it up but she says she can't study with it going. I asked her if she couldn't stop it and she said no, that if it didn't bother her why did it have to bother me. I told her it still did and she said that's too bad. Lately I've been doing all my studying at the library but that's pretty inconvenient. Well, I've been thinking about frustration and how it may affect my stuttering and I know her sniffing makes me jittery so I said to myself, "All right, let's see if you can learn to bear it." Ruth's a very nice girl in other ways and we have lots of fun together. So I said to myself, "Let's measure how many sniffs you can count before you get nervous and then you can give her one stutter for every five sniffs." That made me grin to myself. Well, I stuttered eleven times to her before we went to bed, ten for her sniffs and one for myself. It actually took fifty sniffs and three hours of studying before I couldn't stand it any longer. I guess I can get used to it if I can only use a little psychology on myself.

Anxiety, Guilt, and Hostility. For some stutterers only professional counseling can help to ease the pressures of these emotions. There are therapists who are qualified to do such counseling. Others cannot and should not do it and must seek help elsewhere. Professional psychotherapy for the stutterer whose disorder is primarily neurotic in nature is a must. But most stutterers, in our opinion, do not fall in this category. Yet they all have some anxieties and guilts and hostilities which need ventilation and release. Fortunately, the speech assignments devoted to other factors usually bring about the expression of many of these feelings which the therapist must permissively accept and reflect. Usually in this early phase of therapy we do not use many direct assignments in exploring these factors but some illustrations may be given.

Interview some friend and try to discover what anxieties he possesses. Report which ones you also have.

Here is a list of behaviors (list is provided) which create feelings of guilt in children. Which of these do you remember experiencing?

Keep stuttering to strangers until you have a clear experience of hostility. Describe this as vividly as you can.

For what things other than stuttering do you tend to punish yourself? Watch yourself all this day and see what you might discover.

Communicative Stress. Here we confront the stuttering directly. In this phase of treatment, the case explores and identifies the types of communicative stress to which he is most vulnerable. Again he is *seeking* speaking experiences instead of avoiding them, which is healthy in itself and a reversal of old practices. Here are some typical assignments.

Which of these two audience reactions seems to produce more stutterings: (1) interruption by having the listener finish what you are trying to say or (2) having him look away when you're stuttering? Collect two experiences of each kind and report.

Read a passage aloud to some other stutterer very swiftly; then another of equal length at a normal rate; then another at a normal rate; and finally a fourth at a fast rate. Using hand counter, have him count how many blocks you have under fast and ordinary speaking rates, averaging the two trials for each. How much of a factor is speed in producing more stuttering? Report your findings.

Tell a joke to some friend. Do you have more stuttering on the words that carry the key meaning, or on the punch lines? Why?

Analyze four speaking situations which produced different amounts of stuttering and attempt to identify the kinds of communicative stress present in each.

Read aloud the names on one page of the telephone directory to some other person and have him indicate which ones you stuttered on most severely. Were some of these strange unfamiliar combinations of sounds such as occur in foreign names?

What kinds of attitudes shown by your parents when you were trying to talk to them seemed to produce the most stuttering when you were a child?

Collect an experience of each of these types: Interrupt another person when he is talking. Ask a favor. Repeat in other words what someone has just said. Arrange these, if possible, according to a progression of decreasing stress. Talk aloud to yourself when alone, answering the phone, and making a phone call.

Situation Fears.   In exploring these, the stutterer should not only identify those of the present and the past but also attempt to assess their intensity. He should also try to discover what he specifically dreads. Many very important insights come from this sort of investigation. He may even find that he doesn't know what he is afraid of. The stutterer should also study the relationship between situation fears and the amount of actual stuttering which does occur. He may find that the correlation is not as high as he thinks it is. We find that experiences of this sort are very salutary because they weaken the *fear of fear.* Often these people seem to be more afraid of the fear than of the stuttering itself. By seeking out that which is dreaded, by exposing and analyzing it, the evil subsides a bit.

Some typical assignments are as follows:

> Before you enter five different speaking situations, predict on this five-step scale how severely you will stutter. Then, after you have left the situation, record how badly you actually did stutter.
>
> What three speaking situations in your whole life do you remember as being the worst? Why were they the worst?
>
> Apply for a job at some restaurant. On your way down town, try to identify and remember the kind of thinking you were doing and what you were especially dreading. Report this in writing.

Word Fears.   This factor, as we have said, includes not only fears of specific words but also the phonetic fears of sounds. It might be objected that by focusing the stutterer's attention on them, we only make them that much worse. All we can say in this regard is that any increment of this sort is negligible. They already have their full strength based upon a thousand memories. Stutterers also fear these phonetic fears; they attempt to distract themselves from them, to repress them, to escape from them. We have found it healing to look them plumb in the face.

Here are some typical assignments:

> When a stutterer reads and rereads a given passage, the number of stutterings decreases through adaptation. Usually those words on which stuttering persists longest are the most feared. Therefore, to discover them, read a given passage four times and have someone else underline all words on which you stutter each time. Then take the fourth reading's underlined words and try to tell why they resisted adaptation.
>
> Underline all the words of a reading passage on which you expect to stutter and then read it aloud to some other person. Have him underline all words on which you actually do stutter. What percentage of correct prediction did you show?
>
> Take two of the sounds which you feel are your "Jonah sounds," those most feared, and prepare a reading passage which is full of them. For example, if you usually fear S words and M words, prepare a passage which has many sentences such as this one: "Many snakes must search such marshes as may be seen by the seashore." Read this aloud to some other person and have him underline all words on which you stutter. Compute the percentage of S words and M words on which you actually stutter.
>
> Before you make a phone call, prewrite what you plan to say. Underline all feared words and predict the severity of stuttering on each. Use a five-step scale of severity. After you have finished, score each

underlined word in terms of how severely you did actually stutter on it.

What kind of rehearsals do you use when fearing a specific word? Investigate and report on five of these.

The M Factor. We also feel it very important for the stutterer to study his own variable feelings of self-worth. As we have said, stutterers are focused so much on their stuttering that they fail to see their other difficulties. In much the same fashion, they are also unable to evaluate with any objectivity the other assets they possess. In this phase of the treatment they learn objectivity and it is important that they apply it to the favorable factors as well as to the unfavorable ones. While much of the increase in ego strength comes from the sense of achievement gained by working on their stuttering and from the identification with a strong therapist, nevertheless we find that certain assignments can have a real effect. Here are some samples.

Prepare a list of all your personality assets and liabilities. Shyly we suggest that you include stuttering among the latter.

Write up an account of all the things for which you have received approval from others.

Keep a mood chart in which you assess your feelings of morale four times a day: after breakfast, lunch, and dinner and before you go to bed. Make a graph of your mood swings for an entire week on a five-step scale with these values arranged on lines from top to bottom: 1. Whoops! 2. Feeling good. 3. Uncertain. Don't know. 4. Depressed. 5. Mighty, mighty lowdown.

Who are the people who have evidenced some faith in you? Why do you suppose they evidenced this faith?

The Fl Factor. Only the stuttering seems to have stimulus value for the stutterer, never the quite evident amount of fluency he also possesses. Again we must help him assess the real state of affairs. At this stage he has become morbidly conscious only of his abnormality, not of his normality. Also, most secondary stutterers have an exaggerated concept of what constitutes normal fluency. They do not realize that normal speakers are also nonfluent, at times of stress very nonfluent. This area must also be investigated.

Here is a tape recording of one of ex-President Eisenhower's press conferences. Record how many hesitancies he demonstrates.

On what percentage of words do you stutter? Make tape recordings of yourself (1) reading to another person, (2) explaining something to a friend, and (3) making phone calls. Count the words spoken and the stutterings and find out how fluent you are in each.

Listen to the conversations of other people and be able to show us all the different kinds of nonfluencies they demonstrated.

In this section describing the *identification* phase of therapy we have tried to show how we help the stutterer recognize the scope of his problem as expressed in terms of the various factors which make his stuttering better or worse. We would like to re-emphasize here that this exploratory phase by itself often produces immediate decreases both in the amount of stuttering and in the intensity of the fear and avoidance. As in motivation, identification experiences will continue throughout therapy. We find, however, that we have more success when we stress it early in the treatment.

Desensitization Phase of Treatment

The third major phase in the treatment of secondary stuttering we have termed "desensitization" because our major goal in this part of the therapy is to toughen our case to those factors which normally increase the frequency and the severity of his stuttering. It should be pointed out at once, however, that the methods used are not the same as those used in desensitizing the stutterer in stages one and two. We now work directly, rather than indirectly. We do not use basal fluency levels and introduce the stress without the case's knowledge that we are doing so. Instead, we enlist his cooperation and provide him with challenges. His task now is consciously to learn to endure the stresses which formerly threw him into inadequate and abnormal behavior. He seeks them deliberately and the therapist, with the case's cooperation, deliberately provides them. His goal is to remain integrated despite forces which tend to cause disintegration. His task is to decrease his hypersensitivity, in short, to toughen himself.

Human beings are wondrously adaptable. They can exist in the Arctic Zone and on the equator. They can even live in big cities. They can endure anything once they put their minds to it. Rats can be trained to bear electric shocks of great intensity with proper schedules of reinforcement. Surely, we can hope that our stutterers can improve in their ability to resist and endure the stresses they must encounter. In this phase, we are raising the thresholds of breakdown. It is very necessary that the stutterer understand why this is being done. But there are immediate rewards from desensitization. He will soon learn that as he becomes more hardened, he stutters less and suffers less. As he becomes tougher, he finds that penalties do not throw him so quickly; that frustration has less evil effect; that he can tolerate more anxiety, guilt, and hostility than he could before; that communicative disruption and fear do not precipitate stuttering as frequently as once they did. And the morale factor rises, as any soldier knows, once he has learned he can endure.

It is obvious that the administration of this phase of therapy takes some skill and empathy on the therapist's part. By now he should have gained a clear picture of his case's sensitivities and the energies the latter might marshal to modify them. He must not overload. Indeed, often the therapist must keep the case from overloading himself. But there must be always present the faith that comes from realizing the enormous potentials which all humans seem to possess, and the support which only a loved and respected therapist can give. Evidence must be provided that the therapist can also share these experiences, can also bear the stress, can also suffer but endure. Often he must become the accepting receptacle for the hostile attacks that result from the hurt the stutterer experiences when he tries and fails. But the therapist knows that if he can accept these, the stutterer can try again. And he knows, as does Britain, that you can lose a hundred battles and still win a war.

Again, assignments are given which provide opportunities for desensitization to occur. Again, the stutterer is prevailed upon to construct his own assignments and to bring to the therapist for sharing and analysis the trophies and the failures which result. Group therapy provides an excellent situation for sharing these accounts, and the stutterers vie with each other and support each other. For example, we have found, in such a group, that if one girl shows she can make progress, all the males have to do more. Also, as they often do assignments together, there is built up a sense of comradeship which relieves the feeling of isolation so many stutterers know so well.

Usually, we begin fairly gradually to introduce the stress challenges and the therapist sets models for the case to follow. We have found it wise to enter a store or similar speaking situation and to fake a very long stuttering block in the presence of the stutterer or stutterers. And we show we are not upset, that we remember exactly what the clerk did and how he reacted. We also verbalize our own feelings honstly. And then we do it again. We have found this often to be another crucial experience in the stutterer's life. The fact that another human being, a normal speaker perhaps, would be able to undergo such an experience and remain well-integrated and relatively unperturbed, seems to impress the stutterer greatly. After a few of these demonstrations, he is willing to try himself. We now list just a few illustrative assignments and experiences.

Penalty.

Keep making phone calls and fake one long repetitive block until one listener hangs up on you. Time the faked stuttering with a stop watch and report how many people you called before one did hang up.

Ask one of the other stutterers to yell at you "Stop that damned stuttering!" every time you do so as you read a paper aloud.

Ask one of your friends to laugh at you every time you stutter in a conversation. Explain that you are trying to be able to resist going to pieces when such reactions occur.

Keep your collar buttoned but do not wear a tie all morning. Report all actual and suspected penalties.

Irritate some other person until he attacks you. Then explain why you did it.

Frustration.

Prewrite everything you say before you say it for an entire morning. Report your feelings of frustration but try to hold to the assignment despite the desire to talk without the annoyance of putting it down.

Do not smoke at all today.

During the noon hour, before you say the first sentence of any conversation, tap your toe once for each word within it.

Do some cumulative reading aloud. Read the first word; then the first and second; then the first, second, and third; and so on.

Have real or faked stuttering on every word of (1) a reading passage, (2) a conversation, and (3) in asking a stranger to direct you to the nearest movie theater.

Anxiety, Guilt, and Hostility.

Deliberately stutter to one person in a mildly hostile fashion, and then to another in a very hostile fashion. Smear him with a little of it, then with a lot of it. Report his reactions and your feelings.

Verbalize some of your worries about the future to five different listeners, one at a time. Say the same things each time. Report your feelings.

After each of five faked stuttering blocks, stop and say this to your listener, "I'm sorry I stuttered so hard. I'm sorry I took so much of your time." Report your feelings.

Using a hand counter, click it every time you feel ashamed during your conversations at meal times. Do this for three days in a row and see if the number doesn't decrease.

Communicative Stress.

Find someone who habitually interrupts your attempts to speak or finishes the words for you on which you are stuttering. Every time he does either, go back to the beginning of your sentence and repeat the whole thing. Report what happened.

Ask your roommate to heckle you as you explain something. Try to keep from hurrying or getting upset. And do not stop moving forward even though you stutter. Do not stop or repeat. Have him heckle only a little at first, then turn on the heat.

Interrupt another person three times in one conversation but do not hurry when you do so. Wait till he stops to take a breath but then interrupt him. Report your feelings.

Find one listener who seems to stop listening or who always says "What?" or "What did you say?" Keep talking to him till he has done this five times.

Situation Fears.

Make twenty-five phone calls before you go to bed tonight.

Stop at every residence in one block; go up to the door and ask if someone with your own name lives there. Stutter at least once, real or faked stutterings, at each house.

Smile and say hello to every girl you meet on your way to school.

Remembering one of the worst speaking situations you've ever had in the past, try to invent another which has some resemblance to it, and enter it.

Apply for a job at every store in one block downtown.

Ask a policeman how to get to the railroad station.

Word Fears.

Prepare a reading passage containing your most feared words and make a tape recording of four readings of this material to the same listener.

In speaking to a friend, repeat each stuttered word either until you no longer stutter on it, or until you have tried it ten times.

Make a list of five of your most feared words and deliberately introduce them into conversations. Write each word on a small slip of paper and hold each of these in your hand until it has been used.

Prepare prewritten phone calls in which you load what you have to say with words beginning with your feared sounds. Example: "Sammy Smith speaking, is my sister Sue staying with Sandra this evening?" Keep calling till you've got it all out and without going haywire.

Purposely fake repetitions of the first feared sounds of words until you find yourself calm, then say the word. Collect ten of these.

Hold the silent posture of the feared sound of a word until you have tapped your toe five times. Collect another for ten toe taps, and, if you can bear it, another for twenty toe taps. Be sure to count the toe taps.

In making a phone call, time your deliberate prolongation of the first sound of one feared word for two seconds. Then do it again to another listener for three seconds; and if possible, to another for four seconds. Don't count any who hang up.

Let us repeat that these are merely illustrative speech assignments, any one of which might be entirely inappropriate for certain stutterers. Moreover, we have not indicated—and cannot indicate—the wide variety of assignments possible under each heading. Each therapist and each stutterer must invent his own. We have found it wise to keep the busywork at a minimum, to ask for as little performance as possible and yet enough to produce some impact. Assignments must be so structured that an objective report can be produced. They must provide enough stress to permit desensitization to occur. For any given case, their difficulty must be so tailored that more success than failure ensues, but failure is not to be avoided entirely. Indeed, in the sharing period with the therapist and other stutterers, often the failures when expressed and accepted do more good than even the successes. But there must be therapist approval and reward for meeting these challenges. And constantly we must emphasize the basic purpose these desensitization experiences are designed to fulfill: the building of a thicker hide on the stutterer's sensitive soul.

The Variation Phase of Treatment

It is not enough to motivate, to identify, and desensitize, although these bring reductions in the frequency and severity of stuttering. In this new phase of therapy we begin to change, to modify the reactions to the factors that determine stuttering. Our purpose is to break up the stereotypy of the stutterer's responses, to attach new responses to the old cues. Much of the strength of habitual compulsive reactions lies in their stereotypy, in the consistency of their patterning. Varying them weakens them. Until new responses are made available, the stutterer has no choice except to yield to the old ones. We must help him to know that he has this choice. We cannot persuade him through intellectual argument. Only by behaving differently can he know that it is possible to behave differently.

This variation phase of treatment is usually short in duration because it passes directly into the next one of approximation, in which we seek to help the stutterer learn not just *new* responses to old pressures, but *good* responses. By "good" we mean only that new responses can be learned which will facilitate fluency rather than reduce it. There are always better ways of responding to penalty, frustration, word fear, and all the other evil factors than those the stutterer has habituated to compulsive automaticity. We must help him learn new responses which do not continually reinforce his stuttering as his old responses do. But before these new ways of behaving can be learned, the old ways must be weakened. Variation must precede approximation. The stutterer must realize that he has a choice of responses before he can pick out and master a better one.

Again we seek to provide for the stutterer experiences in which this learning may occur and to motivate him to seek such experiences himself. Let us reverse our usual sequence of presentation and begin with the factor of word fear.

Varying the Reactions to Word Fear.

Read a passage omitting all words on which you anticipate any stuttering.

On every other word on which you stutter, be sure to stutter repetitively but slowly on the first syllable. Do this to three listeners.

Underline the feared words in a reading passage and substitute (or add) a tremor in your right leg for each one that you find in your lips or tongue.

In a phone call, when you find yourself using such stallers as *a* . . . *a* . . . *a* . . . , vary them so that you also use *um, uh, ub, oops,* and *Ozymandias.* Your job is to vary the way you usually postpone.

During three moments of stuttering attempt to shift the focus of the tension from where it usually resides to some other parts of your body. Report what you did.

Instead of gasping as an interrupter of your tremors, try blowing out a puff of air on four of your stuttering blocks.

Since you usually lower your head whenever you stutter, watch yourself in a mirror with an observer, and make it rise instead.

Instead of shutting both eyes as you usually do when stuttering, try shutting only one. Work before a mirror until you get ten successes.

Varying the Reactions to Situation Fears.

You have said that when you enter a phone booth to make a call, you hurry too much and go all to pieces. Today, enter five phone booths, stay in each for two minutes before you call me. When I answer, just make noises and hang up. Report your feelings.

You report that when you must do an errand, you rehearse over and over again what you plan to say, picking out easy words and revising sentences. Today, do three such errands with a friend but you are to say only what he tells you and to say it exactly as he does. He is not to tell you what to say until the last minute. Report your experiences.

Ordinarily you walk around the block several times before entering a store to ask for something. Today, ask questions in three stores, but stand absolutely still looking in the display window for as long as it would take you to walk around that block. Then go in and ask for it. Report your introspections.

In your trigonometry class today, sit in the front row for a change. Get there in time so you can.

Varying the Reactions to Communicative Stress.

Get a companion and hunt for the noisiest places you can find. Try not to speak more loudly to your friend but speak more slowly and distinctly.

Ask some acquaintance to do you a favor you know he will not grant. Do not apologize or appear uncertain. Just ask him.

Criticize your roommate for some of the behavior you do not like and return to it until he gets angry. Speak very slowly as you do so.

When one of your listeners looks away while you stutter, speak more loudly or do something different so he will look at you.

Varying the Reactions to Anxiety, Guilt, and Hostility.

You say you find yourself worrying vaguely about everything and find it hard to get to sleep. Tonight, assign yourself to worry on purpose and do so aloud in self talk just before you hop into bed. Worry aloud about everything you can possibly think of.

You've reported that when you've felt ashamed about something you did or didn't do, you found yourself biting your fingernails to the quick. Keep a pocketful of peanuts and remember to bite one of them (only one) instead whenever you start to nibble a fingernail or find yourself feeling guilty or ashamed.

You've reported how frequently you keep reviewing your wrongs and hates. This evening before you go to bed, write out as many of them as you can on toilet tissue, read them again, then flush them down the drain.

At the beginning of each hour, by your watch, verbalize to yourself a statement of one anxiety, one guilt, and one hostility. Try not to repeat yourself. Do this for each hour of the afternoon.

Varying the Reactions to Frustration and Penalty.

Every time you feel frustrated this evening, smile and continue to smile until the frustration has subsided.

Whenever a listener interrupts you or finishes a word on which you are stuttering, say to him, "Don't interrupt me. I've got a hard enough time talking anyway."

Collect three instances in which a moment of stuttering causes you feelings of frustration or evokes listener penalty and in which you repeated the same word over and over again at least three times.

You say your stuttering often produces smiles on the faces of your listeners. Suddenly ask one of them why he's smiling.

As we write this chapter we are constantly aware of the inadequacy of our presentation of such assignments in reflecting what actually occurs in therapy. These assignments by themselves have no value. Only when shared with the therapist and when feelings are expressed and when rewards are appropriately timed, do the experiences they evoke have potency in modifying the attitudes and outward behavior of the stutterer. It would be easier and perhaps safer to resort to statements of vague general principles, but students seem to profit more from specific examples. So be it!

The Approximation Phase of Therapy

Once the stutterer has learned that his habitual reactions to the factors which make stuttering worse can be varied, we try to help him learn *new responses which will diminish that stuttering.* We now seek not just different responses but the best responses, those which tend to extinguish stuttering rather than reinforce it. Why do we call this phase the approximation phase? Because we feel that new responses are acquired, not by sudden exchange, but by gradual modification. You just don't stop stuttering severely and suddenly begin to stutter easily. Again, it's like learning to target-shoot. You shoot and miss; then you change a bit of your behavior and shoot again. Your attempts result in a coming closer, in an approximation to the behavior needed to hit the bull's-eye consistently. By approximation we mean the progressive modification of behavior toward a goal response. It is operant conditioning.

The basic goal then of this phase of therapy is to learn how to stutter and to respond to stress in such a fashion that the disorder will not be reinforced. The therapist's responsibility is to see that rewards are felt whenever the stutterer moves closer to this goal. Approval is contingent upon progress, not merely upon performance. Happily, the relief from communicative abnormality seems to follow the same course, and provides even more powerful reinforcement. The goal is getting nearer now.

In our discussion of this phase of therapy, we will confine ourselves to the exposition of what we do with the fears and experiences of stuttering itself. It must be remembered, however, that the characteristic responses to penalty, frustration, and all the other disturbing factors must also be modified in the direction of nonreinforcement of the stuttering. There are better responses to penalty, to communicative stress, than those the stutterer first brings to us, and these he can also learn by progressive approximation. However, here we will concentrate on the stuttering behavior.

Stuttering in Unison.   One of the best ways we have discovered to help the stutterer learn an easier, nonreinforcing kind of stuttering is to do it with him. He watches us and hears us as we join him in his stuttering, duplicating the first of his behavior, but then we ease out of the tremors, cease the struggling, and smoothly finish the word. Often at first, the contrast between his continued struggles and our smooth utterance tends to shock him, but gradually he begins to follow our lead and to stutter as we do. He finds us sharing his initial behavior but then diverging. We make the changes gradually, at first setting models of minor changes which he may be able to follow, and rewarding them when they appear. Once he can make these minor changes (e.g., stuttering with his eyes open rather than closed), he gets no more approval until a further change occurs (e.g., lips are loosened from their tensed closure), and so on. We move only as far as the case is ready and able to go in any given session. It is vitally necessary that this training be done under some stress, stress that can be felt but not stress which overwhelms. To sum it up, we share and show him how to shift, how to change his responses. Verbalization of feelings is always encouraged, and this phase of therapy often produces some new storms. But the mere fact of the sharing, the fact of the therapist's faith, the fact of his patient acceptance of failure as a necessary part of learning—all these create a favorable climate for change and growth.

Cancellation. As soon as any change in the stuttering behavior has been learned, the stutterer is encouraged to use it in cancellation. By this term we mean that the stutterer stops as soon as a stuttered word has finally been uttered; pauses; and then says it again, this time using the modification he has learned in unison stuttering with his therapist. He still stutters this second time, faking, if he must, a duplication of the same stuttering he has just experienced but now he modifies it in accordance with the new behavior he has learned. Then he finishes his sentence. Communication stops once he stutters and it continues only after he has used a better stuttering response. This also is powerfully reinforcing.

Pull-outs. This awkward term, stemming from the stutterers' own language usage, refers to the moment of stuttering itself and what the stutterer does to escape from his oscillations or fixations. Evil pull-outs are the jerks, the sudden exhaling of all available air. These only increase the penalty and all other factors that make for more stuttering in the future. There are better ways of terminating these fixations and oscillations, and once these new ways have been learned in unison speaking with the therapist, and practiced frequently in cancellations in all types of speaking situations, the stutterer should begin to incorporate them within the original moment of stuttering itself. Any change for the better should be incorporated as often as the stutterer can manage it. Thus the new behavior moves forward in time, from the period just following the stuttering into the moment of stuttering itself.

Preparatory Sets. Our next step is to move it even further forward, into the period of anticipation, into what has been called the "pre-spasm period." Usually, in response to word or phonetic fears, the stutterer actually makes little covert rehearsals of the stuttering abnormality he expects. These preparatory sets to stutter often determine the kind and length of abnormality which result. Therefore, once the stutterer has shown that he can incorporate the new change not only in cancellation but also during the actual stuttering behavior, he is now challenged to incorporate it within his anticipatory rehearsals, to plan to stutter this new way. Often we help him by rehearsing for him and by getting him to duplicate our model before he attempts the word he has indicated he will stutter upon. Again we reward the successes and disregard the failures. Again we reward progressive change.

As each new modification of stuttering is learned and starts up the series of experiences in cancellation, pull-outs, and preparatory sets, new modifications are being born, either with the help of the therapist through unison stuttering or through self-discoveries. With each new change comes a decrease in the severity and often in the frequency of stuttering as well. Fears of words, then of situations, lose their intensity. The stutterer's self-confidence begins to grow with each new achievement. The fluency factor grows larger. He becomes able to tolerate more communicative stress. It is also interesting to watch how he applies the same therapeutic principles to his other inadequate behaviors. He begins to modify his old inadequate reactions to penalty and frustration, and the ways he handles his anxieties, guilts, and hostilities improve. Progress comes swiftly on all fronts. Instead of avoiding stuttering experiences, he hunts for them so he can try out his new skills. Avoidance declines.

Perhaps some glimpses of the actual interaction between therapist and case would be helpful here, although it is impossible to indicate the changes in behavior which occur. The student will have to use some imagination.

> This stutterer, when he attempted a feared *p* or *b* or *m* word, characteristically assumed a wide-open-mouthed posture, invested it with a strong tremor, then attempted to release himself from it by a sudden movement in which the head went up but the jaw went down. The final utterance of the word always emerged from one of these jerks. Often he would have to use two or three of the latter before release occurred, and if one failed, he then returned instantly to the tremorous highly tensed open mouth posturing.

Therapist. Today, let's see if we can't learn to stutter a bit more easily than you've been doing it on that feared *p* sound of yours.

Subject. GGGGGGGood. I'm rrrrready.

Therapist. On these cards I have written some *p* words that you have often stuttered on and I'm hoping that you'll stutter on a few of them at least.

Subject. (*Opens mouth and has his characteristic abnormality*) . . . (*jerk*) Probably!

Therapist. Well, I won't need the card, I guess. I'll ask you a question now, and if you stutter on the answer, I'll join you, do just what you do at first, but then do something differently too. Try to follow my lead. Here's the question: Do you think you'll have some stuttering on these words?

Subject. (*Opens mouth in same tremorous posture, which the therapist duplicates almost exactly, but therapist slowly closes mouth while continuing the tremor so that finally the tremor is occurring on the lips alone. The stutterer also closes his lips as he watches and follows the model, but just before he says the word "Probably" his mouth again opens suddenly and the head-and-jaw jerk of release precede its utterance. The therapist's utterance finally emerges from the closed lip position, so the two performances, at first fairly identical, later diverge.*)

Therapist. Good. You made some change. Not enough but at least you managed to produce the only posture that the first sound of "prob-ably" can use. Here's what you did . . . (*demonstrates*) and here's what you always have done in the past . . . (*demonstrates*) so you can see that you made some change for the better. Nobody can say "probably" with his mouth as far open as your Grand Canyon of the Colorado. Now show me both ways. Show me, by faking if you must, how you usually stutter on the word, and then how you just changed it a bit.

Subject (*Demonstrates old way*) . . . (*jerk*) Probably . . . Hey, that . . . (*jerk*) bbecame real! (*Therapist grins, and the stutterer then demonstrates the changed stuttering pattern.*)

Therapist. Pretty good! Now let's try some of these *p* words and be sure to get your mouth closed and hold it closed a bit before you jerk it out. Remember I'll be joining you every so often . . . not always.

They work on eight different *p* words this way. The therapist gives approval intermittently but only for lip closure during the stuttering. Then he says:

Therapist. Now let's hear about that job you have with the *Gazette*. Forget about doing anything about any other stutterings, but if you have one of your old unchanged blocks on a *p* word, stop immediately, pause until I give you the signal, and then cancel it by stuttering again on the word but in the changed way.

Subject. OK. Well, I, I, I ddddddelivered ffffffffforty . . . (*jerk*) papers . . . (*Therapist signals and case stops. Therapist pantomimes changed stuttering pattern, then nods and case cancels in the new way*) . . . ppppppp . . . (*jerk*) papers. How's that?

Therapist. Attaboy. Good. Let's do some more cancelling. Tell me some more about your deliveries. (*The stutterer begins but forgets to cancel on the first* p *word.*)

Subject. Oooops, I fffffforgot.

Therapist. It's hard to remember when you're interested in what you're saying. (*The stutterer gets some more cancellations, and then he uses the new change in the first attempt on another* p *word.*)

Subject. (*Surprised*) Hey, I used it in the mmmmmmmmmiddle.

Therapist. Good. Good! How about trying to get some more of those in the middle of your stutterings? Look, here's how you did it. . . . (*Therapist demonstrates.*) You don't *have* to keep your mouth open when you try to say a p word.

They collect several more experiences, some successful, which the therapist rewards, and some failures, which he ignores. Several times the case failed but then cancelled. This was reflected and rewarded. Once, he successfully rehearsed it before succeeding.

Therapist. How do you feel about this experimenting?

Subject. MMMMMan! It's ffffffffffascinating. I, I, I, I think I'm gggggetting the idea. MMMMaybe I can do it easier, hey?

Therapist. Want to try changing it a bit further?

Subject. Sure.

Therapist. OK. Now, let's see if you can stop jerking just before the word comes out. Look, here's what you do (*demonstrates*). . . . Can you also do this? . . . (*Demonstrates the elimination of the jerk release and shows how the utterance could come directly from the tremorous lip posture.*)

They then work on this new change in the same way. Now the therapist only rewards the new changes. The session ends in some fairly potent expression and reflection of feelings revolving about the stutterer's fear of hoping too much and his many doubts about the future.

We cannot end this section on approximation without reminding the student that most of the progress made must be due to the stutterer's solo efforts. Many speech assignments are devised to provide the necessary opportunities for progressively modifying the stuttering behavior under stress. But this is how we begin.

Stabilization. The final phase of stuttering therapy we have called stabilization. For lack of a clear-cut program of this sort, many stutterers have experienced frequent relapses and despair. It is not enough to bring the stutterer to the point where he is fluent, where he can speak with little struggle or fear. We must stabilize his new behavior, his new resistances to stress, his new integration. Anxiety-conditioned responses are very difficult to extinguish entirely. New adjustments must be made, new responsibilities undertaken now that the stuttering excuse is no longer valid. Terminal therapy must be done carefully. It must be done well. We always keep in fairly close touch with our secondary stutterers for two years after formal therapy is terminated. Many of them occasionally avail themselves of our counsel for many years, often on matters other than stuttering.

Often stuttering seems to go out the same door it entered. More of the easy and unconscious repetitions and prolongations appear; periods of fairly frequent small stutterings alternate with periods of very good fluency. Sudden bursts of fear and even avoidance occur. Under moments of extreme stress an occasional severe blocking may be evident. It is important that the stutterer understand this and accept it as part of his problem. Often the therapist must be available for the verbalization of these traumatic episodes and receive the confession of avoidance and compulsive behaviors with accepting reassurance and remedial measures. However, it is possible to prevent much of this stress by an organized program of terminal therapy.

Fluency. Even when the stuttering disappears, there remain gaps in the flow of speech where the stuttering formerly occurred. These people have had so little experience in smooth flowing speech that some training is needed to provide it. One of the best ways we have found to do this is through echo speech or shadowing, in which the stutterer, while watching TV or observing some fluent speaker, follows in pantomime the speech that is being produced, saying it silently as it is being spoken aloud. Often we train the stutterer to repeat whole sentences exactly as the speaker spoke them. We also ask him to cancel whole sentences of his own in which gaps or hesitancies appeared so that they can be made to flow more smoothly. We persuade him to do much self-talk when alone. We emphasize display speech of all types so that he can get the feel of fluency. At the same time we also show him that even excellent speakers have some nonfluencies and that these are different from the residual breaks which come from a long history of broken speech.

Faking. We also train our stutterers to fake easy repetitive or prolonged stutterings, to put these into their fluent speech casually in certain situations every day. We ask them, too, to demonstrate an occasional faking of a short block of the old variety and then to follow it with a cancellation. Occasionally it is wise to fake a pull-out or some of the modifications of postures and tremors so that these basic skills may remain fresh for use in emergencies. Most stutterers dislike doing these things and they will not do them unless the activities form a basic part of the stabilization phase of treatment.

Assessment.   The practice of taking an honest daily inventory must be encouraged. In this phase of treatment, we help the stutterer to learn to survey his own personal stuttering equation, to assess the variations in strength of the various factors, and to be honest in his evaluations. Here the accepting attitudes of an understanding therapist are most essential. He hears the confession and turns it into an inventory, for these are not sins but the natural residues of a severe disorder of communication.

Resistance Therapy.   In this final phase of active therapy, we work especially hard to help the stutterer learn to maintain his new methods of fluent stuttering and fluent speaking in the face of pressures of all kinds. When he first comes to us the stutterer has but two choices: to stutter on the feared words or to avoid them. We now have given him a third choice, the ability to stutter in a relatively fluent and unabnormal fashion. It is necessary not only to stabilize his new behavior of this third choice under conditions of stress but also to give him a fourth choice—to resist stuttering.

In helping the stutterer to resist communicative stresses of all kinds and yet maintain his new ways of short, easy stuttering, we (both stutterer and therapist) deliberately create conditions in which the pressures to stutter in the old way are strong, and then the stutterer does his utmost to resist them. We seek out and enter the feared situations of the past; we look for more and more difficult situations. By programming this stress so that the stutterer is largely (not always) able to beat it and yet can stutter easily when he does stutter, we enable him to strengthen the new behavioral responses to the old cues, to the old stresses which once set off the old abnormal responses of avoidance and struggle. This stress strengthening is even good for concrete beams; it is good for stutterers in the terminal stages of therapy.

But there is another form of resistance therapy which goes further and which holds the promise of curing stutterers and not merely making them fluent. It provides the fourth choice we mentioned earlier. Stutterers have long known a curious experience, namely, that occasionally they are able to summon up their powers and just refuse to stutter. It sounds unbelievable but most stutterers will so testify, and often this occurs under conditions of great stress. They do not know what happens, nor do we. However, we have found that in the terminal stages of therapy, when avoidance has been pretty well eliminated, and when, if difficulty does come, it can be handled without great distress, we can train the case to resist his urge to stutter. Let us illustrate.

A simple procedure is to have the stutterer read in unison with the therapist. Under these conditions he will be very fluent. He is also very fluent in automatic echoing or shadowing. But then the therapist deliberately introduces some stuttering into his own speech and challenges the stutterer to resist him, in other words, to continue to speak the words as fluently as when the therapist was using fluent speech.

This is a strange and a new challenge. It is possible to resist the therapist's behavioral suggestion that he must stutter! There is no avoidance of feared situations, words, or sounds here. There *is* the resistance to suggestion, a resistance which stutterers need badly. Why should they always yield? By judiciously using the principles of desensitization therapy and introducing just enough stuttering in the model so that the case wins more often than he loses, it is possible to teach him to battle rather than succumb. There's no virtue in stuttering if you can resist the influences which tell you that you must. In this technique there is no avoidance, no running away. The challenge is proffered and accepted. No postponement, starting tricks, or other devices are permitted. The stutterer is simply to say the word if he can without stuttering at a moment when the therapist is trying to make him have some stuttering. Once the principles of this resistance therapy have been mastered, the stutterer, through speech assignments and self-therapy, continues to battle the suggestion that if he has fear, he must stutter.

Treatment of the Young Secondary Stutterer. In order to spell out exactly how we treat the secondary stutterer, we have described our therapy as it would be administered to a person who is relatively adult. With slight modifications—especially those in which the therapy is done with the therapist in the safety of the speech room —the suggestions made are useful with the person of high-school age. But there are secondary stutterers in the elementary school. Indeed, we have had to treat children as young as three and four years who showed all the overt and covert behavior characteristics of the fourth and terminal stage of the disorder. Most of them begin to come to the speech therapist later, when they are at least in school and in the third grade or above. How do we treat these children?

The general pattern of treatment is the same. It also follows *MIDVAS*. We begin by identifying with the child during his stuttering, sharing it, helping him confront it without shame. We teach him to watch it, feel it, try to change it so that when he does stutter he does not avoid or struggle. We give him models and have him imitate us directly as we show him how to ease out of his tremors, his hard contacts, his hypertensed mouth postures. "Watch me," we say. "Look! Here's how you stuttered just now. Now see how I can start the way you do but ease out of it . . . like this. Try it again." Fortunately, in these younger children, the disorder is as yet not too deeply rooted. They unlearn more easily. Once they put their trust and love in you, they will follow your demonstrations and directions most willingly. We almost always use play therapy along with the speech work to relieve the pressures of *PFAGH*. We provide situations in which there is little communicative stress. We do desensitization therapy often, as though the child were still in the earlier stages. We give him many experiences in being completely fluent through the use of echoing, unison speaking, rhythmic talking, and relaxation. We do our utmost to build his ego strength in every possible way. We use no speech assignments but, through parental counseling and home and school visits, we gradually incorporate his new ways of talking into his entire living space. We can help these children.

Summary

The three different methods for treating stuttering in the secondary stage have been presented: psychotherapy, distraction, and modification through operant conditioning. Each of the factors determining the frequency and severity of stuttering have been defined and methods for their reinforcement or extinction have been given. The therapeutic activities and experiences for each of the four developmental stages have been described. Finally, we have outlined the course of therapy in terms of motivation, identification, desensitization, variation, approximation, and stabilization.

1. Write a letter to the mother of a child who is in the primary stage of stuttering, giving her some of the basic information she should possess.

2. Make a list of some of the common frustrations experienced by any boy aged three.

3. Invent a story to be told to a stuttering child which may help to relieve his fears of thunderstorms.

4. A child is very fearful of going to bed at night. How can you reduce this fear?

5. What are some of the ways in which parents may increase guilt feelings in their children?

6. How can you help relieve a child's feelings of hostility through play therapy? Invent a play-by-play account which will answer this question.

7. Invent a dialogue with the mother of a young stuttering child in which you attempt to relieve her feelings of anxiety over his primary stuttering.

8. Invent an anecdotal account of a group therapy session with the parents of three young stutterers.

9. Keep track of all the moments of broken fluency you experience during a half-day and attempt to determine what caused them.

10. Invent a dialogue with a young stutterer in which you speak very simply in an effort to set easy models for him to follow.

11. Explain, as to the mother of a stuttering child, why she should ask him few questions.

12. Explain, as to the mother of a primary stutterer, why she should not ask him to stop and think or to relax, or to talk more slowly.

13. Invent some "speech play" activities in which there will be little communicative stress and much fluency.

14. Invent a dialogue showing how you would help a child in the third stage of stuttering to confront his stuttering and to stutter more easily.

15. Demonstrate with a classmate who pretends to have some secondary stuttering, one bit of therapy typical of each of the three major treatments of this stage of the disorder.

16. Practice stuttering in unison with some stutterer so that you can duplicate his behavior very closely. Then both of you put on a demonstration before the class.

17. Demonstrate some resistance therapy.
18. Demonstrate (with commentary) cancellations, pull-outs, and preparatory sets.
19. Invent a desensitization speech assignment for a secondary stutterer.
20. Demonstrate four different types of faking and explain why they are used.

REFERENCES

1. Ainsworth, S. "Present Trends in the Treatment of Stuttering," *Journal of Exceptional Children*, Volume 16, 1949, pages 41-43.
2. Baldwin, M. "Notes on Play Sessions with Two Stammering Boys," *Speech* (London), Volume 18, 1954, pages 17-23.
3. Belgum, D. "Stuttering," *Hygeia*, Volume 22, 1944, pages 346-347; 391.
4. Bleumel, C. S. *The Riddle of Stuttering*. Springfield, Ill.: The Interstate Printers & Publishers, Inc., 1957.
5. Boome, E. J., and M. A. Richardson. *The Nature and Treatment of Stuttering*. New York: E. P. Dutton & Co., Inc., 1932.
6. Bryngelson, B. "Prognosis of Stuttering," *Journal of Speech Disorders*, Volume 6, 1941, pages 121-123.
7. ———, M. E. Chapman, and O. K. Hansen. *Know Yourself—A Worldbook for Those Who Stutter*. Minneapolis: Burgess Publishing Co., 1944, page 53.
8. Cypreason, L. "Group Therapy for Adult Stutterers," *Journal of Speech and Hearing Disorders*, Volume 13, 1948, pages 313-319.
9. Despert, J. L. "A Therapeutic Approach to the Problem of Stuttering in Children," *The Nervous Child*, Volume 2, 1943, pages 134-147.
10. Dow, C. W. "Stuttering: A Tentative Outline of an Hypothesis and Therapy," *Journal of Speech Disorders*, Volume 6, 1941, pages 40-45.
11. Freund, H. "Reflections on Subconscious Phenomena in Stuttering," Current Problems in *Phoniatrics and Logopedics*, Volume 1, 1960, pages 184-189.
12. Froeschels, E. "Pathology and Therapy of Stuttering," *The Nervous Child*, Volume 2, 1942, pages 146-161.
13. Glasner, P. J., and M. F. Dahl. "Stuttering—A Prophylactic Program for Its Control," *American Journal Public Health*, Volume 42, 1952, pages 1111-1115.
14. Gottlober, A. B. *Understanding Stuttering*. New York: Grune & Stratton, Inc., 1953.
15. Harle, M. "Dynamic Interpretation and Treatment of Acute Stutter-

ing in a Young Child," *American Journal of Orthopsychiatry,* Volume 15, 1946, pages 156-162.

16. Hejna, R. F. *Speech Disorders and NonDirective Therapy.* New York: The Ronald Press Company, 1960.

17. Honig, P. "The Stutterer Acts It Out," *Journal of Speech Disorders,* Volume 12, 1947, pages 105-109.

18. Jameson, A. "Stammering in Children," *Speech* (London), Volume 19, 1955, pages 60-67.

19. Johnson, W. "An Open Letter to the Mother of a Stuttering Child," Chapter Two in *Speech Handicapped School Children.* New York: Harper & Row, Publishers, 1948, pages 443-451.

20. ———. *Stuttering and What You Can Do about It.* Minneapolis: University of Minnesota Press, 1961.

21. Kent, L. R. "A Retraining Program for the Adult Who Stutters," *Journal Speech and Hearing Disorders,* Volume 26, 1961, pages 141-144.

22. Kinstler, D. B. "Covert and Overt Maternal Rejection in Stuttering," *Journal Speech and Hearing Disorders,* Volume 26, 1961, pages 145-155.

23. Klingbell, G. M. "The Historical Background of the Modern Speech Clinic: Stuttering and Stammering," *Journal of Speech Disorders,* Volume 4, 1939, pages 115-131.

24. Kopp, G. A. "Treatment of Stuttering," *Journal of Speech Disorders,* Volume 4, 1939, pages 166-168.

25. Lemert, E. M., and C. Van Riper. "The Use of Psychodrama in the Treatment of Speech Defects," *Sociometry,* Volume 7, 1944, pages 190-195.

26. Louttit, C. M. *Clinical Psychology.* New York: Harper & Row, Publishers, 1936, pages 446-450.

27. Matis, E. E. "Psychotherapeutic Tools for Parents," *Journal Speech and Hearing Disorders,* Volume 26, 1961, pages 164-170.

28. McAllister, A. H. "The Problem of Stammering," *Speech Pathology and Therapy* (London) Volume 1, 1958, pages 1-8.

29. Murphy, A. T., and R. M. Fitz-Simons. *Stuttering and Personality Dynamics.* New York: The Ronald Press Company, 1960.

30. Murray, F. P. "Observations on Therapy for Stuttering in Japan," *Journal Speech and Hearing Disorders,* Volume 23, 1958, pages 243-249.

31. Pollitt, J. "A Review of Cases of Stammering," *Speech* (London) Volume 15, 1951, pages 33-41.

32. Sander, E. K. "Counseling Parents of Stuttering Children," *Journal Speech and Hearing Disorders,* Volume 24, 1959, pages 262-271.

33. Schultz, D. A. "A Study of Non-Directive Counseling as Applied to

Adult Stutterers," *Journal of Speech Disorders,* Volume 12, 1947, pages 421-427.

34. Sheehan, J. G. "An Integration of Psychotherapy and Speech Therapy through a Conflict Theory of Stuttering," *Journal Speech and Hearing Disorders,* Volume 19, 1954, pages 474-482.

35. ———. "The Modification of Stuttering Through Non-Reinforcement," *Journal Abnormal and Social Psychology,* Volume 46, 1951, pages 193-195.

36. ———. "Theory and Treatment of Stuttering as an Approach-Avoidance Conflict," *Journal of Psychology,* Volume 36, 1953, pages 27-49.

37. ——— and R. B. Voas. "Stuttering as Conflict: 1. Comparison of Therapy Techniques Involving Approach and Avoidance," *Journal Speech and Hearing Therapy,* Volume 22, 1957, pages 714-723.

38. Van Riper, C. "Do You Stutter?" *Atlantic Monthly,* Volume 164, 1939, pages 601-609.

39. ———. "Experiments in Stuttering Therapy," in J. Eisenson (ed.), *Stuttering: A Symposium.* New York: Harper & Row, Publishers, 1958, pages 275-390.

40. ———. "Symptomatic Therapy for Stuttering," in L. E. Travis (ed.), *Handbook of Speech Pathology.* New York: Appleton-Century-Crofts, 1957, pages 878-896.

41. ———. "Treatment of Stuttering," *Speech* (London) Volume 17, 1953, pages 17-20.

42. Wedberg, C. F. *The Stutterer Speaks.* Redlands, Calif.: Valley Fine Arts Press, 1937.

43. Whitten, I. E. "Therapies Used for Stuttering: A Report of the Author's Own Case," *Quarterly Journal of Speech,* Volume 24, 1938, pages 227-233.

44. Will, N. "A Six-month Report on the Personality Development of a Thirteen Year Old Stuttering Boy," *Quarterly Journal of Speech,* Volume 30, 1944, pages 88-95.

45. Wingate, M. E. "Calling Attention to Stuttering," *Journal Speech and Hearing Disorders,* Volume 2, 1959, pages 326-335 .

46. Wolpe, Z. "Play Therapy, Psychodrama, and Stuttering," in L. E. Travis (ed.), *Handbook of Speech Pathology.* New York: Appleton-Century-Crofts, 1957, pages 991-1023.

CHAPTER THIRTEEN

Cleft Palate Speech

At least one baby in every thousand born possesses a cleft lip or palate or both. The moment this happens, a complex rehabilitation problem also comes into being, often requiring the cooperative efforts of a team of specialists comprised of the oral surgeon, the prosthodontist, the orthodontist, the plastic surgeon, the psychologist, and the speech therapist. The cleft must be surgically repaired or an artificial palate constructed. Teeth must be straightened or repositioned. Scars must be removed and nose straightened. Adjustment problems, not only those of the child but also those of the parents who must pay for all this and care for a deviant child, may need counseling. Most important, probably, of all these is the need to make sure that the child can talk without the honking, snorting unintelligibility which characterizes cleft-palate speech when untreated.

Types of Clefts. Although classifications differ, there are three major problems involved: clefts of the prepalate, clefts of the palate, and clefts which include both palate and prepalate. All of these stem from embryological failure, or more rarely, from accidents. The two halves of the lip, or of the bony upper gum ridge (alveolar process), or the two halves of the hard and soft palate fail to grow together and unite as they do before the third month in normal children. As a result, when the baby is born, it shows clefts of the upper lip, the upper gum ridge, the hard palate, or the soft palate. These clefts may be complete or incomplete, but the right and left sides of these structures have not come together as they should have done.

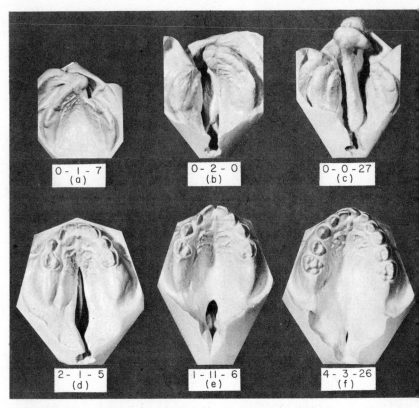

FIGURE 29. *Representations of the Most Common Clefts of the Lip and Palate.*
All of these casts (of the upper surface of the mouth) were obtained from infants prior to any surgery. The numbers refer to the child's age in years, months,
and days. They may be interpreted as follows: A. Complete unilateral cleft of
the lip and alveolar process; B. Complete unilateral cleft of both the lip and
palate; C. Complete bilateral cleft of the lip and palate; D. Cleft of the hard
and soft palate; E. Cleft of the soft palate; F. Bifid uvula.[*]

Clefts of the Prepalate. These include clefts of the upper lip and
also those of the alveolar process (upper jaw bone beneath the
upper gum). They may be unilateral and show a cleft on one side
which if *complete* extends up into the nostril on that side. Or they
may be bilateral or double clefts, each of which (if complete

---

[*] From Samuel Pruzansky, "Description, Classification and Analysis of
Unoperated Clefts of the Lip and Palate," *American Journal of Orthodontics*,
Volume 39, 1953, pages 590-611. By permission of the author.

rather than incomplete) runs up into the nostril above it. These clefts of the lip in some children are also accompanied by similar clefts in the alveolar process; in other children the rift is in the lip alone. Although the majority of clefts are right sided, left sided, or both, a few rare median clefts (in the middle) are found.

Clefts of the Palate. Clefts in both the soft and hard palates are included in this category. The opening in the muscular soft palate may show itself merely in a split (bifid) uvula or may extend upward and forward all the way to the edge of the bony hard palate. In this case we speak of a complete velar (or soft-palatal) cleft. There are also soft-palate clefts which extend only partially toward the hard palate.

Clefts of the Hard Palate. The bony roof of the mouth cavity formed by palatal shelves which grow together and join long before birth, also may be cleft, creating an opening up into the nasal cavity. These clefts are along the midline, but one of the edges of the cleft may be attached to the base of the *vomer* (the bony partition that separates the right and left chambers of the nasal passages above). Usually, if the hard palate is cleft, the soft palate is also, since in the embryo the two halves of the roof of the mouth unite in stages proceeding from the front toward the rear.

Submucous Clefts. Some children show no apparent signs of clefts when their mouths are visually inspected and yet clefts may be present under the mucous linings of the mouth cavity. Those of the soft palate may be felt by palpating them; those of the hard palate at times cannot be discovered except by radiography. The child's speech can be affected by such submucous clefts.

Clefts of Both Palate and Prepalate. Unfortunately frequent are these clefts that run through both the palate and prepalate. There are some children who show total clefts: bilateral complete clefts of the lip and upper gum ridge and an opening which runs from these all the way back to the division of the uvula. Some cases show no uvula. These babies with total clefts are not pretty to look at when they are born.

Causes. When the cleft is in the prepalate or in both prepalate and palate, the cause seems to lie mainly in heredity. When the palate alone is cleft, we find other causal factors such as malnutrition, certain drugs such as cortisone, fetal anoxia (lack of oxygen in the blood, probably due to incompatible blood groupings), and mechanical injuries. The genetic factor is probably recessive. Other types of congenital abnormalities often seem to be found in the same familial lines, but it should be stressed that all clefts do not show hereditary influence. The inability of the embryonic structures to unite has also been explained in terms of the failure of the tongue to descend from the nasal cavity in which it resides before the embryonic palatal shelves begin their growth toward the midline. Not only humans, but mice, lambs, dogs, and goats have been born with clefts. Scientists have been able to produce clefts along with other abnormalities by depriving the animal mothers of riboflavin, a vitamin found in large amounts in the liver, by inducing calcium deficiency, and by irradiation. The exact origin of clefts is as yet not completely understood.

Effects of Clefts. As we have indicated earlier, when a baby is born with a cleft, special services are required to combat the many problems which arise. Among other problems are those involving feeding. The baby must be fed more carefully, held in a special position, burped more often, and fed more frequently. The family must finance trips to all the special services and spend the time necessary. Many psychological problems arise, silent accusations leading to friction between the father and mother, sacrifices of the needs of other siblings to the cleft-palate child's needs, problems in social adjustment. Since often the speech therapist must serve as a general, long-time counselor for these families, she should know the nature of these difficulties.

Surgery. Surgery for the prepalate is accomplished early, within the first three months in a healthy baby. Scars remain which will diminish as the child grows and these can often be removed or concealed by later plastic surgery. The double and complete pre-palate clefts present more difficulty than the incomplete or uni-lateral ones and may require more than one operation.

The age for palatal surgery is still the subject of conflict. Critics have shown that early surgery has sometimes been responsible for distortions of head growth and for some of the facial, dental, and palatal malformations which contribute to the cosmetic handicap and that of speech. The defenders of early surgery have attributed such failures to poor surgical technique or to insufficient tissue or other reasons and they point out that with proper surgery, no head malformations occur and the child is enabled to learn his initial

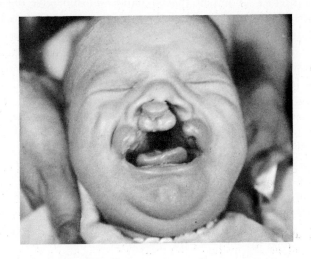

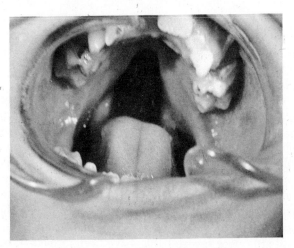

Figure 30. *Clefts of the Lip and Palate*

speech without the handicap of the open cleft which otherwise
would produce abnormal speech habits. Fortunately, the speech
therapist is able to stay out of these arguments. His job is to help
with surgical failures at any age. While some surgery is now being
carried out as late as four and five years, often after a temporary
prosthesis has enabled the child to have a chance to develop good
speech from the beginning, the majority of initial operations take
place early.

In cases of extensive clefts, the surgery is performed in several
stages, necessitating two or even three operations. The first is to
effect closure or partial closure of the cleft palate, the others to
create a muscular mechanism capable of shutting off the pharyngeal
(throat) passageway to the nose. Several different types of operations are employed, which need not be described here since this
information is available in other texts and articles, but the student
should at least know that the "push-back" operation requires an
incision along the inside of the gum ridge so that the tissue can be
moved rearward to effect a better closure, and that the "pharyngeal
flap" operation creates a living bridge of tissue taken from the rear
wall of the throat and joined to the soft palate in front. In other
operations, the side walls of this part of the throat are narrowed.
It should be kept in mind that what is intended in all these operations is the provision of a mechanism which can direct the airflow
and sound through the mouth rather than the nose.

Prostheses.   There are certain cases of cleft palate for whom
surgery is not the wisest course. Certain clefts are so large or the
tissue remaining so scant or poorly developed that the prognosis
for good speech, easy swallowing, and a good facial appearance is
very poor. A real controversy has raged for many years between
the dentists (prosthodontists) and the surgeons. Surgeons claim
that living tissue is always preferable to any artificial means for
closing the mouth from the nose. They point to the unsanitariness
of prostheses, the inconvenience, the difficulty of fitting, the lack of
a movable-at-will valve, the inability of small children to tolerate
them until after poor speech habits have been formed. The prosthodontists, on the other hand, point to the numerous instances of
surgical failure, the interference with facial growth and the poor
cosmetic appearance, the pain and mortality, the short palates which
do not work, the tearing of tissues and perforations, and the de-

fective speech which often results from surgery. The argument still rages in many quarters, but recently the development of teams of specialists to fit the treatment to the needs of the particular child rather than to the disorder has resulted in a most hopeful com-

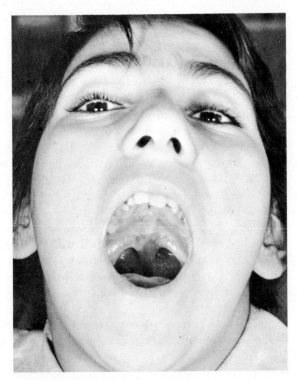

FIGURE 31. *Pharyngeal Flap*

promise. Often the speech therapist is called upon to referee, and so he had better know enough about prostheses to play his part.

Essentially, prostheses, are artificial substitutes for a missing part. In the past the term was synonymous with "obturator" but so far as cleft palates are concerned, obturators are now used to mean fixed appliances which are more or less permanently inserted into clefts of the hard palate, whereas prostheses are detachable appliances consisting of an artificial hard palate (perhaps bearing also some artificial teeth) and a bulb. The latter is designed to close the nasopharynx (partially rather than completely), and to serve as an object to be gripped by the constrictor muscles of the pharynx to create a valve.

Prostheses have been made of many materials. There are accounts in ancient Greek literature of cleft-palate individuals filling their clefts of the hard palate with fruit rinds, cloth, leather, tar, and wax so that they could eat and drink. Passavant made a stud-shaped obturator which he inserted into a slit in the palate after it was sewed up, but it did not work too well. Others injected wax or inserted silver plate projections into the back wall of the pharynx. In the late 1800's artificial hard palates anchored to the teeth were provided with hinged gates, rubber bulbs, rubber tubes, silver balls, and other devices to plug or narrow the nasopharyngeal airway. All of these were very unsanitary, often prevented nasal breathing or interfered with it, and at times produced marked denasality on some sounds while failing to eliminate the nasality on others. Some of these devices were painful and caused gagging and choking. Ear infections were common.

The first modern appliance used an acryllic resin which can be molded and worked by the designer so that it will fit any opening. It is highly sanitary, easily cleaned, and is very light in weight. Plastics opened the way for truly effective cleft-palate prostheses. They can even be modified without the need for new impressions to be taken or new casts made.

Design of Prostheses. There are two parts to the usual prosthesis, the palatal part and the bulb. The former is designed through the taking of impressions to conform to the contours of the hard palate. Frequently, if there is a cleft in the hard palate, the palatal part of the appliance is raised to fit into this cleft to provide some of the retention. Besides this, clasps to fit around the teeth are provided. Even in very small children, as soon as their first teeth have been cut, small orthodontic bands on the molar teeth can be used to keep the prosthesis in place. In most instances, the palatal part of the appliance is made first and fitted into place to close the cleft. Gradually an extension is added to the rear part of this palatal section as the individual learns to tolerate it and larger and larger bulbs are used until finally the desired size and shape has been reached. Some very young children are thus fitted with these prostheses when study of their case indicates that surgery should be postponed until they are five and six years old.

The location of the bulb in the nasopharynx often is critical. In general, the bulb should be placed in the area of greatest naso-pharyngeal constriction. This is usually determined by taking X-rays in the production of a sustained (u) vowel, or by observation in a dental mirror, which is less satisfactory. Often the fitting of these

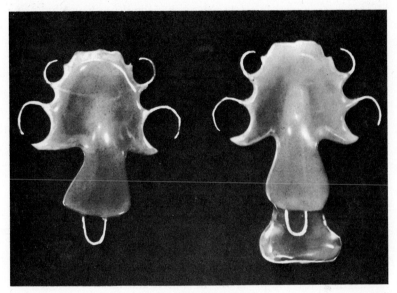

Figure 32. *A Prosthesis*

bulbs is tedious and the speech therapist is sometimes called upon to use his critical ear to determine the extent of nasality and nasal emission in the various trial positions. If the bulb is placed too high, some denasality may appear and reducing the size of the bulb will not affect the amount very much. Instead of shaving the bulb it is sometimes wiser to change its position.

It is often difficult to predict the shape or size of bulb required and only patient fitting with judgments of speech adequacy and tolerance in swallowing, yawning, and blowing will help. At times altering the shape of the bulb may be even more important than the cross sectional area, since the constrictor muscles may require a larger vertical surface to grip for adequate closure. Usually the first bulbs used are larger than those required later since the bulb itself stimulates muscle activity and as these muscles develop, the bulb may need to be shaved if denasality or interference in breathing is to be prevented.

In the fitting of the prosthesis it is sometimes unavoidable that a secondary operation be performed to create a better shaped cleft so that the prosthesis can be made suitable to the needs of the case. Many surgeons tend to oppose this but if the tissue is not functioning and the scar tissue or perforations are preventing the proper positioning of the appliance, it is wise to accept the necessity. There are also times when some of the taut musculatures may move along with the constrictor muscles which squeeze upon the bulb and displace the palatal part of the appliance with their residual movement. In these instances, operations on the tensor muscles may eliminate this movement, though care must be taken to insure that they not be cut completely since their upper ends seem to play a part in the opening of the Eustachian tube to the middle ear.

With regard to the cost of prostheses, it seems that they are seldom any less expensive than surgery. Repeated visits are necessary, and when the prosthesis is fitted to a small child, the costs mount up. However, if costs are calculated in terms of pain, the appliance certainly will win. We should not expect that the use of a prosthesis will immediately produce normal speech, though some reduction in nasality and nasal emission usually does occur. The patient must be taught to use the prosthesis in speech and in swallowing.

Summary:

When should a prosthesis be recommended?

1. In cases of unilateral and bilateral clefts of the palate which have been surgically closed anteriorly but the constrictor muscles left unscarred and still functional.
2. In cases of postsurgical failure in which excessive scar tissue or loss of tissue or perforations have produced a nonfunctioning closure so far as speech or swallowing are concerned.
3. In cases of acquired clefts.
4. Where any operation would be likely to interfere with the centers of

growth or tend to produce marked malformations of the maxillary bone.

5. Where operations cannot be performed because of health conditions or psychological hazards.
6. When three stages of operations have already been performed.

When should we refuse to recommend a prosthesis?

1. Where there is a floating premaxilla, which will dislodge the appliance until it is removed. Also a protruding premaxilla.
2. Where the hard palate is depressed or so full of scar tissue that the palatal part of the appliance would be unlikely to be retained.
3. When there are not sufficient teeth in good condition to hold the appliance.
4. When surgery seems to be the better course.

What are the requirements of an adequate prosthesis?

1. It should be so designed as to create sufficient closure for good speech.
2. It should have good retention, bracing, and support.
3. It should be comfortable after adaptation.
4. It should improve, where necessary, the facial appearance. (27)

Speech Therapy with Prostheses. When the prosthesis is finally finished, the speech therapist's work has just begun. If the case has been properly prepared, he will realize that the appliance itself will not solve his speech problem but that he must learn to use it. If the prosthodontist is wise he will have made the acryllic bulb so it can be temporarily detached, though it will be fixed later.

The speech therapist will begin with warming up exercises for pharyngeal constriction and oral airflow, then insert the bulb and duplicate these. We use silent air sucking through the mouth in the supine position first, then gradually raise the head. Then we run through all of the other activities which involve no phonation but airflow control. Next we use pantomimic speech while holding the breath; then whispered (soft) vowel sequences, omitting the *i* and *u*. Then we use the same with soft voice, often returning to the silent air-flow activities between trials. Then we begin with the consonants, first of all the loose-contact *p* and *t*, then the *b* and *d* sounds. Then the *f* and *v*, and then the *ch* and *j*, the *l* and *r*, and only finally the *z* and *s*.

Only after the case has worked with each of these sounds successfully with the prosthesis and has used them not only in isolation but in nonsense syllables and in isolated words, should he be permitted to begin to speak short phrases or simple sentences, and these at first should have no *m, n,* or *ng* sounds in them. Much checking with a recording device and amplification of nasal air flow or voice should be used during the training sessions.

Gradually, the muscle control will improve and better closures will be obtained. We have seen cases who made steady gains for more than two years. But the beginning of therapy is vital. Unfortunately, many prosthodontists do not understand how important it is to build new habits from the start. If the first speech attempts with prosthesis in place are done without guidance of a trained speech therapist, the case may learn how to continue his habitual nasality and nasal emission despite the appliance.

Evaluation of Velopharyngeal Competency. Surgery and prosthetic appliances unfortunately do not always guarantee that normal speech can be obtained even with the best of speech therapy. The person may come to us with a closure mechanism that will not close sufficiently to permit adequate speech no matter how long and hard we work. We may be able to improve the person's articulation and intelligibility but he will still sound hypernasal and abnormal. We have known therapists and cases who struggled for years to do the impossible, years which might better have been spent in designing better prosthesis or in new surgery. How can we be sure that this case of ours can really close the rear passageway to the nose? How can we know that he has a competent velopharyngeal valve?

In the past, speech therapists have used such simple tests as the ability to suck liquids up a straw or to blow a horn or a feather or to say a series of isolated vowels to determine this capacity for closure. Or they visually observed the uvular movement or the constriction of the pharyngeal wall. Unfortunately, tests of this nature are far from being adequate. At times it is possible to procure from the cleft-palate clinic some evidence from X-ray films that the closure is sufficient. Still pictures, however, are not as good as those procured by fluoroscopic movies, since the former require the prolongation of sounds and do not show what happens in a plosive sound such as *p* or *k.* It is also possible to determine the competency of velopharyngeal closure by comparing the amount of air pressure which can be produced with the nostrils open and with them closed. A crude test of this differential pressure can be obtained by having the case blow into an uncoiling carnival blower as the therapist alternately pinches the nostrils and releases them. If the closure is sufficient the uncoiling will move evenly.

However, we can also get some impression concerning the adequacy of the closure mechanism by analyzing the speech itself. First of all, we should check the articulation errors. If we find key words in which all of the defective sounds or most of them are used correctly, we can be pretty sure that enough closure is present. Again, if at times these errors are not accompanied by nose twitching or nasal emission of air, we can feel that the valve is all right. If the person can speak very well with his nostrils closed but has much nasal distortion when they are open, we would suspect inadequate closure. Finally, if the consonants which require extra mouth pressure (*p-b; t-d; k-g; s-z; ch-j*) are those which are nasally distorted while the *r* and the *l* or *f* and *v* are quite adequate, we would feel that the closure was poor.

It is impossible to outline a program of speech therapy techniques which would be applicable to all cleft-palate cases, or even a majority, since the problems presented by the cases are so different. Individual diagnoses are absolutely essential. We deal with speech that reflects the personality of the case, with his concept of self. The basic attitude of a case who feels that, because he has an organic disability there is nothing which can be done to alter the speech which is affected by that disability, has a profound effect upon therapy. Often little speech therapy can be accomplished until psychotherapy has produced some reality testing, until some hope has been provoked, until the case can trust the therapist when he cannot trust his own parents or closest friends. Most of these cases know little about the nature of their problem, the possibilities for improving speech. They come as passively and as unenthusiastically as they go to the surgeon, the prosthodontist, or the orthodontist, because they have been told they should. Few of them feel any powerful urge to accept some of the responsibility for their speech improvement. Like the stutterer, the cleft-palate case has detached himself from his speech because it is too painful to confront. As in stuttering, we meet with strong resistances when we are forced to demand the active cooperation of the cleft-palate person in confronting his nasal emissions, his nasality, and his poor articulation. Without this control, without this monitoring, it is almost impossible to make any but perfunctory gains. Like the normal speaker, the cleft palate person does not hear himself speaking; he hears his expressed thoughts. It is difficult for the normal speaker to concentrate on self-hearing. In the cleft-palate person, this self-hearing is not only burdensome but also painful. Unless the speech therapist understands this basic psychology, he can hardly hope to be effective.

It is also necessary, quite apart from the individual's attitudes toward his speech and its therapy, to take into account the actual organic disability which may be present. Some cleft-palate persons with very defective speech may have complete closures and the potential for completely normal speech. Some of these are already using their closures in activities other than speech or on other speech sounds save those which are defective. Others of the same group may have the potential to use their soft palate or pharyngeal musculatures but have not learned to do so. But we must also recognize that there are some cleft-palate cases whose structures or prostheses are not adequate for normal speech, and for whom we may be able to do very little except in the improvement of intelligibility. Again, let us state our melioristic philosophy of speech therapy: We make the person's speech better and we make him a happier person. We do not have to make his speech perfect or make him a completely happy human. Within the limits of our time and energy and knowledge, and with an awareness of the limitations which the case also possesses, let us do our utmost and be content with that. They must learn to speak as well as they can, with as little interference to communication as possible and as little abnormality as possible.

Aims of Speech Therapy for Cleft-palate Speech. Our basic points of attack are these: We must decrease the nasal emission, the hypernasality, and the defective articulation. We must improve the oral air pressure and oral airflow. We must eliminate abnormal foci of tension and abnormal nostril contractions. We must activate the tonguetip, lip, and jaws. We must improve the respiratory rhythms of speech, its rate, and control. We must improve velar and pharyngeal contraction.

We once examined a complete, unilateral cleft of both the hard and soft palates who had completely normal speech. How he managed this we were unable to tell, but he did use wide jaw move-

ments, slow speech, short phrases, and dentalized most of his
frontal sounds. All plosives were made with very loose contacts. He
spoke softly and did become nasal when he spoke loudly. So far as
we could ascertain, this person operated his speech with very little
air pressure and it flowed out of the larger mouth opening rather
than the smaller nasal opening merely because it was larger. He
was not tense but very relaxed and perhaps this accounted for his
lack of hypernasality, since certain authorities feel that the characteristic tone of nasality is due to a *constricted* open ended tube rather
than to the open tube itself. At any rate, he demonstrated how much
we might be able to do in speech therapy. This case also illustrates
an important principle. We should work for altering the direction of
airflow so that it flows outward toward the mouth rather than upward through the nose. And we should teach the cleft-palate person
to articulate with a minimum of oral air pressure.

Air Pressure Controls. Air pressure within the mouth varies with
the various speech sounds. The plosives and the sibilants require
the most air pressure. Voiced sounds require less than do the unvoiced sounds due to the increased audibility of the former. The
t and d require less than k and g. People vary widely one from
another in the degree of closure used in producing the plosives and
the fricatives. Certain individuals use very tight closures and sudden
releases; others do not. Cleft-palate cases often use very tight
closures and sudden releases. This is very unwise since much more
air pressure is required for such plosives than for the loose contact-
slow release type. We experimented once by inserting a small air
hose into the corner of the lips and had the subjects, both normal
and cleft-palate, articulate a series of plosives and fricatives. They
then held their breath and pantomimed the various sounds both with
tight contacts and with loose ones. Less air pressure was required
to produce clear sounds when the loose contacts were used. In the
cleft-palate cases, little air escaped from the nose when loose contacts were used but it was very evident when tight contacts were
used. The cleft-palate person whose velum is functioning also reacts
very characteristically to a tight contact either of tonguetip or lips.
These tight contacts almost seem to act as triggers to cause a
lowering of the palate and a relaxation of the superior constrictor,
in much the same way as they tend to set off stuttering tremors in
the stutterer.

Not only does this occur with the plosives. The fricatives, which employ a narrow opening or channel for the airflow, are also produced differently by different people. Certain ones use a very narrow channel; others a broader one. Cleft-palate individuals tend to use the narrower ones which require a greater air pressure, and so nasal emission tends to occur. We therefore should teach them differently.

Much of the stimulus value of a sound can be increased by prolonging its duration. If cleft-palate persons are to soften their contacts in order to make use of the lessened air pressure in the mouth due to the palatal airleak, they must prolong these sounds somewhat, to gain the same intelligibility. Weaker *s* sounds should be held longer. A slightly prolonged *f* in the word *fish* even if weaker in airflow will be understood as readily as a quicker, stronger one.

Concentration in therapy upon these factors also emphasizes the direction of airflow through the mouth rather than the nose. Cleft-palate people are nose-conscious as the contraction of their nostrils demonstrates. By concentrating on the longer, slower, looser contacts and the shallower channels of articulation, the airflow tends to go mouthward. This emphasis upon the mouth rather than the nose as the major channel for speech and airflow is among the major objectives of any speech therapy. It is in large part a psychological problem as we have indicated. We have known cleft-palate children to speak much better as soon as they held a megaphone to their lips or thought that we were going to hold their noses. We have had several cases who were able to blow trumpets very well and yet could not manage a simple *p* sound without having it come through their nose. For this reason, most speech therapists do much lip and tongue training along with blowing exercises. We have given lip exercises with profit to cleft-palate cases who already had perfect lip control, primarily so that they would become mouth-conscious. We have had them talk through fringed holes in a sheet of paper, through various sizes of slits and blowing tubes, with their fingers in their mouths, with their mouths to ears, through fringed paper mustachios, into the vibrator mouthpieces of toy musical instruments, with their mouths held under water, into cones whose apex flickered a candle flame. One of our children spoke much better when he put on a clown's mask which had a monstrous big mouth which he watched in a mirror. He just became more mouth-conscious and the air came out of that opening. We have improved the speech of cleft-palate cases by teaching them to read lips and to help in training deaf children in lip reading. One of our majors got better speech from a cleft-palate girl by putting lipstick on her mouth and having her watch it in the mirror. We have darkened a room and put a little flashlight focused on the outside of the mouth in a narrow beam and also within the mouth and improved the speech by having the case watch it in the mirror. Cleft-palate cases must think of speech as coming out of the mouth.

Many speech therapists teach their cleft-palate cases to open the mouth widely in speech, as far as they can without appearing abnormal. This is often difficult to teach and resistance is almost sure to be found, but when it can be used it does seem to improve speech markedly. It does this first because any larger opening attracts airflow. Air must take a tortuous course when it must go upstairs, through the filters of the nasal caverns and then down and out through the narrow slits of our nostrils. It would much rather come out of a side door, especially if that side door is open. Moreover, larger mouth openings for the vowels tend to produce looser contacts of lips and tongue, and they certainly increase the consciousness of the mouth rather than the nose.

The source of the air pressure and airflow is of course in the contractions of the muscles which lower the chest and contract the abdomen which, with a relaxing diaphragm, create a condition of pressure upon the lungs. Many cleft-palate cases require training in breath control for speech. Their breathing records show many instances of air wastage, speaking on residual air, opposition, and staircase breathing. They often start speaking with a very strong pulse of air which goes up through the pharynx or cleft because of its pressure and then creates the path for whatever air is left to follow. They often inhale too deeply prior to utterance (which causes tension all along the airway) to produce this initial strong blast or pulse. With much of the air wasted in the first few syllables, the person then must speak on residual air or opposition breathing, both of which increase tension everywhere. It is possible to improve the speech, the nasal emission, and the hypernasality, by teaching the case to inhale a normal amount of air and to start his utterance gradually rather than suddenly and to monitor the amount of air used. Cleft-palate speakers must learn to watch their phrasing, which means their breathing.

Muscle Training. It is also possible of course, in many cases, to improve the state of air pressure within the mouth by shutting off the air leak, by improving velo-pharyngeal closure. Many of the muscles are weak and can be strengthened through appropriate exercises if surgery or prosthesis has been successful in creating the conditions for a possible closure. If the cleft-palate case can blow up a balloon or whistle, or inspection with a dental mirror shows good occlusion of the nasopharynx, we should be able to help him use some closure in speech. Even when this is not possible but when, in phonation, yawning, or other activities, we can see the velum lift or the side walls of the pharynx contract or the rear wall come forward slightly, we must presume that we can improve this functioning until we find otherwise. (This last statement may not be true if the velum is too short or taut or the pharynx so enlarged that no closure seems possible.)

Such muscle training requires two major items besides devoted practice: location of the musculatures by the patient and perception of their movement. In physical therapy where comparable tasks are present, the physical therapist, through massage, positioning, and passive movement, is often able to get movement of muscles as inert as those of the cleft-palate patient's repaired velum. Unfortunately a limb is easier to manipulate than is a palate. Nevertheless, speech therapists have employed some of the same principles of physical therapy in activating the velar and pharyngeal muscles. Light massage with a finger cot (covering of rubber), first along one side of the uvula, then on the other, and then with two fingers straddling the midline, has helped to localize the area. The stroking must be done very lightly and both away from the midline in a horizontal direction, and anteroposteriorly. Care must be taken that the child does not gag or bite your fingers off. These exercises must also be done with caution lest tissues be injured, but when they are done lightly and the patient attempts to feel and predict the location and direction of movement, they can be very effective. Only a little of this can be done at a time since the patient tires quickly. Another procedure involves the tapping of these structures in the same areas, the patient being requested to tell the number of taps and their intensity. We also may slightly depress the surface of the palate or tickle it or the pharyngeal wall if the gag reflex is not present or is weak. These techniques all involve the location of the structures by the tactual sense.

We may also use the visual sense. Many cleft-palate cases have no visual imagery of their palates with which to correlate movement. They should study and describe the action of the therapist's palate in action. They should watch both their own and their therapist's palate in mirrors. They can be shown large pictures of the palate on charts and be taught to point to the area which the therapist touches. Where there is residual movement, it should be viewed visually, and then imagined. A very clear picture should be possessed by every cleft-palate patient of the nature of his problem. Even little children can be given this in imaginative terms: "the little red gate or door."

Since most repaired cleft-palate cases have some movement of the levator and tensor muscles as well as of the constrictor muscles in certain activities, they must be taught to isolate and to identify the experience. Certain key words should be conditioned to palatal activity: "up . . . down . . . squeeze . . . let go . . . open . . . shut." These must be used by the therapist only when the activity actually occurs. They should first be used by the case when observing the therapist's palatal movements, then when observing his own, then with intermittent eye-closing with attention to kinesthesia.

It is also possible to become aware of palatal movement by other sensations. With the mouth open, try to get the case to feel some air pressure in his middle ear, to feel it click or pop. This must be done while holding the breath. The palatal tensor, when it contracts, has some effect upon opening the Eustachian tube. Also in yawning, the palatal muscles tend to contract and can be felt in action. Closed-mouth yawning is especially effective in developing kinesthesia, and it can be combined with the middle-ear pressure cues. Also use different mouth openings.

Some of the tactual sensations can also be achieved with a syringe by blowing a stream of air or "warm water" against certain parts of the soft palate. The child may also explore his own mouth with his own finger, using the fingers cut from sterilized rubber gloves. Loud snoring with the nose held so that all inhalations are made through the mouth will vibrate the uvula, and research has shown that in this snoring the palate is raised. It is possible to snore on the various vowels and with different tongue positions or lip postures. Tight closures of the tongue and velum in silence as in the position for a *k* sound will, if the release is very sudden, provoke some upward movement of the palate at the same time that the tongue is jerked downward. The sound-play known as "gibbegadong" is also effective when the case can do it, since it is based upon the last mentioned principle.

Weak palatal movements when present can be made more effective in closure by having the patient lie on a cot with his head held far backward so that the force of gravity aids rather than resists the palatal movement. Where there is asymmetrical pull on the palate, turning the head or the jaw to one side seems to be of some assistance.

Dry swallowing, when repeated, often helps the patient to activate and localize the velo-pharyngeal contractions. Often a state of localized strain or fatigue may help the case to become aware that he has such muscles. Very slow chewing may also produce certain muscular contractions of the pharynx and velum. Sudden sucking of air through various sizes of tubes will also initiate velar activity. Tubes of different sizes and shapes will produce more palatal contraction than others, but the sucking must be sudden.

Blowing Exercises. Perhaps blowing exercises have been used more frequently than any other single device for strengthening the palate. Blowing takes air pressure, and if the air is to come out of the mouth, a velo-pharyngeal opening will reduce that pressure enough to reduce the airflow through the mouth to a considerable degree. We must be certain, however, that we are having an increasingly greater ratio of mouth airflow to nasal airflow if we can hope that the palate is being strengthened. Various devices have been employed to demonstrate this ratio: double shelves to be placed under nose and mouth openings with feathers or fringes to indicate airflow, tubes from the nose to the ear, contact microphones, the phonodeik and phonoscope, polygraphic recording, candle flames affected by tubes from nose and mouth, clouded mirrors, and many others. Usually it is necessary that the patient become familar with the two air channels by sucking air in through the nose, then through the mouth, then exhaling alternately through each channel. By using different mouth openings and palpating the nostrils during the blowing or interrupting the oral airflow with vibrating palms across the orifice, the case can come to have a clear idea of these channels. We must not expect that he already has such a concept. Also by having the case alternate nasal and oral airflow while he holds his fingers in his ears, he can hear a difference in the pitch of the two blowings. The oral airflow can be made to vary markedly in pitch by changing the lip protrusion or mouth opening; the nasal airflow is pretty well fixed in pitch. By attending to the different palatal and pharyngeal sensations during the different airflows, a more adequate control of the velo-pharyngeal musculatures can be achieved.

We should emphasize that blowing exercises performed with great tension and the constriction of the nostrils are most unwise. They merely inform the case that palatal contraction is too laborious to be used in speech. Besides they often can cause ear infections. We also doubt the efficacy of blowing air out of the mouth while holding the nose shut, since we may raise the air pressure too high in the middle ear and make the case too nose conscious, and in any event, closure of the nostrils does not help the velo-pharyngeal valve to shut. Indeed, there seems to be a sort of inverse reciprocal reaction in the action of the nares (nostrils) and the velar musculatures. Even in normal speakers, voluntary contraction of the nares often produces an increase in nasality. As the front door shuts, the back door opens. Kantner (19) claims that there is very little transfer of training from blowing to speech. This is especially true if the blowing is too strained, if air pressures far exceeding those used in normal speech are used, and if set mouth openings and passive tongue postures are employed. We could hardly expect much transfer with so many variables in the training. Nevertheless, others have shown that the palatal and pharyngeal activity in blowing (especially in soft blowing) is more like that used in speech than is shown in such activities as yawning, swallowing, and so on. We must not throw the baby out with the bath. Blowing exercises can help the case to become mouth conscious; they can help him discriminate the two airflow channels; they can help him to increase the amount of oral air pressure needed for good articulation; and they can improve the contraction of the velar and pharyngeal muscles. But they must be used wisely rather than indiscriminately.

Many ingenious devices and activities have been invented by speech therapists to make the blowing activities interesting to children. Paper boats have been blown across pans of water. Ping-pong balls have been blown across miniature football fields or golf courses. Balloons have been blown up and burst. Bubble-pipes, huffer-puffers, bean shooters, uncoiling paper tubes, flame throwers, vibrating wind instruments, mouth organs, holding tissue paper against a mirror with the breath, air-writing on the therapist's hand, cooling wet fingers, drying nail polish, blowing dry cereal or feathers on a string—all these are but a few of the activities used.

While many of these may be used for motivation or as transitional techniques, we feel that the most effective types of blowing exercises are those which alternate oral and nasal blowing done at fairly low levels of pressure; which have a greater fraction of oral rather than nasal emission; which are combined with phonation, tongue protrusion and movement, or lip protrusion and movement. These transfer much more adequately to speech, and improve velo-pharyngeal closure. All blowing exercises under pressure may tend to cause dizziness and must not be maintained for more than short periods of time.

We conclude this section on velo-pharyngeal closure training by mentioning two other techniques which we have used with some success with adults. In the first, a large balloon is blown up (preferably by the case while holding his nose) and then held shut by the therapist's fingers on the stem as the case holds a tube leading from the stem with his lips. The therapist gradually releases his grip and allows some of the air to escape into the case's mouth. The latter tries, while holding his breath, to keep from letting the balloon collapse; this requires velar closure or the air will leak out of the nostrils. Another variation of this technique has the outlet to the balloon enter a Y-tube, the arms of which are attached to nasal olives inserted into the case's nostrils. He tries to retard the collapse of the balloon as he produces various vowels or merely contracts his palate in silence.

Articulation Problems.   The backward playing of samples of speech of various degrees of nasality has demonstrated that the listener judges a given sample as being more nasal if it has poorer articulation. The voice quality itself seems more nasal when it is played forward than when it is played backward. Thus, the improvement of articulation can produce a decrease in perceived nasality. We have also seen that the majority of cleft-palate speakers have speech sounds which are defective.

The basic problems in articulation are three: lalling, the substitution of glottal stops and fricatives for the standard stops and fricatives, and the nasalization or nasal emission of most of the consonants.

Lalling. The treatment for lalling requires training in increasing the mobility of the tonguetip, in raising the points of anterior contact for the *t, d, n, l, ch,* and *j* sounds, and the differentiation of tongue-lifting from simultaneous jaw movement.

Exercises for increasing the mobility of the tongue include sensitization of the tonguetip, curling, grooving, lifting, lowering, thrusting, arching, tapping, sustaining postures, pressing, scraping, fluttering, and many others. These should not be practiced while holding the breath but while blowing gently both voiced and unvoiced air if the training is to generalize to speech. Undue tension is to be avoided. Speed gains should be made in terms of rhythmic patterns. Different sizes of mouth opening and lip postures should be also practiced with the tongue-training. Many of these cases have never explored the many possibilities of tongue movement or action. It is wise to use these exercises as warm-up periods for consonant practice. Often the production of certain consonants is sandwiched between two tongue-training exercises.

The localizing of the focal articulation points higher and more forward in the mouth than those normally used can be done only by identifying those ordinarily used and searching for higher points while continuously articulating the sounds. This "stretching" of the phonemes in terms of height of contact will at first seem unpleasant and will seldom be used at their extremes, but practice will cause the necessary compromise. Most cleft-palate persons also have certain scar tissue, indentations, or bulges on the alveolar ridge which can be used as landmarks, but they must be found and localized. Tactual feedbacks must be sharpened. The teeth, especially the lower teeth, must come to lose their function as the basic contact point. Silent practice in touching these new focal articulation points should be done. With one of our cases, we inserted a bit of toothpick or dental floss between the upper incisors and used this as the guide. An immediate improvement in speech occurred.

The differentiation of tongue movement from the accompanying jaw movements can be done by immobilizing the jaw with various heights of tooth props until enough independence is achieved to permit the activity without this aid. Frequent checking is necessary. Visual feedback from a mirror is also useful. Lateral movements of the mandible during tongue tapping and consonant production will also be useful. The use of the first two fingers forked to monitor the location of both lips will help. Also, if the case will place one finger on his nose and his thumb under his chin, any accompanying movement of the jaw will be noticed immediately. Ventriloquism often provides an interesting motivation for these cases, and aids in the freeing of the tongue.

Glottal Stops. The use of the glottal stop or fricative substitutions requires a state of localized tension in the larynx and some relaxation in this area often provides the optimal conditions for retraining. The use of slight coughs to teach a *k* sound is therefore very unwise. The back of the tongue must be raised, and this can be accomplished more easily on the *k* and *g* sounds by pressing hard with the tongue-tip against the lower teeth and closing the jaws partially. Ear training is essential. We have also been able to eliminate this difficult error by having the case produce the consonants on inhalation, a procedure which improves much of the articulation of cleft-palate cases. The subsequent use of donkey breathing (inhaled, then exhaled) in the production of the sounds often solves the glottal problem.

Decreasing Nasality and Nasal Emission. While much of the success of articulating the consonant sounds without nasality or nasal emission will depend upon the success of establishing oral air flow and better velo-pharyngeal closure, we find that by teaching the plosives with very loose contacts, great improvement can be made. Too hard contacts seem to trigger off a lowering of the velum and a relaxation of the superior constrictor.

For the fricatives, the use of wider mouth openings on the following or preceding vowels tends to decrease the nasality. We also suggest the prolongation of these sounds with decreasing air pressure, thus using the duration rather than the clear quality of the fricative as the message-carrying feature.

It is important, of course, to use the usual ear-training to identify the defectiveness of a given sound and to contrast it with the correct sound. Then we must teach the proper production of the isolated sound, strengthening and stabilizing it. We have mentioned before that cleft-palate cases often speak very rapidly so as to conserve the breath pressure. Slowing down the speed of utterance, with proper phrasing and breathing, often produces immediate improvement in all of the articulation even when little attention is paid to the isolated sounds.

Perhaps the most pronounced of all the ticlike mannerisms which characterize cleft-palate speech is the nostril contraction or flaring. This often serves as an equivalent for velar contraction, and often prevents the latter from taking place. It is cosmetically unattractive, often interferes with the utterance of the labial plosives, and helps to produce the snorting snuffling which is so unpleasant in these cases. It has no effect upon nasality or nasal emission except to make them worse. We therefore always do as much as we can to eliminate this habit. We first attempt to bring this nostril tic up to consciousness, to help the case to become aware of its unpleasant stimulus value, and then through negative practice, canceling, pull-outs, and preparatory sets to eliminate it. Usually it is responsive to this treatment, especially when mirror work is used. In the more severe cases a nucleus of non-nostril-contraction speech can be achieved by contracting the lips in a wide tight smile, stretching them so far that the upper teeth are bared. The therapist must be sure that he does not penalize contraction and thus suppress it before it is weakened.

Many cleft-palate cases have as poor eye contact as do stutterers, a behavior which makes the speech and condition more noticeable. They also may have unusual head postures, lip bitings, or cover their mouths in speaking. All these should be reduced.

Speech therapy with cleft-palate cases is usually long-term therapy. Few of these children show any dramatic improvement in a short time. There are many problems to be solved and many avenues to be explored. The work is time consuming and often difficult. Nevertheless we can do much to help the person with cleft-palate speech to speak better.

PROJECTS

1. Make clay models of heads showing the various clefts of the lip.
2. Make clay models of the upper surface of the mouth showing the various clefts of the palate and alveolar process.
3. Make a large wall chart showing what is done in the pharyngeal-flap operation.

4. Make a series of models or drawings showing the embryological development of the palate.

5. Explain, as to a high-school boy, the essential information he should possess concerning his cleft palate.

6. Interview some orthodontist concerning his methods as they might apply to a child with a cleft palate.

7. Construct a clay model of a prosthesis.

8. Make a wall chart showing what is done in a palatal operation.

9. A high-school girl with a repaired cleft palate is worried about the prospect of having a cleft-palate child some day. Invent a dialogue in which you show what you would do to help her.

10. Construct a device to help the case know *visually* the amount of nasal snorting he is having.

REFERENCES

Cleft Palate

1. Baker, H. K. Cleft palate habilitation—present tense, *Children,* Volume 2, 1955, pages 94-97.

2. Buck, M., and R. Harrington. "Organized Speech Therapy for Cleft Palate Rehabilitation," *Journal Speech and Hearing Disorders,* Volume 14, 1949, pages 43-52.

3. Dalrymple, L. H. "Our Child Had a Cleft Palate," *Hygeia,* Volume 27, 1943, pages 136-187; 199-200.

4. Eckelmann, D., and P. Baldridge. "Speech Training for the Child with a Cleft Palate," *Journal Speech Disorders,* Volume 10, 1945, pages 137-148.

5. Fomon, J. "Pathologic Conditions and Surgery of Maxillofacial and Oropharyngeal Areas," in N. M. Levin (ed.), *Voice and Speech Disorders,* Chapter 22.

6. Hahn, E. "Speech Therapy for the Pre-School Cleft Palate Child," *Journal Speech and Hearing Disorders,* Volume 23, 1958, pages 605-609.

7. Jaynes, H. D. "Cleft Palate—Report of a Case," *American Journal Orthodontistry,* Volume 38, 1952, pages 258-288.

8. Johnson, W. (ed.). *Speech Problems of Children.* New York: Grune & Stratton, Inc., 1950, pages 115-157.

9. Kantner, C. E. "Diagnosis and Prognosis in Cleft Palate Speech," *Journal Speech and Hearing Disorders,* Volume 13, 1948, pages 211-233.

10. Koepp-Baker, H. "Speech Problems of the Person with Cleft Palate

and Cleft Lip," in L. E. Travis (ed.), *Handbook of Speech Pathology.* New York: Appleton-Century-Crofts, 1957, Chapter 20, pages 597-607.

11. Laing, J. M. "Therapy Techniques for Better Nasal Resonance," *Journal Speech and Hearing Disorders,* Volume 23, 1958, pages 254-256.

12. Law, F. E. "Unoperated Oral Clefts at Maturation; 1. Study Design and General Considerations," *American Journal of Public Health,* Volume 49, 1959, pages 1517-1574.

13. Lillywhite, H. "Teamwork in the Oregon Cleft Palate Program," *Journal Speech and Hearing Disorders,* Volume 21, 1956, pages 18-24.

14. ———. "counseling with Parents of Children with Cleft Lip and Palate," *Cleft Palate Bulletin,* Volume 7, 1957, pages 3-5.

15. McDonald, E. T., and H. Koepp-Baker. "Cleft Palate Speech: An Integration of Research and Clinical Observation," *Journal Speech and Hearing Disorders,* Volume 16, 1951, pages 9-20, Volume 16.1.

16. ———. *Bright Promise.* Chicago: National Society for Crippled Children and Adults, 1959.

17. McWilliams, B. J. "Cleft Palate Management in England," *Speech Pathology and Therapy,* Volume 3, 1960, pages 3-7.

18. Morimitsu, K. J. "A Review of Prosthetic Therapy of the Cleft Palate Patient," *Cleft Palate Bulletin,* Volume 8, 1958, pages 7-10.

19. Morley, M. E. *Cleft Palate and Speech.* Baltimore: The Williams & Wilkins Co., 1946.

20. Palmer, J. M. "The Pharyngeal Flap Operation: Role of the Speech Therapist," *Journal Speech and Hearing Disorders,* Volume 23, 1958, pages 601-604.

21. Phair, G. M. "The Wisconsin Cleft Palate Program," *Journal Speech Disorders,* Volume 12, 1947, pages 410-414.

22. Rosen, M. S. "Prosthetics for the Cleft Palate Patient," *Journal American Dental Association,* Volume 60, 1960, pages 715-721.

23. Pirruccello, F. W. "Primary Surgical Correction of Congenital Clefts of the Lip and Palate," *Journal American Dental Association,* Volume 60, 1960, pages 699-703.

24. Schwartz, R., "Familial Incidence of Cleft Palate," *Journal Speech and Hearing Disorders,* Volume 19, 1954, pages 228-238.

25. Slaughter, W. B., and G. M. Phair. "A Complete Cleft Palate Program," *Journal Speech and Hearing Disorders,* Volume 17, 1952, pages 123-128.

26. Snyder, C. C., and N. M. Levin. "General and Surgical Aspects of Cleft Lip and Palate," in N. M. Levin. *Voice and Speech Disorders.* Springfield, Ill.: Charles C. Thomas, Publisher, 1962, Chapter 21.

27. Spriestersbach, D. C. "Criteria for Establishing the Need for a Speech Appliance," *Journal Speech and Hearing Disorders,* Volume 21, 1956, pages 365-370.

28. Subtelny, J. D. "The Significance of Early Orthodontia in Cleft Palate Habilitative Planning," *Journal Speech and Hearing Disorders,* Volume 20, 1955, pages 135-147.

29. Van Thal, J. H. "A Typical Cleft Palate Speech," *Speech* (London) Volume 15, 1951, pages 10-12.

30. Van Riper, C. *Speech Therapy.* Englewood Cliffs, N.J.: Prentice-Hall, Inc., 1953, pages 181-205.

31. Wells, C. "Improving the Speech of the Cleft Palate Child," *Journal Speech Disorders,* Volume 10, 1945, pages 162-169.

32. ———. "Practical Techniques in Speech Training for Cleft Palate Cases," *Journal Speech and Hearing Disorders,* Volume 13, 1948, pages 71-73.

33. ——— and G. M. Phair. *Speech Training for Cleft Palate Children: A Teacher-Parent Guide.* Madison, Wis.: Dept. Public Instruction, 1957.

34. West, R., M. Ansberry, and A. Carr. *The Rehabilitation of Speech,* Harper & Row, Publishers (revised edition, 1957), pages 180-193; 450-455.

35. Westlake, H. "Understanding the Child with a Cleft Palate," *Quarterly Journal Speech,* Volume 39, 1953, pages 165-172.

CHAPTER FOURTEEN

Aphasia

The Disorder.   Aphasia is the general term used for disorders of symbolization. The aphasic has difficulty in (1) formulating, (2) comprehending, or (3) expressing *meanings.* Often there is some impairment in all of these three functions. Along with these difficulties there may be associated problems in defective articulation, in inability to produce voice, and broken fluency, but the basic problem in aphasia lies in handling *symbolic* behavior. Aphasics not only have difficulty in speaking, they also find it hard to read silently, to write, to comprehend the speech of others, to calculate mathematically, or even to gesture. Let us illustrate some of this behavior in a severe case of aphasia.

Mr. A. was fifty-five when he had his "stroke." Some blood vessels in his brain had ruptured. As a result of this injury, his right arm and leg became paralyzed, his face pulled to one side a little, and he had many symptoms of aphasia. For example, he was unable to tell time even when he looked at his watch. He was still able to speak a little but often he spoke a gibberish or his meanings were very difficult to understand. Here is how he asked for a cigarette: "Me me my . . . ah . . . go come . . . no . . . me go . . . no no no . . . um . . . suck now . . . suck, smuck, smoker . . . . scum . . . oh my . . . smoker me smoker . . . oh dear . . . goddamm . . ."

And this is how he wrote to his wife. We found that this was the best of his methods for communicating although the script was very poor because he had to use his left hand. "I want you you come now see mmy. Butter I am. (He meant "better.") I love tell John. I come well sssssn."

But Mr. A. could not write his name, not even in his checkbook, not even from copy. He could print from copy but the letters were often reversed. He seemed unable to read and had no interest in doing so but he spent much time looking at the pictures of an illustrated magazine and enjoyed the television. Most of the gestures, and he gestured a lot, were fairly easy to understand but at times he would shake his head vertically when he really meant "No!"

We had known Mr. A. before his stroke and knew him as an extrovert, a pleasant, highly verbal person. He was a crack salesman for a life insurance agency. When we saw him some six months after the stroke, he seemed markedly different. He cried frequently and did not seem to be able to stop crying once he had begun. Often he was profoundly depressed, confused, and withdrawn. Occasional bursts of profanity and vile language appeared in many inappropriate situations, and this behavior was very unlike his former manner.

There are some terms which are commonly used to describe some of this behavior. Mr. A.'s inability to write is termed "agraphia"; his inability to read, "alexia"; his inability to handle mathematics, "acalculia"; his jumbled sentences, "paraphasia." The inability to stop crying, the repetition of words in speaking or letters in writing, is called "perseveration." His inability to remember or find a necessary word is called "anomia." Recovered aphasics tell us that often they can see the letters but that they appear to have no meaning, or they see the picture of an object but cannot tell what it is. This is termed a "visual agnosia." Or they can hear someone talking to them but cannot comprehend. The speech sounds "jumbled." This is called an "auditory agnosia." There is one other major term we must, reluctantly, provide you: "apraxia." This refers to an inability to command a part of the body to make a willed movement. An aphasic who may understand perfectly what you mean when you ask him to protrude his tongue or to pick up a pencil may not be able to command his tongue or hand to do so. Perhaps he lacks the inner speech that determines voluntary movement. At any rate, this inability to make a voluntary movement is termed "apraxia." There are many other technical words, but these are the most common.

Different aphasics show different patterns of impairment. The case we cited, Mr. A., was severely affected not only in the *expressive* and *receptive* aspects of handling meaningful symbols but also in their *formulation*. Most aphasics show some general loss in language ability and it becomes more marked under fatigue or stress. However, certain aphasics may show their difficulty *primarily* in only one area. One of our cases after an automobile accident could speak fairly well but she could not read even a child's primer. Another could read magazines and newspapers readily but had much paraphasia in speaking. It is necessary to explore each case individually to determine the areas of language and symbol functioning which are impaired. Generally speaking, the aphasic can handle concrete concepts better than abstract ones. Aphasics may be able, for example, to tell what a cup is named, yet be unable to *tell* you what it is used for, though they may show they know by going through the gesture for drinking. One other characteristic should be mentioned. Aphasics often seem to be able to handle what is termed "automatic speech" and social gesture better than speech which is highly communicative. For example, they can sing the words of a simple song when they cannot say them meaningfully. They might be able to say "Hello" and "Fine" or "Nice day," when they can't tell you the names of their children. They may be able to count only if they begin with "one, two, three"; never if they begin with "five" or have to count backward. They can often curse when they cannot talk at all. Aphasia is a complicated disorder because it deals with symbolic meanings, the most complex of all human achievements.

Causes. In the adult, the most common causes of aphasia are strokes caused by hardening of the arteries, blood clots which block off the nourishment of the nerve cells in the brain, or hemorrhages of the blood vessels in the brain. Aphasia is also caused by severe head injuries such as those caused by automobile accidents, brain surgery needed to remove tumors, or gun-shot wounds. Diseases which affect the brain may also be numbered among the causes.

Prognosis. Immediately after the injury, the patient often shows a picture of extreme helplessness and impairment which may subside within three or four months when what is known as "spontaneous recovery" occurs, though it is seldom complete and residual signs of aphasic disturbance can usually be found even in those who apparently have become well. Spontaneous recovery seldom can be expected after six months, and any improvement thereafter must be viewed as due to the relearning efforts of the patient himself or the teaching efforts of his therapists. The younger and the more intelligent and the more motivated the person is, the better are his chances for regaining his place in a communicative world. Wise handling of these patients immediately after the injury is absolutely essential if the effect of the terrific frustration in producing depression and defeatism is to be avoided. Often the attitudes of the members of the family, doctors, and nurses, can create unfavorable prognoses. With professional speech therapy and the cooperation of all those who tend the patient, many individuals suffering from aphasia can regain much of their ability to communicate.

*Treatment.** It is difficult to outline the treatment for aphasia in general terms because the patterns of disability vary so much from case to case. When we begin, we concentrate on the functions which show the least impairment, so that the aphasic can begin to hope that he can make progress. But we also work hard on the whole general language disability, building a foundation for improvement in all areas. We begin and end each session with things he can do. We try as soon as possible to teach him the basic communicative tools he needs: to call the nurse, to ask for a drink, to write his wife, to say hello and goodbye, to say yes and no.

Parallel Talking. We emphasize stimulation with simple materials, not complex ones. We speak simply and clearly, supplementing with gesture or written or pictured materials when needed. We do a great amount of parallel talking in this stimulation, telling him, simply and in short phrases or sentences, what he is doing, feeling, or perceiving. We use not only this sort of commentary but also prediction and recall. Often, as we do this parallel talk, we find the patient will almost unconsciously join in and say a word for us on which we fumble or postpone the utterance. This technique we have come to make the basic part of our therapy. It is a bit difficult to learn to do this well, for the therapist must make sure that he does the appropriate verbalization and hesitating at exactly the moment when the patient is experiencing the thought expressed. It is also necessary to keep from making too much of the case's spontaneous utterance when it does occur under these conditions. We merely say yes, and then restimulate him with what he has spoken in the context of the entire utterance. This is especially effective with the *expressive* aphasic, but we have also used a whispered or pantomimed form of parallel talking to help those who have trouble understanding spoken speech to read our lips. Often these individuals, if they learn to pantomime the speech they *see*, can then comprehend it, and some of the auditory

---

* In this chapter we are concerning ourselves with the adult aphasic, since we have described the problem in childhood in our chapters on Delayed Speech.

agnosia subsides. Wives and other associates of the patients can be taught to do much of this parallel talking. We have found it most useful.

Basic Program. Some of the activities used in working with aphasics in general are now listed in terms of their major aims:

Stimulation. The world of an aphasic must be a most confusing place. Depending upon the particular functions affected, he may hear sounds or people talking to him but be unable to comprehend them; he may pick up the morning paper and see only meaningless squiggles running across the page. He may try to write his name in his checkbook and be unable to do so. He tries to ask for a cigarette and either he cannot remember its name or he speaks gibberish. He looks at the clock and cannot tell the time. He puts his hand in his pocket and feels something but does not know that what he feels is a coin. It is a blooming, buzzing confusion without rhyme, reason, or meaning. Here and there are moments of clarity but they flit by too swiftly or are lost in frustration and depression.

One of the major tasks of the therapist is to provide islands of consistency in this sea of uncertainty. Patiently she explores her case to determine the things he can do. Perhaps he can copy letters from the alphabet; or if he cannot, perhaps he can trace over those she provides. Very well, she begins with this activity and continues with it until he knows that this function at least is within his powers. Then she stimulates him with other things. She may have him echo her words, or animal noises or gestures. They (therapist and patient) may put their spoons in their coffee cups in unison and stir the sugar and cream. She may ask him to point predictively to which one of the objects—knife, fork, or spoon—she will use in a moment to spread his bread. She may ask him to read her lips as she stimulates him with the number "three" for the three peanuts in her hand, then help him count them aloud. She may guide his hand in writing a few sentences to his wife. She will take his hand and touch it to his nose, his ears, his mouth, his feet, saying these names as she does so. Always she uses self-talk and parallel talk in very simple words, phrases, or sentences, providing the spoken symbols for every experience, for every activity. Day after day, she reviews this patient stimulation, tolerant of failure and happy when success comes. For success will come as the confusion subsides and the aphasic begins to find the functions he has lost.

Inhibition. Brain injury makes it hard to inhibit oneself. The lower centers of the brain miss their old brakes, as we see in the frequent overflow of emotion in the form of crying and laughing spells or catastrophic responses. Perseveration continues too long. One of our aphasics, once he had begun a sentence with "I think" could not stop saying these two words, over and over, over and over, over and over. Another was unable to speak what he desired to utter because all speech attempts began with "Yes, yes, yes" and the broken record went round and round on that single word. Accordingly we train our cases to inhibit themselves, to stop doing what they are doing, first upon our command, and then upon their own. We train them to inhibit any attempt to speak until we give the signal, or until they tap their foot five times. We teach them to wait, to pause, to say "No more that." We give them time to reorganize. We have them wait until we smile before they try again. We ask them to rehearse silently or in a mirror or in pantomime what they are about to do or say. We have them duplicate on purpose their crying or laughing jags and to stop them when the second hand of the watch points down. For the aphasic who can read, we provide "inhibition cards" which might, for example, read as follows: "Stop laughing!" "Wait!" "Whisper first!" We have them confess and cancel the perseveration which does occur.

Translation. The aphasic often gets blocked in formulating, receiving, or sending messages because he keeps going up the same blind alley over and over again. We must teach him to shift when he meets these dead ends, to try another tack. Basic to this is translation training. By this we mean that we train the aphasic to shift from one type of symbolization to another. We may ask him to spell aloud, then print the name of the animal he hears meowing on the tape recorder. We have him count to three by the taps, again by drawing vertical lines, again by clapping hands, again by tracing the numeral, and finally by saying it. We say "Sit down!" and he must try to point to the appropriate picture, then to pantomime it with his lips silently, then to act it out, then to find the phrase on a card. We don't overwhelm him with too many translations at first; we let him lead us; but we always work to give him experiences in shifting from one set of symbolic meanings to another.

Memorization. One of the best ways of creating islands of consistency in the hurly-burly world of the aphasic is to teach him to memorize. They often resist this at first but if you will read reference 12 by Dr. Rose at the end of this chapter you will come to realize how important memorization can be. Often we begin by having them memorize sequences of movements as in a calisthenic exercise or a sequence of lines to be drawn or the selection of a set of objects in a definite order. We demonstrate such sequences as opening the window, then closing the door, then saying "Too hot!" and then ask them to duplicate our performance. We have them find us three desired objects in a catalogue in the order in which we write them on the board. We arrange wooden-block letters in a row on the table so that they spell his name. We have him memorize the cards of different sizes and shapes which have written upon them such phrases as: "Good morning," "Nice day," "How are you?" "Goodbye," so that he can show them to us appropriately long before he can say these things. We have him write from memory, draw from memory, using flash cards to stimulate him and varying the exposure and delay time so he succeeds more than he fails. Finally, we ask him to learn by rote such passages as this:

> I have been sick. I had a stroke. I must learn to read and write and speak again. Getting better. Takes time. Must work hard. No use feeling sorry. Get to work now.

Later on, we have the aphasic memorize poems and prose passages of increasing complexity. These not only help to provide associations between words, but also help in relearning the basic syntax of language.

Scanning and Concentrating. The aphasic is like a man who suddenly finds himself in a strange country. He is overwhelmed by strange sights and sounds. He may hear people talking and be unable to understand what they are saying. He cannot write their language. He does not know what purposes some of the objects about him serve. Even a spoon is not a spoon but something strange. What he must do, in such a situation, is to learn to observe, to scan for meanings, for consistencies. He must come to concentrate on things that look alike or on meaningless words which always seem to appear in the same contexts. Only in this way can such a person, suddenly transported to a strange land, come to find a place in it. But it is difficult for him to concentrate and difficult for him to observe closely. He needs help in scanning and concentration.

Accordingly, the therapist assists him to create order out of his chaos by training him in sorting out things that look alike, feel alike, sound alike. She may give him a magazine and ask him to find all the pictures in which shoes are portrayed, to tear them out and to put them under one of his own shoes. She may say some words for him and ask him to signal every time he hears one which begins with an *s* sound. She may have him feel a series of objects with his eyes closed and select those which are smooth to the touch. She may work with opposites: big things and little things; hot foods and cold foods. She asks him to choose, to match, to classify. He needs categories. She helps him acquire them again.

Organization. The aphasic needs order in his disordered cosmos. He needs definite routines of daily living, consistent schedules of events. When we come to our daily sessions with an aphasic, we use the same greeting each time and begin our therapy with the same sort of activity before we try something new. The other people about him must help in this same ordering of his life so that a portion of it will become familiar and organized rather than confused.

But he must also learn to organize his own life, his own thoughts and outward behaviors. He needs help in patterning his consciousness. Accordingly we train him to make patterns of all types. We may begin by merely asking him or showing him how to set the table, or to turn the pages of a magazine left to right, or to arrange a few scrambled numbers in the proper order. We may have him raise his arm in a series of gradual steps. We may ask him to count the number of windows in the room, to draw a house, to roll a clay model of the cigarette he cannot ask for. We give him form boards to assemble. We ask him to arrange a series of boxes according to increasing size. We give him some cards, each with a word on it, and ask him to place them serially so they make a sentence which commands us to do something. We get him to sing some old tunes. We ask him to read aloud a sentence through the window of a shield which exposes only one word at a time. We ask him to correct our mispronunciations, our use of wrong words, his own mistakes. All these activities require scanning and concentration. The therapist helps, always using her self-talk and parallel talk to provide a running commentary for his thinking.

Formulation. The aphasic often has trouble not only in sending his messages or in receiving them; he also cannot formulate them with precision. Sometimes he cannot find the exact word he needs and instead of searching for another almost as good, or revising the whole utterance, he stops right there, helplessly, fixed on the thorn of his frustration. Basically, what he needs is the freedom to make new wholes, to try it again in a different way so that this different way also makes sense.

Although, as we have indicated, we use self-talk and parallel talking constantly throughout all of these various approaches to therapy with the aphasic, in helping him to formulate we use these techniques with great effectiveness. Here is a brief excerpt from such a therapy session:

> Therapist: All right, John. Let's begin. Talk to yourself. Say what you do. Like this. (*Therapist opens her purse, takes out pencil, writes his name. As she does so, she speaks in unison with her activity.*) Open purse . . . here pencil . . . write name. (*She hands him the purse and signals him to repeat her behavior.*)
>
> Aphasic (*opens purse*): Open puss . . . no . . . poos . . . no . . . oh dear oh my . . . (*gives up*).
>
> Therapist: OK. You got mixed up on "purse" . . . Purrrrrse . . . Never mind. Say the whole thing. (*She repeats action.*)
>
> Aphasic: Open puss . . .
>
> Therapist: And here pencil . . .
>
> Aphasic: Pencil . . . and now I write mame . . . no . . . mama . . . no . . .
>
> Therapist: Write name . . . name . . . like this. (*Demonstrates.*)
>
> Aphasic: Write name like . . . (*writes John*) . . . John . . . John . . . Write no good . . .
>
> Therapist: Fine! You did it. Now let's do it again. Talk to yourself. Say what you're doing.

A thousand experiences of this sort, based on the experiences of daily living, cannot help but aid the patient to improve in formulation. His wife and his children can easily learn to do these things. They should use simple self-talk whenever he can hear them so he knows what they are doing, perceiving, or feeling. Through parallel talking, they can put the words in his ears at the moment he needs them, thus reauditorizing his thinking, giving him the verbal symbols that have become lost or scrambled. Sooner or later, the aphasic will begin to talk to himself as he does things, sees things, or feels things. This should be highly rewarded by all about him. He may even begin to use parallel talk as he views the behavior of others. We have found no difficulty in having this vocalized thinking persist in inappropriate situations because later, as he becomes facile in their use, we have him learn to do his self-talk and parallel talking in a whisper or in pantomime.

We may also help him to formulate in other ways. We ask him to complete unfinished figures, to assemble toys, to repair a broken electric cord, to weave a rug, to complete the writing of unfinished sentences, to pre-write what he is about to say, or to rehearse it in pantomime. We have him do simple description and exposition on paper or aloud. We teach him to fill in the hands of a series of blank clock faces to indicate the hours. We teach him to make change; to do mental arithmetic, or if he cannot do so, to do the operations on paper. We give him simple problems to solve. We teach him to paraphrase, to tell us what he has read in the paper or heard on the radio. The fascinating thing about all of this is to discover how each new achievement seems to unlock the doors to new achievements. If this therapist could begin over again, he would specialize in aphasia.

Body Image Integration. It is not only the outside world which is strange to the aphasic. He also is a stranger to himself. He has changed. He is not the person he used to be. The various members of his family often show this by their reactions. They treat him like a child or as a nuisance or as though he were an imbecile. Good counseling can prevent much of this but it is difficult for a family to become adjusted to a handicapped stranger in the house.

We have said that the aphasic is also a stranger to himself. Often there is paralysis of the arm or leg. A part of him will not obey his bidding; he has suddenly sprouted a dead limb. Any one of us who has lain too long on an arm in bed and awakens to find it "gone to sleep," a strange inert thing there in bed with him, will vaguely understand how important this experience must be. But there are a thousand other changes in the person too. He has trouble reading, writing, talking, telling time, comprehending, counting. Who is this person who suddenly has come to inhabit his skin? It is the therapist's job to help him become acquainted, to introduce him to his new self and to get him to like this new person. It isn't easy but it can be done.

We begin by introducing him to his body. We massage his feet and name them as we do so. We lift his arm and tell him what we are doing. We have him stroke his face and find his eyes and ears and mouth. We get him to move his lips and his tongue as we do. We do much of our work with the body image in front of the mirror. We command the helpless hand to squeeze on the exercise ball, and we squeeze it. We take his picture in all sorts of therapeutic activities and show them to him. We look together in old albums at the snapshots of his childhood and youth. Perhaps all the king's horses couldn't do it, but a good therapist can put Humpty Dumpty together again.

Psychotherapy. It should be obvious by now that these patients need psychotherapy. They meet many penalties, experience frustrations so intense they would break up almost any physically normal person. They find their cups overflowing with anxiety, guilt, and hostility. They worry about the hospital bills, about the paycheck that is no more, about their possible future in a nursing home. They become furious with anger, often over trifles. And yet, fortunately, the same brain injury which creates these storms of emotion also makes them transient. They do not last, do not reverberate. Furious one moment, the next moment he is laughing.

Such an outline of therapeutic activities is far from being comprehensive but it may provide a starting platform. It does not indicate how the therapist works especially on the functions of one area in which progress seems most likely to occur. And it does not show, except by implication, the need for ingenuity and, above all, the patient perseverance needed to rehabilitate these persons. Personally, we have found our work with aphasics to be more fascinating and rewarding than that with many other communicative disabilities. This is true not only with children with aphasia but also with the many adults who have been brought to us for help. To see a person, who has been stricken down at the entrance to the valley of death, rejoin the human race, and to feel that perhaps you have had a humble part in that rejoining, is reward enough for all the failures and frustrations aphasia therapy brings.

REFERENCES

Aphasia

1. Baker, E. E. "Teaching Aphasic Patients to Talk Again," *American Journal of Nursing*, Volume 52, 1952, pages 831-832.

2. Barry, H., *The Young Aphasic Child*. Washington, D.C.: Alexander Graham Bell Association for the Deaf, 1961.

3. Berry, M. E. *Speech Disorders*. New York: Appleton-Century-Crofts, 1956. Chapters 16, 17, 18.

4. Bixby, L. "Comeback from a Brain Operation," *Harper's*, CCV, November, 1952, pages 69-73.

5. Butfield, E. "Acquired Receptive Dysphasia," *Speech Pathology and Therapy* (London) Volume 3, 1960, pages 8-12.

6. Eisenson, J. "Aphasia in Adults—Classification and Examination Procedures," in L. E. Travis (ed.), *Handbook of Speech Pathology*. New York: Appleton-Century-Crofts, 1957, Chapters 12 and 14.

7. ———. *Examining for Aphasia* (revised edition). New York: Psychological Corporation, 1954.

8. ———. "Prognostic Factors Related to Language Rehabilitation in Aphasic Patients," *Journal Speech and Hearing Disorders*, Volume 14, 1949, pages 262-264.

9. Morley, M. E. "Developmental Receptive-Receptive Aphasia," *Speech Pathology and Therapy*, Volume 3, 1960, pages 64-76.

10. Myklebust, H. R. *Auditory Disorders in Children*. New York: Grune & Stratton, Inc., 1954, pages 143-180.

11. Pfaff, P. L. "The Moto-kinesthetic Method Applied to Aphasics," *Journal Speech and Hearing Disorders*, Volume 5, 1940, pages 271-274.

12. Rose, R. H. "A Physician's Account of His Own Aphasia," *Journal Speech Disorders*, Volume 13, 1948, pages 294-305.

13. Schuell, H. "Auditory Impairment in Aphasia: Significance and Retraining Procedures," *Journal Speech and Hearing Disorders*, Volume 18, 1953, pages 14-21.

14. Silverman, M., and K. Holliday. "Half Your Brain is a Spare," *Saturday Evening Post*, Volume CCXXI, 1948 (December 11), pages 26-27.

15. Smith, M. "Teaching an Aphasic How to Write Again," *Journal Clinical Psychology*, Volume 4, 1948, pages 419-423.

16. Turnbloom, M., and J. S. Myers. "A Group Discussion Program with Families of Aphasic Patients," *Journal Speech and Hearing Disorders*, Volume 17, pages 393-396.

17. Van Riper, C. "Speech Disorders," in L. A. Pennington, and I. A. Berg (eds.), *An Introduction to Clinical Psychology* (second edition). New York: The Ronald Press Company, 1954, pages 353-356.

18. Wepman, J. M. *Recovery From Aphasia*. New York: The Ronald Press Company, 1951.

19. Wood, N. D. "Language Disorders in Children," *Monographs of Social Research in Child Development*, Volume 25, 1960, pages 15-23.

CHAPTER FIFTEEN

The Speech Therapist

For many students this text will have been their first introduction to speech therapy as a professional field. We hope it has not been an unpleasant experience. We hope also that some of them may be interested in entering this new profession. But even those who have no personal interest in speech therapy as a career should know something of the qualifications required of those who do. They may desire to refer some child or their own child to a speech therapist some day.

Speech Therapy as a Profession.   First, we must make it very clear that speech therapy is a very young newcomer to the family of the healing professions. Its professional organization, the American Speech and Hearing Association, is not even forty years old, whereas medicine, dentistry, and nursing have long histories. Nevertheless, this young profession has shown astounding growth both in membership and in its standards. Speech and hearing specialists are now to be found in almost every country of the world. The journals of this profession publish articles in many languages containing basic research and clinical methods. Certification standards require stringent preparation both in academic courses and in supervised casework and they are constantly being raised. Parents who now refer their speech defective children to a certified speech or hearing therapist can feel confident that they are in well-trained and competent hands.

The demand for trained workers in this field has constantly exceeded the supply and seems destined to continue in this accelerating fashion for some years. Training centers are finding it increasingly difficult to meet requests for newly trained clinicians to staff the many positions available. In part this is due to the fact that many college students still in search of a satisfying career never hear about this professional field, or, if they do, they hear about it too late. Speech and hearing therapists have probably been too busy with their cases and their research to blow their horns loudly enough to be heard over the masking noise of the other older professions. If the student who reads this finds some interest in such a career, or knows of other students who are still searching, he will find a cordial response from those who are actively engaged in the work. We have personally known speech therapists from all over the world. They form a devoted clan, still too young professionally to have become cynical or hardened to the troubles of those they serve. They are a bit idealistic. They are concerned about their cases. They care! They are still pioneering and exploring, still hungry to learn from each other and from their cases. A comradeship exists among them which is very warming.

Perhaps this spirit is due to the appreciation which speech therapists get from those who through them have finally become able to join the human race in that uniquely human function of speech. Teachers get affection and respect but not much appreciation. Businessmen get money—and ulcers. Speech therapists are paid more than teachers and less than businessmen, but they get more appreciation and have more fun than either. This is an intriguing profession in many ways. It uses information from many professional areas. The speech therapist, for example, who works with cleft-palate cases will need to know something about surgery, dentistry, orthodontia, prostheses, psychological counseling, family problems, and a host of other things. It is difficult to become bored in this field; there are too many new challenges. Indeed, each new case presents a different one. There are always new things for the therapist to discover, new skills to acquire, old skills to perfect, new roles to play. And, throughout the days of his professional career, the speech therapist enters many lives, shares many burdens, and heals many old wounds. In this life of ours there are belly pleasures and other pleasures. There are values of status and material possessions. But we know of none so thoroughly good as that of seeing some twisted life become untangled as the result of our efforts.

Perhaps another major feature of the attraction which speech therapy holds for its practitioners is that the work itself is usually pleasant work. These children we serve have been hurt in the mouth —and even deeper. They come to us feeling that speaking is unpleasant, that communication holds threat and rejection. Accordingly, one of the first tasks in therapy is to change this attitude; we must make speaking pleasant. No child can confront a speech defect long enough to modify it until he finds not only a permissive therapist but a pleasant one. With little children, much of our work is done through play. Even with adults, the interaction is usually flavored with humor and good natured comradeship in experimentation. Relationships are close and warm. We deal with growth and change. We help the buds of potential to bloom.

To some people speech-correction work is very distasteful, and there seem to be certain personal qualifications which make all the difference between success and failure. In general, the nervous, impatient, high-strung individual does not make a good speech correctionist. Neither does the person who falls into routine, stereotyped methods and remains there contentedly. Successful teachers of speech correction possess the majority of the following traits to a high degree: a sense of humor, patience, curiosity, social poise, ingenuity in inventing and adapting techniques, professional enthusiasm, a sensitive and discriminating hearing, interest in the personalities of others, industriousness, objective attitude toward their own insecurities, calmness, ability to recognize subterfuge and mental mechanisms, and self-respect. Few people, of course, are born as virtuous as the above list of traits might imply, but speech correction puts such a premium upon such characteristics that those who do not possess them try to acquire them as soon as possible. Speech therapists constantly seek to improve themselves in all of these traits. There is also one other highly essential qualification which must be developed if it is not already possessed: *empathy*. By empathy, we mean the ability to identify with the case, to understand how he feels, to predict his reactions—in short, to be able to get temporarily inside his psychological skin. The therapist must be secure enough herself so that she can do this identification and share the outward and inward behaviors of the case. She should understand herself, accept herself, and seek to improve herself.

All of these personal pronouns need some qualifying. Throughout this book, the author has referred to the therapist in the feminine gender, using the pronouns *she* and *her*. This was done, not because speech therapy is a female profession, but merely as a literary convenience because the majority of the cases we had to mention were male. Speech therapy is rapidly attracting more men than women, perhaps because the latter get married and leave the profession until their children are grown, or they do private practice in their own homes while the men stay on the job. At any rate, a noticeable trend toward male personnel is apparent. And the males marry the female speech therapists and put them to work teaching their own children to talk.

Varieties of Professional Experience. One of the author's former students is employed by the State Department, teaching officers in the Turkish army to speak English. Another runs a Crippled Children's Speech and Hearing Clinic in Alaska. Another operates a private pre-school nursery for very young children with speech defects. Another is the speech therapist tutor of the stuttering son of a multimillionaire. Another works as a hospital therapist specializing in the diagnosis of aphasia. Another does nothing but laboratory research in voice science. Another manages a cleft-palate speech clinic in conjunction with a team of surgical, orthodontic, and other specialists. Another has a mobile speech clinic in a Western state financed by the Elks and travels continually with her trailer clinic over the hills and far away. Still another does her speech therapy in an orthopedic school for children with cerebral palsy. Another has shifted from speech therapy into audiology and heads up that department in a university. Another has become a psychiatrist specializing in children's problems including those of speech. Another does private practice primarily with actors who have voice problems. Many of them are directors of college speech clinics. But most (and we almost said "the best") of them are doing speech therapy in the public schools.

Speech Therapy in the Public Schools. In the setting of the public schools, speech therapists find not only real interest and financial support but also an opportunity for service which is almost unique. A public school speech therapist is employed as a teacher but she (remember again, please, that many are men) is a very special sort of a teacher, a teacher-therapist. Her job is more like that of the school nurse than like that of a classroom teacher. Children are referred to her for help, or she discovers them through screening testing. The case loads seem (and often are) very large. Many public-school therapists see one hundred children each week and they therefore work with most of them in groups ranging from three to about seven children in a group. Fortunately, the majority of these children do not present very difficult problems. Most of them have mild articulatory defects and improve swiftly. A few of them need individual therapy and parental counseling. Usually one day each week is set aside for these purposes and for general co-ordination of the therapist's program with other school activities. One of the basic advantages of this setup is that it permits the child to have therapy in a natural rather than a clinical setting, and it makes possible a transfer of new skills from the therapy room into the child's daily life in the school. For the speech therapist, too, there are advantages. She is not frozen in the same room of the same school with the same children under the same principal day after day and month after month. She moves from school to school, often shifting midmorning from one to another. She prepares her own schedule, selects her own cases, designs her own therapy and does not have to put on overshoes or collect the milk money. Some- how, her regime keeps her from having to wear the teacher's mask. She remains a pretty free agent. A good therapist can usually dis- miss over a third of her cases each year and most of the rest show improvement. Thus she has a sense of real achievement which is augmented by the appreciation of parents, teachers, and the chil- dren themselves.

Speech Therapy in the Hospital Setting. It is difficult to describe any typical program for this type of practice since programs vary widely. The hospital therapist generally sees the more severely im- paired cases, especially those of organic origin. She works with patients such as those with aphasia, cleft palates, cerebral palsy, laryngectomies, stuttering, voice problems, and dysarthrias. A por- tion of her work is solely diagnosis; the rest is therapy, both indi- vidual and in small groups. The case load is small. Therapy is usu- ally difficult, however, and often the prognosis may be poor. At times the amount of real improvement may be slight. Hospital ther- apy demands real competence on the part of the speech therapist. He (or she) must show that professional competence in the white glare of the hospital walls under the scrutiny of other specialists in rehabilitation. But hospital speech therapy is also very rewarding. One constantly learns more and more about the human being. There are ward rounds and staffings of cases of all types. There is close collaboration with the psychologist, the social worker, the occupational therapist, the physiotherapist, as well as with the medical profession.

Speech Therapy in Schools for Crippled Children.   In the orthopedic schools, we find a blend of the two types of therapy settings described above. The case loads are small and the problems are usually difficult. Much of the work is individual therapy although small groups are also employed when socialization is needed. The therapist often must coordinate her own therapy with that of the other special teachers. For example, if the classroom teacher is having a social science project on the farmer's life, the speech therapist will use this theme in the communication used to work on smooth breathing in a child with cerebral palsy, or on the final sounds of the words *cows* and *chickens* as spoken by a post-polio child with a partially paralyzed tongue and a lateral lisp. Each child is studied very intensively from every angle by the staff members of such a school and the speech therapist is a member of a teacher-therapist team.*

Private Practice.   Once a speech therapist has satisfied the clinical certification requirements of the American Speech and Hearing Association (not only certain strict academic requirements but also therapy experience under the sponsorship of a designated professional therapist) he may do private practice in this field. In this setting, the speech therapist often works with cases referred by physicians or other speech therapists and is paid for his work by the patient. He may have an office in a medical arts building or clinic, or may do the work in his own home. Many female speech therapists do some private practice in their own homes once they are married and have small children of their own. There also seems to be a growing trend for private summer speech clinics operated by public-school speech therapists in which they offer intensive therapy to the more severely handicapped children they could not adequately serve during the school year. The majority of the cases seen in private practice are those with delayed speech, stuttering, or the organic speech disorders. There are many problems that arise in pri-

---

* An excellent account of some speech therapy casework in a school for crippled children is found in the article by George O. Egland, "An Analysis of an Exceptional Case of a Retarded Speech," *Journal Speech and Hearing Disorders,* Volume 19, 1954, pages 233-243.

vate practice which should be seriously considered by individuals who plan such a career.* It is no bed of roses.

Audiology. We have already indicated that there are many other settings in which speech therapy is flourishing. However, most professional speech therapists begin their work either in the clinic or the public schools and then diverge later. So we will not describe these other types of work here. However, we must not forget to describe the way in which speech therapy serves as a beginning to other careers, especially those of audiology and special education. All speech therapists take some courses in hearing during their undergraduate preparation, and they take more when they continue in graduate school. Some of them find in audiology a smell of scientific certainty (illusory or not) which contrasts markedly with that of speech therapy where one must constantly deal with probabilities and the intangible. They find in audiometry and the research on hearing loss a definiteness which they crave. Audiology is a very fast growing field and the demand for workers is even greater than in speech therapy. All beginning students should give it serious consideration.

Special Education. In much the same way, beginning speech therapists usually take courses in special education as part of their undergraduate preparation, and those who later work in the public schools often come into close contact with other special teachers. As a result, some of them (the male therapists especially) find themselves active in such professional organizations as the Council for Exceptional Children, which serves all the fields of special education including the gifted child. Perhaps because of his experience in organizing and administering the speech therapy program and the public relations work which it often entails, the speech therapist becomes a marked man in the school system. He knows all the principals and the superintendent. He works with all the special teachers. Moreover, he already has an extensive academic background in not one but two fields of rehabilitation: speech and hearing. These experiences and qualifications often lead superintendents to encourage the speech therapist to do graduate work in special education

---

* See Paul D. Knight. "Advantages and Disadvantages of Private Practice," *Journal Speech Disorders*, Volume 12, 1947, pages 199-201.

See also "Private Practice in Speech Pathology and Audiology," in *ASHA*, Volume 3 (November), 1961, pages 387-407.

in the areas in which his preparation was scanty so that he can be promoted to the directorship of all special education services. Those of us in speech therapy often regret our profession's loss when a competent therapist becomes an administrator but, when this occurs as it has been happening more frequently each year, at least his newly hired replacement can find sympathetic understanding and support.

So we end this book with an invitation. We have helped you explore a portion of the forest of speech pathology. Strange at first, some parts of this forest are now familiar to you. Yet, there are many parts of this forest no man has entered. Perhaps you would like to join us in blazing a trail.

REFERENCES

1. Ainsworth, S. "Suggestions for a Successful Speech Correction Program in Public Schools," *Quarterly Journal of Speech,* Volume 31, 1945, pages 471-477.
2. ———. "The Profession Devoted to Speech and Hearing Disorders," *ASHA,* Volume 2, 1960, pages 388-402.
3. ASHA Committee. "Private Practice in Speech Pathology and Audiology," *ASHA,* Volume 3, 1961, pages 387-406.
4. Berry, M. F., and J. Eisenson. *Speech Disorders.* New York: Appleton-Century-Crofts, 1956, Chapter 19.
5. Gorman, T. "North Dakota's Clinic on Wheels," *Today's Health,* Volume 28, 1950, pages 23-24, 44.
6. Johnson, K. O. (ed.). "Abstracts of the 37th Annual Convention," *ASHA,* Volume 3, 1961, pages 321-373.
7. ———, and P. W. Newman. "A Study of Personal Incomes in the Speech and Hearing Profession," *ASHA,* Volume 4, 1962, pages 59-70.
8. ————, "Trends in the Profession," *ASHA,* Volume 3, 1961, pages 109-114.
9. Kopp, G. A. "Bridging the Gap," *Journal Speech and Hearing Disorders,* Volume 25, 1960, pages 70-76.
10. Lillywhite, H. "Organizing a Hospital Program for Communicative Disorders," *ASHA,* Volume 3, 1961, pages 139-144.
11. ———. "Toward a Philosophy of Professional Behavior," *ASHA,* Volume 3, pages 40-42.
12. Moore, P. "Time Lapse," *ASHA,* Volume 4, 1962, pages 31-35.

13. Powers, M. H. "What Makes an Effective Public School Speech Therapist," *Journal Speech and Hearing Disorders,* Volume 21, 1956, pages 461-467.

14. Sheehan, J. G. "Professional Self-Image in Speech Pathology and Therapy," *ASHA,* Volume 3, 1961, pages 423-425.

15. ———. R. G. Hadley, and G. R. White. "The Speech Pathologist: His Interests, Activities and Attitudes," *Journal Speech and Hearing Disorders,* Volume 25, 1960, pages 317-322.

16. Steer, Mack D. "Public School Speech and Hearing Services," *Journal Speech and Hearing Disorders,* Monograph Supplement 8, July 1961.

17. Streng, A. *Children with Impaired Hearing.* Washington, D.C.: Council of Exceptional Children, 1960.

18. ———. *Hearing Therapy for Children.* New York: Grune & Stratton, Inc., 1955.

19. Summers, R. "Private Practice of Public School Therapists in Indiana," *Journal Speech and Hearing Disorders,* Volume 24, 1959, pages 51-54.

20. Van Riper, C. *Speech Therapy: A Book of Readings.* Englewood Cliffs, N.J.: Prentice-Hall, Inc., 1953, Chapter 9.

※ **Examinations for Voice Disorders**

In order to administer these tests, the examiner should have a normal sense of pitch placement and discrimination and the ability to distinguish the normal from the abnormal. He also needs experience and training.

Pitch Analysis Tests

1. *Ability to discriminate pitch.* This may be tested by whistling pairs of notes at low, middle, and high pitches, and requesting the subject to tell whether the first is higher or lower than the second. Use ten pairs of notes at each of the pitch levels, using a random order. The same test can be given by humming the notes. Do not let the subject watch you, and keep the tones exactly two semitones apart. Record the number of errors at each pitch level. Students should practice giving this test under supervision until they are able to give adequate stimuli.

2. *Ability to produce a given pitch.* This may be tested by humming the nasal *m* at a low, middle, and high pitch. After each stimulus, the subject is required to attempt to duplicate it with his humming. Use different notes at each pitch level and continue the hum for at least five seconds. Score as an error any performance which does not come within a semitone of the stimulus or its octave, but note any tendency to produce a harmonic such as a musical fifth.

3. *Ability to carry a tune in unison or alone.* Tunes chosen should be simple and familiar. Use the unison test first. Use the same tune for both.

4. *Ability to follow inflections.* In this test the student is provided with a pencil and paper and is shown the following graphs of inflection as they are phonated and drawn by the examiner on the vowel *a*: ———↗ ————↘ ——→ ———↘. He is then asked to follow with

his pencil a new series given by the examiner, who phonates the inflections according to the following sequence of graphs: ⟶. The examiner's inflections should not range above a full tone. Record number and type of error.

5. *Normality of inflections in speech.* Use phrases or sentences which ask questions, make statements, give commands, indicate surprise, and express disgust, and have the subject repeat them after the examiner. Some examples are: *What's that noise? I liked that movie. You get out of here! What a* BIG *fish! Oh, I'm sick of this lousy place.* Record marked differences from your own inflections.

6. *Relation between pitch and stress.* Using the sentences in the preceding paragraph, notice whether stress changes are used instead of pitch changes. Underline certain words in sentences and ask subject to emphasize them. Note whether any pitch changes occur. Ask subject to phonate some vowel several times, alternating stressed and relaxed production. Note whether stressed notes are higher in pitch.

7. *Determination of pitch range.* Hum a middle-pitched note as a model for the case to imitate. Then gradually hum down the scale until the case cannot phonate at any lower pitch. Do this several times and note the place at which the individual begins to strain and falter. Locate this note on a piano or pitch pipe. Then, beginning with the same original note, hum up the scale until the voice breaks into the falsetto. Instruct the subject not to use the falsetto if possible. Locate the highest note accomplished without straining or falsetto. The difference between highest and lowest notes may be called the pitch range. If the falsetto keeps breaking in, determine the highest note of its range.

The importance of pitch-range tests is that they help us determine whether the speech defective is using a habitual pitch that is too near the bottom or top of his pitch range. If this is the case, intensity and quality defects may result. Moreover, the optimal or natural pitch at which the subject is most effective is usually located at a point a few semitones above the lowest third of the regular pitch range. If the falsetto is included, the natural pitch is usually located at about the twenty-fifth percentile of the total pitch range.

8. *Determination of habitual pitch.* This is much more difficult for the untrained or inexperienced examiner to determine, since it involves the disregard of inflections and a process of mental averaging of the pitch changes which exist in propositional speech. Nevertheless, the trained ear can spot the average pitch of another individual's voice with amazing accuracy. The subject is asked to repeat over and over, ten times or more, the sentence: "Now is the time for all good men to come to the aid of the party." Disregarding the first and last words, the examiner hums softly up and down the scale until he finds his voice synchronizing with the pitch of the subject's voice. Continu-

ing to hum this pitch, he goes to the piano and finds its notation, which he records. Through similar technique it is also possible to determine the extent of habitual pitch range used by the subject. The reference by Root is recommended if supplementary information is desired.

9. *Determination of natural pitch.* Ask the subject to close his eyes, to begin with a low pitch, and to hum slowly and continuously up the scale, attempting to keep the intensity constant. The observer will note a certain pitch at which the intensity swells. Hum this pitch until it can be identified on the piano and recorded. Repeat the process while humming a descending scale. Give three ascending and three descending trials, and consider the place at which these pitches seem to cluster as the natural pitch. A range of three or four semitones about this note may be considered as optimal for performance. The natural pitch level may also be determined from the pitch range as described in test seven of this section.

10. *Effect of special influences.* By controlling the testing situation in the appropriate manner, study the effect upon the subject's habitual pitch of the following variables: change in quality (have subject speak gutturally, nasally, and so on); changes in intensity (very loud and very quiet speech); relaxation; distraction; imitation of another's speech.

Tests of Vocal Intensity

1. *Maximum duration.* The subject is required to take three deep breaths and then phonate a front, middle, and back vowel. Each is held as long as possible, and the time recorded. Normal individuals should be able to hold any of these vowels for at least fifteen seconds without difficulty. The vowels *i, a,* and *u* may be used, and the series should be given twice if the subject fails the first time.

2. *Breath economy.* The subject should be given a passage to read. Note the first words of sentences to determine whether the subject exhales abnormally prior to speech attempt. Also note the number of inhalations per fifty words of jumbled material, or in reading backward. Over eight inhalations per fifty words is definitely abnormal. It is wise to make a breathing record, if possible, noting attack-exhalation, phonation on residual air, shallow breathing, and disintegrations between thorax and abdomen. These can also be detected by the trained observer without such apparatus. Note also whether clavicular breathing is used.

3. *Muscular tension.* Firm pressure by the experimenter's fingers on both sides of the thyroid cartilage will discover hyper- or hypo-tonicity of the laryngeal musculature.

4. *Effect of special influences.* By controlling the testing situation in the appropriate manner, the examiner can study the effect of the

following conditions on the habitual intensity: strong clinical demand for more intensity, pitch change, change in voice quality, and presence of masking noise, distraction, relaxation, strong physical effort made simultaneously with speech attempt, expression of rage or disgust. It is also wise to determine if the subject can discard speech inhibitions by asking him, for example, to call a dog from across the street in the manner illustrated by the examiner. Determine also whether, in certain speech situations, the person's voice is adequate in intensity.

Voice Quality Analysis

1. Check adjectives which best describe defective voice quality: *hoarse, husky, strident, guttural, breathy, throaty, noisy, pectoral, nasal, denasal.*

2. Make an auditory analysis to determine which vowels are most defective. All vowels are seldom equally bad, and usually only a few need remedial work. Begin by having the subject read until you can be certain to identify the peculiar timbre responsible for the voice disorder. Then have the subject prolong each of the isolated vowels for about five seconds. Check those that are obviously abnormal, making a recheck to determine which of the vowels are most defective. After completing this, go through the articulation test sentences and words which deal with the vowels, underlining all those most defective. Note also whether the defective quality exists all through the prolonged vowel or merely at its initiation, and whether or not it seems to be affected by the consonants which precede and follow it.

3. Make a similar analysis for nasality disorders. With these, one can use a cold mirror held horizontally and placed with the mirror side up beneath the nostrils, but above the mouth. If clouding occurs on the mirror, the vowel has been nasalized. The same test may be used by placing the fingers on each side of the bridge of the nose and determining nasality by the vibration. When using the words of the articulation test, be sure to substitute others for those containing the *m, n,* and *ng* sounds. Note whether nasality is produced on certain vowels when no nasal air is discharged.

4. Once the two or three most defective sounds have been discovered, make a phonetic placement analysis to determine position of lips, jaws, tongue, and velum. Insist upon other methods of producing the same vowel (with tongue and lips in different positions), and note variations in quality.

5. Study the effect of pitch change on voice quality. Use isolated vowels at many different pitch levels, and also use continuous speech.

6. Repeat the preceding test, using variations in intensity.

7. Study the effect of relaxation, both general and specific, on voice quality. Use the vocalized yawn for the worst vowels.

8. Determine the quality of whispered vowels. Is it better than that of phonated ones? If so, try to make gradual transition from whisper through stage whisper to phonation, without letting peculiarity come in.

9. Study the effect of distraction and imitation of other voices.

Examinations for the Articulatory Disorders

Examination for Organic Abnormalities

Examination for Organic Defects. It is wise to make a special examination of the mouth, nose, and throat of every speech case, but such an examination is needed especially for voice and articulatory disorders. While it is true that many normal speakers have organic defects in these speech structures and that such defects therefore cannot be termed essential causes of the speech defect, nevertheless the presence of an overshot jaw or of an excessively long tongue must certainly be a handicapping factor in speech development. Some of us can compensate for these defects because of either training or natural desire for speech perfection, but many others cannot. Hence the presence of these defects is important and must be taken into account in both the diagnosis and the treatment. However, the presence of some anatomical abnormality is of no importance in itself unless it stands in functional relation to defective speech sounds. For example, the presence of a harelip in a child whose sole speech error is an inability to produce the *k* sound is of no causal significance. It is also necessary to caution the inexperienced teacher not to make a hasty diagnosis. Other causal factors may be of far greater importance than the organic defect.

Although a head mirror or laryngoscope is more convenient, an adequate examination may be made by placing the subject slightly to one side of a flashlight or a window and reflecting this light, by means of a little mirror, into his mouth. Tongue depressors, probes, and tooth props are tools easily procured. The examiner should develop a systematic routine involving quick, sure movements and

472

Phonetic Symbol	Key Words English	Phonetics	Phonetic Symbol	Key Words English	Phonetics

Consonants

Phonetic Symbol	English	Phonetics	Phonetic Symbol	English	Phonetics
b	beg, tub	bɛg tʌb	p	paper, damper	pepɚ dæmpɚ
d	do, and	du ænd	r	run, far	rʌn far
f	fan, scarf	fæn skarf	s	send, us	sɛnd ʌs
g	grow, bag	gro bæg	t	toe, ant	to ænt
dʒ	judge, enjoy	dʒʌdʒ ɪndʒɔɪ	ʃ	shed, ash	ʃɛd æʃ
h	hem, inhale	hɛm ɪnhel	tʃ	cheap, each	tʃip itʃ
k	kick, uncle	kɪk ʌŋkl̩	θ	thin, tooth	θɪn tuθ
l	let, pal	lɛt pæl	ð	then, breathe	ðɛn brið
l̩	apple, turtle	æpl̩ tɝtl̩	v	vow, have	vau hæv
m	men, arm	mɛn arm	w	wet, twin	wɛt twɪn
m̩	autumn, wisdom	ɔtm̩ wɪzdm̩	hw	when, white	hwɛn hwaɪt
n	nose, gain	noz gen	j	you, yet	ju jɛt
n̩	sudden, curtain	sʌdn̩ kɝtn̩	ʒ	pleasure, vision	plɛʒɚ vɪʒən
ŋ	wrong, anger	rɔŋ æŋgɚ	z	zoo, ooze	zu uz

Vowels

Phonetic Symbol	English	Phonetics	Phonetic Symbol	English	Phonetics
a*	ask, rather	ask raðɚ	ɒ*	log, toss	lɒg tɒs
ɑ	father, odd	faðɚ ɑd	ɝ	earn, fur	ɝn fɝ
e	make, eight	mek et	ʒ*	earn, fur	ʒn fʒ
æ	sat, act	sæt ækt	ɚ	never, percale	nɛvɚ pɚkel
i	fatigue, east	fətig ist	u	truth, blue	truθ blu
ɛ	red, end	rɛd ɛnd	ʊ	put, nook	pʊt nʊk
ɪ	it, since	ɪt sɪns	ʌ	under, love	ʌndɚ lʌv
o	hope, old	hop old	ə	about, second	əbaut sɛkənd
ɔ	sauce, off	sɔs ɔf			

Diphthongs

Phonetic Symbol	English	Phonetics	Phonetic Symbol	English	Phonetics
[aɪ]	sigh, aisle	[saɪ aɪl]	[ɔɪ]	coy, oil	[kɔɪ ɔɪl]
[au]	now, owl	[nau aul]			

*These sounds are only rarely used in General American speech, but are common in the East and South. General American speech uses [æ] for [a], [ɔ] for [ɒ], and [ʃ] for [ʒ].

FIGURE 33. *The Phonetic Alphabet**

* From Charles Van Riper and Dorothy Edna Smith, *An Introduction to General American Phonetics*, 2nd ed. New York: Harper & Row, Publishers, 1962. Page 8. By permission of the authors.

	Nasals	Glides	Lateral	Fricatives	Affricates	Stops
Bilabial	m	w hw				p b
Labiodental				f v		
Dental				θ ð		
Alveolar	n		l	s z r	tʃ dʒ	t d
Palatal		j		ʃ ʒ		
Velar	ŋ					k g
Glottal				h		b

Location of Highest Tongue Contour
and
Degree of Mouth Opening

Tongue Position	Front	Central	Back	Mouth Opening
High	i		u	Narrow
	ɪ	ɝ	ʊ	
to	e	ə ʌ ɜ	o	to
	ɛ	ɑ	ɔ	
Low	æ		ɒ	Wide

This chart shows the similarities and differences between our vowels according to the positioning of the tongue and, crudely, the degree of mouth opening employed. It does not show the rounding of the mouth opening. All of the back vowels, plus the [ɑ], are rounded; the central and front vowels are not.

FIGURE 34. *Classification of the Vowels of General American English*°

requests. He should examine each structure, not only in quiescence, but also in its relation to the appropriate speech sounds. He must record all evidence of handicapping abnormality, together with a notation as to any evidence of compensatory movements in the

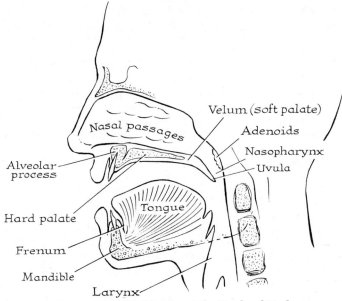

FIGURE 35. *Sagittal Section of the Head and Neck*

production of speech. A convenient sequence for the examination is as follows:

1. Examine lips for presence of scar tissue or harelip. Examine during performance of *p, b,* and *m.*

2. Examine jaws in relaxed occlusion to note overshot, undershot, or asymmetrical jaw formation. Examine during performance of *f, v,* and *th,* and note whether tongue movement is compensatory during performance of *s, l,* and *r* due to the relative displacement of tongue with respect to the upper teeth.

3. Examine teeth to note malocclusion. Record whether it is due to the upper, lower, or both sets of teeth. Record also whether it is on the right, left, or both sides. Note spaced or missing teeth according to a similar scheme. Note whether tongue habitually plugs gaps in silence or in making the following sounds: *s, z, sh, ch, j, zh.* Note relation of teeth to jaws and lips.

4. Note tongue to determine gross abnormality of width and length. Have subject lap tongue several times, finally leaving it out. Note any evidence of atrophy, in terms of area on both sides of midline, and of wrinkling. Have subject touch right and left corners of mouth alternately to determine possibility of unilateral sluggishness or paralysis. Note proximity of frenum to tonguetip. Can subject lick above upper mar-

gin of upper lip without showing bowing effect of frenum? Is there evidence of past tongue-tie? Can subject groove tongue at will? Can subject touch hard palate with tonguetip easily? Have subject touch tongue depressor held one inch out from the teeth as you count rhythmically at a rate of three counts per second for five seconds. Note action of tongue in making *th, s, l, r, d, t, k, g.*

5. Examine roof of mouth to note gross abnormality in height and width of hard palate. Note tongue placement for *r* and *l, k* and *g,* to determine compensatory positions. Note slope of hard palate from alveolar ridge. Note whether any evidence of present or past cleft exists.

6. Examine velum for presence of cleft, shortness, uvular abnormality, atrophy, or asymmetry. Is uvula pulled to one side? Is it so long as to stick to back of tongue? Have subject phonate vowel *a* and note action of velum and pharynx. (A guttural mirror may help in this part of the examination.) Is velum too short for good closure? Note action of velum in producing *k* and *g* sounds. Determine whether gag reflex exists. Note size and condition of tonsils and part they play in velar action. Note injuries or scar tissue on pillars of the fauces. Note inflammation of the velum and surrounding tissues. Ask student to swallow a large mouthful of water. Note if any comes out of the nose. Ask student to blow up a balloon.

7. Examine pharynx as subject nasalizes vowel *a* and as he phonates a normal *a.* Note presence of adenoids, using guttural mirror. Note inflammation and amount of mucosa. Have subject alternate *m* and *ba* sounds as rapidly as possible for five seconds. He should be able to average at least two per second if a child, and three per second if an adult. Note presence and condition of adenoids. Is there a constant nasal drip from the nasopharynx?

In so far as possible it is always wise to examine the articulatory organs (the tongue, lips, teeth, jaws, and soft palate) as the incorrect sounds are being attempted. Occasionally we must insert a tongue depressor between the teeth to observe the action of the tongue or palate. This does not give a normal picture of the manner of sound production, but it does help to identify basically incorrect movements and contacts. Thus, one adult who could not produce a normal *ch* (tʃ) sound was observed beginning this sound from a contact of the tonguetip and the soft palate. A passable *ch* (tʃ) sound can be made in this way but not at conversational speeds. Helping him to locate the normal starting position on the upper teeth or gum ridge soon cleaned up his difficulty. Many cases of lateral lisping will be observed lifting the tonguetip to the contact for an unvoiced *l* as a substitute for the *s*. It is often impossible for these cases to adopt a new correct method of sound production until they can identify the old one. We cannot break an unconscious habit except by bringing it up to consciousness. By studying the action of the articulatory organs as they produce the incorrect sounds, we can plan a much better treatment.

Auditory Memory Span. In testing the articulation cases' auditory memory span, several methods may be used. We may follow the procedure used in intelligence testing and determine how many digits a child can recall. We may use a series of isolated nonsense syllables with two-second intervals (23), or we may use a series of nonsense words in which the syllables are combined as in *goulabi*. Research has not shown any conclusive difference between groups of articulatory cases and groups of normal-speaking individuals on auditory memory-span tests, but certain individuals are found whose auditory memory spans are so short that this factor must be taken into account during treatment. The purpose of these tests is to discover these individuals.

Some norms for auditory memory-span tests are now given:

1. *For repeating digits at one-second intervals* (Robbins):

Age	Number of Digits
3	3
4	4
7	5
10	6
14	7
18	8

2. *For repeating nonsense syllables* (kʌ, pʌ, *and so on*) (Metraux) *at two-second intervals:*

Age	Number of Syllables
5	2.0
6	2.3
7	2.6
8	2.6
9	2.8
10	3.0
11	2.9
12	3.1

3. *For repeating nonsense words* (Beebe[1]):

Age	Number of Syllables per Nonsense Word
4	4
5	3.8
6	4.3
7	4.3
8	4.6

Phonetic Discrimination Ability. Ordinarily we combine our examination of the case's ability to hear differences among the various speech sounds with the general articulation tests. We do this by determining whether he can tell his errors from the correct sounds when both are produced in random fashion by the examiner. But occasionally we find a case who seems to be especially lacking in phonetic discrimination. In order to be certain that this is indeed an important factor, we administer a more formal type of test. The one which we have found most useful is the modification of the Travis-Rasmus test used by Templin (30). It is simply administered by requiring the case to write down on a sheet of paper his judgment of whether or not the two sounds given by the examiner are the *same* or *different*. A short practice session is given to clarify the task. The series of paired syllables used by Templin in the short form of her test are as follows:

SHORT TEST OF SOUND DISCRIMINATION

Examples:	Key: All D Except:
te-de	A. 1, 8
ere-ere	B. 1, 6, 8, 10
os-og	C. 3, 6, 8, 9
	D. 4, 9, 10
	E. 3, 9
	F. 3, 7
	G. 3, 6

A	B	C	D
1. te-te	1. ne-ne	1. fo-θo	1. pe-ke
2. hwe-we	2. dʒe-tʃe	2. vo-ðo	2. tʃo-ʃo
3. ne-me	3. ʃe-tʃe	3. zo-zo	3. ki-ti

---

[1] H. H. Beebe. "Auditory Memory Span for Meaningless Syllables," *Journal of Speech Disorders,* Volume 9, 1944, pages 273-276.

A	B	C	D
4. ðe-de	4. im-iŋ	4. ʃe-ʒe	4. eb-eb
5. fi-vi	5. hwi-wi	5. fi-θi	5. ehwe-ewe
6. he-pe	6. ge-ge	6. ze-ze	6. en-em
7. se-ze	7. dʒi-tʃi	7. mai-nai	7. eð-ed
8. θe-θe	8. fai-fai	8. θe-θe	8. ehe-epe
9. ʒe-dʒe	9. ðe-ve	9. he-he	9. ov-ov
10. vo-bo	10. pe-pe	10. dʒi-ʒi	10. eθ-eθ

Another test of phonetic discrimination is also very useful, the Wepman. The Wepman test[2] consists of forty pairs of words such as *sought-fought, tall-tall, shack-sack* which are read to the child who is then to judge whether they are the same or different. Ten of the choices are the same. The Boston University[3] Speech Sound Discrimination Picture Test consists of a series of cards each bearing three pictures. Each of the pictures has two drawings, one above the other. On one card we find, in picture one, two cats, one above the other; in picture two, a cat above and a bat below; in the third picture of the card we find two bats, one above the other. The examiner says: "Find the cat-bat." Thirty six cards are available, and crude norms are furnished.

TESTS OF PHONETIC ANALYSIS AND SYNTHESIS

These tests, which are often termed tests of vocal phonics, are still far from satisfactory and we do have some research instruments which can be used. For practical use, however, the following tests have some value.

Phonetic Analysis Test

Examiner shows child picture of a rake, shoe, moon, and kite.

Here's a rake. Rake starts with *rrr.* Hear it? *rrrake.*
Here's a shoe. Shoe starts with ʃʃʃ. ʃʃʃu.

---

[2] Joseph M. Wepman. *Auditory Discrimination Test,* 950 E. 59th Street, Chicago 37, Ill., 1958.
[3] W. Pronovost and C. Dumbleton. "A Picture-Type Speech Sound Discrimination Test," *Journal Speech and Hearing Disorders,* Volume 18, 1953, pages 258-266.

Here's a moon. Moon starts with *mmmmm. mmmmmmoon.*
Here's a kite. Kite starts with *k.* (*Whisper the* k).

Now let's see if you can tell me which one starts with *sh.*

(If child is successful, go to Test Plate A, then B. If not try again.)

A. Here's a *chair;* here's a *watch;* here are some *matches.* Which one of these starts with *ch?*
B. There's a *coat;* there are some *dishes;* there's a *sheep;* there's a *fish.* Which one of these starts with *fffff?*
C. Here's a *gun;* here's a *car;* here's a *balloon.* Which one starts with *k* (*whisper it*)?

Other words which may be used in the same way are as follows: *eyes, knife, mouth, face.* Words of one syllable beginning with vowels or continuant consonants are the most satisfactory. Some references concerning these tests are given at the bottom of this page.[4,5,6] It is hoped that standardized tests of these abilities will be soon created.

Phonetic Synthesis Tests

These tests use the same words but a different procedure which may be illustrated by the following example:

I'm going to say some words in a funny way . . . awfully slowly. You must try to guess what I'm saying. Here's one: mmm. . .ow. . . th. Now I'll say it faster—mm. .ow. .th, mm.ow.th, mouth. See I've been saying *mouth* all the time!

OK, now let's see if you can guess this word. *Nnnnn. . . o. . . zzzz* _____
(*Examiner prolongs each sound and has two silent gaps, each of one second. Whether child succeeds or fails, examiner says word after child has made his attempt.*)

OK, now let's see if you can guess this word: sh. . . .oe _____

[4] Charles V. Mange. "The Relationship Between Selected Auditory Perceptual Factors and Articulation Ability," *Journal Speech and Hearing Research,* Volume 3, 1960, pages 67-74.
[5] R. Summers. "Perceptive versus Productive Skills on Analyzing Speech Sounds From Words," *Journal Speech and Hearing Disorders,* Volume 18, 1953, pages 140-148.
[6] O. W. Wensley. *An Investigation of the Vocal Phonic Ability of Children with Normal Speech and Articulation Disorders,* M.A. Thesis, Western Michigan University, 1956.

Tests of Motor Coordination

For the measurement of large motor coordinations we have the Vineland Adaptation of the Oseretsky Tests,[7] which employ such activities as standing on one leg or on tiptoe, hopping, touching the nose alternately with either hand, tapping the foot, patting the head and rubbing the abdomen, and so forth. Or we may use the developmental schedule devised by Gesell and Amatruda,[8] a few of the items of which are now presented: stands on one foot for two seconds (42 months); walks downstairs, one foot to each step (48 months); hops on one foot (54 months); alternates feet descending stairs (60 months); stands on each foot alternately with eyes closed (72 months). Other simple activities which may demonstrate poor general coordination are: walking a straight line, skipping, bringing forefingers together, writing, drawing or copying, and cutting with scissors.

In order to get some further estimate of the coordination ability of the tongue and oral musculature we ask them to swallow, to click the tongue, to whistle, to bite, and to do the activities of this brief excerpt from an examination:

Examiner demonstrates sticking out tongue, moving it from side to side, curling tip upward with mouth open, clicking with little finger and then with thumb between teeth and trilling (with voice). After each activity he asks child to do what he has done.

A. Stick out your tongue like this! (*Examiner demonstrates.*)
B. Now curl up the end of it like this! (*Examiner demonstrates.*)
C. Now move it from side to side like this! (*Examiner demonstrates.*)
D. Now open your mouth wide and then lift your tongue like this! (*Examiner curls tonguetip.*) (Note: *If child has difficulty curling tonguetip within mouth, demonstrate position for L sound silently and ask child to imitate.*)
E. Now put your little finger between your teeth like this and click! (*Examiner demonstrates.*) (Note: *Finger should be held sidewise. Clicking should be done at about rate of three per second. If child*

[7] E. A. Doll (ed.). *The Oseretsky Test of Motor Proficiency*. Minneapolis: Educational Publishers, 1947. This test can also be found in M. F. Berry and J. Eisenson, *Speech Disorders*. New York: Appleton-Century-Crofts, 1956, pages 506-508.

[8] A. Gesell and C. S. Amatruda. *Developmental Diagnosis*. New York: Paul B. Hoeber, 1947, pages 11-14.

fails, try it at slower speeds. Note difference between tongue click and suck click. Note tendency for lips to contract when tongue is lifted. Note tendency for jaws to bite finger when tongue lifts. Is tongue unable to move independently of jaws or lips?)

F. Now put your thumb between your teeth like this and click! (*Examiner demonstrates. Thumb should be held sidewise. Note items given above for finger.*)

G. Now make this sound! (*Examiner trills tongue.*)

Articulatory Test Material

Lip sounds: P—pie, apple, cup; B—boy, rabbit, bib; M—mouse, hammer, drum; WH—wheel, whistle; W—window, sidewalk, sandwich; F—fork, telephone, knife; V—valentine, river, stove.

Tonguetip sounds: TH (*unvoiced*)—thumb, bathtub, teeth; TH (*voiced*)—the, feather, smooth; T—top, potato, cat; D—dog, Indian, bird; N—nose, banana, man.

Back of tongue: K—cup, basket, clock; G—girl, wagon, flag; NG—monkey, swing; H—house, schoolhouse.

Complicated tonguetip sounds: L—leaves, balloon, ball; R—rug, orange, chair; S—Santa Claus, bicycle, glass; Z—zebra, scissors, eyes; SH—shoe, dishes, fish; ZH—pleasure, treasure; CH—chicken, pitcher, peach; J—jelly, soldier, bridge; Y—yellow, onion.

Blends: TW—twenty, between; DW—dwarf; BL—black, bubble; CL—clown, declare; FL—flag, snowflake; GL—glass; PL—please, airplane; SL—slim, asleep; SPL—split, splashed; -DL—cradle; -TL—turtle; -ZL—puzzle; BR—bring, umbrella; CR—cry, across; DR—drop, children; FR—friend, afraid; GR—grandma, angry; PR—prize, surprise, SCR—screw, describe; SHR—shrub; SPR—spring; STR—string, destroy; TR—trip, country; THR—thread, three; SK—school, asking, desk; SM—smell, smoke; SN—snow, sneak; SP—spool, whisper, clasp; ST—stop, upstairs, nest; SW—swing, swim; FS—laughs; -LS—else; NS—once, bounce; -PS—cups, pups; -TS—cats, puts; -STS—vests, tests; -THS—months; -BZ—tubs, bibs; -DZ—birds, reads; -LZ—girls, balls; -MZ—drums, homes; -NZ—pans, runs, rains; -NGZ—songs, rings; -THZ—clothes, breathes; -VZ—lives, moves; -LK—milk, milking, silk; KW—queen, require; SKW—squirrel; -KS—packs, except; -GZ—eggs, rugs; -NG—sing, hang, wrong.

Vowels: i—eat, meant, tree; ɪ—it, pig; ɛ—egg, bread; ɛɝ—bear, pear; æ—at, cat; ʌ—up, cup; ɝ—turkey, mother; ə—away, banana; u—moon, shoe; ʊ—book, cookie; ɔ—all; ɑ—arm, star; eɪ—age, cake, day; aɪ—ice, kite, pie; oʊ—old, boat, snow; aʊ—owl, house, cow; ɔɪ—oil, noise, boy.

Reading Sentences

Lip sounds: 1. *P*—The pig ate his supper with the sheep. 2. *B*—The baby robin is in the tub. 3. *M*—The man hammered his thumb. 4. *WH*—Why is the wheel off? 5. *W*—We found a wagon. 6. *F*—The farmer drank coffee with his wife. 7. *V*—His vest is over by the stove.

Tonguetip sounds: 1. *TH* (*voiceless*)—I think the baby needs a birthday bath. 2. *TH* (*voiced*)—The baby's mother will bathe him. 3. *T*—Take the pretty coat to her. 4. *D*—Get the doll ready for bed. 5. *N*—At night through the window we see the moon.

Back-tongue sounds: 1. *K*—Come and get your broken kite. 2. *G*—Let's go again and find a frog. 3. *NG*—She sang as she was dancing. 4. *H*—He likes horses.

Complicated tonguetip sounds: 1. *L*—Let me bring a tulip and an apple. 2. *R*—The rabbit likes four carrots. 3. *S*—We saw a seesaw on the grass. 4. *Z*—The zoo is the home for bears. 5. *SH*—She washes every dish. 6. *ZH*—It is a pleasure to have a treasure hunt. 7. *CH*—The child went to the kitchen for a peach. 8. *J*—Jack saw a pigeon under the bridge. 9. *Y*—Your dog ran into the barnyard.

Blends: 1. *TW*—The twin stood between the others. 2. *DW*—The dwarf is a little man. 3. *BL*—He blew a bubble from a black pipe. 4. *CL*—The clown climbed a tree to declare he was king. 5. *FL*—The flag flew in the snowflakes. 6. *GL*—He broke the big glass. 7. *PL*—Please let me have an airplane ride. 8. *SL*—The slim little boy fell asleep. 9. *SPL*—I will splash some water on you. 10. *-DL*—Put the baby in the cradle. 11. *-TL*—See the little turtle. 12. *-ZL*—I like a puzzle. 13. *BR*—Bring me a brown umbrella. 14. *CR*—You could hear him cry across the room. 15. *DR*—The children dropped their balls. 16. *FR*—My friend is afraid of the dark. 17. *GR*—Grandma was angry with me. 18. *PR*—Won't the prize surprise her? 19. *SCR*—The screw is described in the book. 20. *SHR*—There is a shrub by our barn. 21. *SPR*—Spring is coming. 22. *STR*—The string has been destroyed. 23. *TR*—A trip to the country will be nice. 24. *THR*—She has three spools of thread. 25. *SK*—I am asking for a new desk at school. 26. *SM*—Do you smell smoke? 27. *SN*—Let's sneak out and play in the snow. 28. *SP*—They whisper about the lost spool. 29. *ST*—Stop upstairs and see the robin's nest. 30. *SW*—We will swim over to the dock. 31. *-FS*—She laughs at all the jokes. 32. *-LS*—Give me something else. 33. *NS*—You can bounce my ball once. 34. *-PS*—The little pups can drink out of cups. 35. *-TS*—She puts the cats to bed in the barn. 36. *-STS*—He slipped the tests in one of his father's vests. 37. *-THS*—It took him two months to read the book. 38. *-BZ*—Mother washed the bibs in the tubs. 39. *-DZ*—He reads about birds every day. 40. *-LZ*—The girls took our balls away. 41. *-MZ*—They have drums in all the children's homes. 42. *-NZ*—The water runs over the pans when it rains. 43. -*NGZ*—Teacher rings the bell for us to sing more songs. 44. -*THZ*—I have some new clothes. 45. -*VS*—The fish lives and moves in water. 46. -*LK*—Don't wear a silk dress when you are milking a cow. 47. *KW*—The queen requires that we obey her. 48. *SKW*—That squirrel has a bushy tail. 49. -*KS*—Bring all the packs except one. 50. -*GZ*— Mary dropped the eggs on the rugs. 51. -*NG*—We all sang the wrong song.

Vowels: 1. i—The dog can eat his meat under the tree. 2. ɪ—Give the rest of it to the pig. 3. ɛ—Let's eat an egg with the bread. 4. ɛɚ—That bear went up our pear tree. 5. æ—Don't throw a tin can at the cat. 6. ʌ— Take the cup up from the table. 7. ɝ—Mother put the turkey on the platter. 8. ə—Throw away that banana skin. 9. u—Can you look in the moon and see a shoe? 10. ʊ—I like to eat a cooky when I read a book. 11. ɔ— All of us like corn. 12. ɑ—Point your arm up at the biggest star. 13. eɪ— At the age of ten I will have a cake on my birthday. 14. aɪ—If the ice doesn't freeze overnight, I will make you a pie. 15. oʊ—The old boat was lost in the snow. 16. aʊ—The owl hooted from the house and the cow was afraid. 17. ɔɪ—The oil lamp made so much noise that the boy couldn't sleep.

The following passage may be used for a quick survey of the student's ability to produce correct speech sounds. It includes all of the speech sounds, and may either be read by the student or be repeated phrase by phrase after the examiner.

My Grandfather

You wished to know all about my grandfather. Well, he is nearly ninety-three years old; he dresses himself in an ancient black frock coat, usually minus several buttons; yet he still thinks as swiftly as ever. A long, flowing beard clings to his chin, giving those who observe him a pronounced feeling of the utmost respect. When he speaks, his voice is just a bit cracked and quivers a trifle. Twice each day he plays skillfully and with zest upon our small organ. Except in the winter when the ooze or snow or ice prevents, he slowly takes a short walk in the open air each day. We have often urged him to walk more and smoke less, but he always answers, "Banana oil!" Grandfather likes to be modern in his language.

Initial Examination for Stutterers

It is always wise to observe the child below the age of twelve in an informal situation to determine whether or not he is in the first or second stages of the disorder. We do not wish to make such a child highly aware of his speech difficulty. Avoid interviewing the parent in front of the child but attempt to overhear some of the child's speech when he is speaking to the parent. You may need to play with him a bit, helping him become interested in some toy or machine. Perhaps the tape recorder itself. Use some casual conversation, self-talk, or natural questioning to evoke some speech—enough to make a preliminary diagnosis. If you are pretty certain that he is not in the third and fourth stages, and that he has little awareness of his stuttering—if any—just continue to play and talk with him as you survey his speech in terms of the following report blank:

Report Blank for the Primary Stutterer and for the Transitional Stutterer

1. Locate this person on the scale of development by indicating with √ the most commonly exhibited responses and by × those which occur occasionally.

_____ 1. Repetition of whole words and phrases.

_____ 2. Seems to lose train of thought; hesitates.

_____ 3. Repeats one-syllable words or single syllables less than three times per word.

_____ 4. Repeats sounds and syllables more than three times. Approximate no. times per word on the most severe example:_____ Average number:_____

_____ 5. Some syllable repetition in every other sentence or oftener.

_____ 6. Prolongation of consonants or consonant postures. Duration of worst example: _____

_____ 7. Prolongation of vowels without pitch rise. Duration of worst example: _____

_____ 8. Prolongation with pitch rise. Extent of shift _____

_____ 9. Were the repetitions at the normal rate of speed or faster?

_____10. Were the repetitions regular or irregular?

_____11. Did the repetitions end in prolongations or silent postures (blocks)?

_____12. Did you notice any tremors? Where? _____

_____13. Were there any facial contortions?

_____14. Did you notice any deliberate avoidance of speaking, in attempting words?

_____15. Did you notice any recoil or retrial? Describe:

_____16. Was there any evidence of frustration *due to the stuttering?*

_____17. Was there any evidence of anxiety *due to the stuttering?*

_____18. After a moment of stuttering did he hurry on? Or stop speaking? Or flush?

_____19. Did he seem to use any behavior to escape from his repetitions or fixations? What?

_____20. Was his voice normal in pitch, in inflection, in loudness, and quality. If not, describe:

_____21. Did you notice any starters or rituals of attempt?

_____22. Did the stuttering come in volleys or was it scattered?

_____23. Did he have periods of completely normal speech for as long as five or six consecutive sentences?

_____24. Did he watch you closely to see how you were reacting to his stuttering?

_____25. Did he look away when he stuttered?

2. You should be alert to the various influences which precipitate the stuttering. Try to determine which reactions on your part seem to produce more stuttering—or more fluency. Whenever the child starts to stutter after a period of fluency you should endeavor to discover why this stuttering was precipitated just then. Note your own behavior just before this change occurred. Were you hurrying him, failing to listen, threatening an interruption, questioning, demanding. Stuttering frequency and severity varies with many conditions. Try to determine what they are.

Similarly, you should attempt to create conditions which will produce more fluency. Talk a bit more slowly or simply or casually. Move slowly. Distract the child. Ease excitement or demand. Often by using parallel talk or self-talk, you can create a basal level of fluency which may be pretty solid. Try to do so. Echo games, puppet speech, talk-and-do activities, creating characters and roles, nonsense speech or Scamboolian or animal talk, rhythmic speech—all of these if used as play can create this basal level of fluency. Once you have achieved it, see how long it can be sustained. Find out what disturbing influences upset it (sometimes you should create these disturbing influences so that you can find out), and see how soon you can get him fluent again. *Use the rest of this sheet and the back of it to report this important information.*

EXAMINING THE STUTTERER WHO IS SECONDARY

Here the problem is a bit different. You should start with the assumption that he knows and that you know that he stutters. You should introduce yourself and as quickly as possible show him that you know a lot about the disorder of stuttering. One of the best ways is to do some stuttering yourself, using several of the common varieties of stuttering reactions, and asking if he has ever stuttered in that fashion. Take down his answers but don't believe him without checking the stuttering he does show. Next it is wise to ask him to show you some samples. Have him say suddenly: "banana-banana-banana." Ask him his name, his middle name, his teachers' names. Have him read to you or tell you about his father's job, or some favorite TV program. Ask him questions which he must answer with more than a yes or no. And during his responses you should imitate his stuttering in unison, telling him that you must learn to stutter just like he does if you are to help him. Make an occasional comment which tells him that you know how it feels to get blocked or to fear words or speaking situations. Ask him about these feared things. Ask him about those situations in which he is free from stuttering. Ask him about the ways he has tried to conquer his problem or the ways other people have tried to help him.

As you listen to him, fill in the items of the Summary Report Blank for Secondary Stutterers. If the parent is unable to be present, and the case is old enough, use the items of the Parental Interview to procure the necessary information.

Summary Report Blank for Secondary Stutterers

1. Frequency: Two or three per sentence or more _____
   One per sentence on the average _____
   Volleys of stuttering with periods of free speech between _____
   An occasional stuttering after a pause or in beginning an utterance _____
   Very infrequent _____
2. Severity: Very little tension, short blockings, little struggle _____
   Occasional forcing and struggle but duration is usually short _____

Avoidance, retrials, tremors; duration about one second _____

Avoidance, retrials, tremors, struggle; 2-4 seconds _____

Marked struggle or prolonged repetitions or pauses; occasionally 4-6 seconds _____

Completely stuck, helpless, struggling or avoiding; very long pauses _____

3. Check the appropriate item, using √ to indicate the common reaction and × the rare reaction.

_____ 1. Uses synonyms or rephrasing to avoid feared words. Example: _____

_____ 2. Uses postponement tricks. Of what types: _____

_____ 3. Uses tricks to get started: What types: _____

_____ 4. Hides and disguises his stuttering. How? _____
_____

_____ 5. Forcing and tremors during block. Where? _____

_____ 6. Stops and tries again after tremor.

_____ 7. Uses timing jerk or contortion with release. How? _____

_____ 8. Uses release on residual air. _____, uses gasping _____, uses opposition breathing _____.

_____ 9. Uses the glottal fry. _____

_____10. What else? _____

4. What are his feared situations?

5. What are his feared sounds or words?

6. Which of these reactions do you sense? anxiety _____, guilt _____, frustration _____, hostility _____, disgust _____, depression _____, helplessness _____, other _____.

7. How swiftly does he adapt in repeated reading of the same material? In terms of frequency: very swiftly, slowly _____, does not adapt _____ In terms of severity: very much adaptation _____, some _____, very little _____.

8. In repeating *words* upon which he stutters, how many retrials are required before he is fluent?
   a. When he has blocked severely on the word for the first time _____
   b. When he has had an average amount of stuttering _____
   c. When he has had a short block the first time _____

9. How did he respond when he heard his stuttering on the tape recorder?

10. How did he respond when he watched his stuttering in the mirror?

11. What comments did he make about his stuttering?

12. On the back of this sheet describe your trial therapy and his response.

13. How fluent was he at his best?

14. To what listener reactions is he most vulnerable?

Interview with the Parent of the Stutterer

The essential information we need is that concerning the possible causes of the stuttering, its course of development, the reactions of the stutterer and his associates toward the stutterer and his speech difficulty, the penalties and traumatic experiences associated with his speech, the ways in which he has been treated for his stuttering therapeutically, his other assets or liabilities, the way in which he reacts to penalty or frustration or approval, and other emotional conflicts or behavior problems which he may have had.

We must realize that many parents feel guilty because their child stutters, and many of them have marked anxiety. They will seek reassurance; they may prefer to talk about other siblings or other things. They will ask for premature opinions, may try to get you to take their part in family conflicts. They will try to blame the stuttering on the child down the block or a frightening experience. Just listen and get your information. We suggest you prepare yourself by reading the material on the case history and interview in Van Riper and Gruber: *A Casebook on Stuttering.* New York: Harper & Row, Publishers, 1957.

But be sure you get some information on each of the following:

1. Onset of speech. Difficulties in learning to talk. Excessive approvals for early speaking.
2. Competition for speech in the home.
3. Policies in the home about the right to talk.
4. How swiftly do the other members of the family speak? Any difficulty here? Any stuttering?
5. Excessive demands for speech.
6. Penalties upon speech: cursing, dirty talk, demand for confession, etc.
7. Onset of stuttering. Age of child. Circumstances surrounding onset. Did it begin gradually or suddenly? In what form did it first occur?
8. What does the parent think caused the disorder?
9. At what point did the child become aware that he stuttered?
10. What changes in the form of stuttering have occurred?
11. Evidence for avoidance, fears of situations, fears of words or sounds.
12. What penalties has the child experienced in the home, at play, at school?
13. How does he and how did he react to these penalties?
14. What methods have been used in the home to help him overcome his stuttering?
15. Who else has tried to help him and how and with what result?
16. What other problems has the child had? What other difficulties at home or at school?

17. Have there been certain times of stress in the family home life?

18. What are the relationships between the child and the other children in the home?

19. Have there been conflicts between the parents? Is this a happy home? Has it been?

20. How close are son and father, daughter and mother?

21. Do the parents desire our help? Just want information? Or counseling? Or therapy?

22. If they want therapy, are they prepared to bring the child in for appointments for at least a semester and perhaps a year? Do they have transportation?

23. Is this parent able to accept counseling? What is the probability that he can change his behavior or attitudes (or she hers) or alter the environmental influences which may be harmful to the child?

You will doubtless find other information even more important than what this list contains, so be alert. We suggest that you take notes (brief hinting notes) as the interview proceeds but do not record items of highly loaded significance. Remember these. Summarize your information and impressions on the back of this sheet and on other sheets if needed.

Do not forget to procure the basic case-history data. See General Case History Form and also the Special Case History Form for Stuttering.

The Case History

Administering the Case History. While most of the information is usually obtained from the parents or the case himself, it is generally necessary to interview other associates of the speech defective. Former teachers, the family doctor, welfare investigators, and neighbors or friends may be called upon. The speech defective is often asked to get the cooperation of his former associates in determining the early symptoms or reactions toward his speech defect. These individuals often provide more information than the parents. While the majority of questions should be made as pointed as possible, a few general questions appropriate to the material in each major section should be used. Questions should be phrased so that the influence of suggestion will not prejudice the answer. An exception to this rule, however, is found in the recommendation that delicate questions be asked so as to favor an affirmative answer. Answers should be recorded immediately, and the examiner should master a system of abbreviations or shorthand so that there will be no delay. He should always distinguish in the recording between the person's actual answers and his own interpretation of those answers. The examiner should perfect himself in the art of interrupting irrelevant vocal wanderings and bringing the parent back to the point in question. It is unwise to have the child present during questioning of the parent, and except when the relationship between parents is being studied, it is wiser to question only one at a time. The summary of important case-history findings should be written up as soon as possible.

The case histories given here are phrased in the form of direct questions. This policy was chosen because the text is intended for beginning students in speech correction, and experience has shown the author that such students require this guidance. It must be emphasized repeatedly that each question is merely the first of a series of supplemental queries when the answer indicates that vital information may be forthcoming. No examiner will ask all the questions, nor will he confine himself to these alone.

The general case history may be considered the device used to procure a picture of the individual's background and physical, mental, personality, and speech development. A shorter form of this history may be obtained by using only the starred items for exploration. Demands upon the teacher's time and the overwhelming case load frequently experienced in public-school work occasionally necessitate this compromise, but the short case history is seldom used except for certain simple types of articulatory or voice cases. In addition to the general case history, an appropriate special case history should be used. Even as the general case history is used for exploration of the person having the speech defect, so the special case history is used to tap the parent's fund of information concerning the causes, development, and consequences of the speech defect itself.

GENERAL CASE HISTORY

Person Interviewed_____ Interviewer_____
Name of Case_____ Date of Birth_____ Sex_____
Address_____ Telephone Number_____
Rapport_____

1. Father
   °Name_____
   Age (if dead, date and cause of death)_____
   Handedness_____ Education_____ Occupation_____
   Religion_____ Health_____ Nationality_____
   °Type of speech defect, if any_____
   Type of physical defect, if any_____
   Nervous diseases _____ Excesses (liquor, drugs, etc.)_____
   Marital history (separation, divorce, previous marriage, etc.)_____
   _____
   _____
   Attitude toward child's defect _____

2. Mother
    °Name ....
    Age (if dead, date and cause of death) ....
    Handedness .... Education .... Occupation ....
    Religion .... Health .... Nationality ....
    °Type of speech defect, if any ....
    Type of physical defect, if any ....
    Nervous diseases ....
    Marital History ....
    Attitude toward child's defect ....

3. Other relatives (Write number of people having the following disorders)

	Physical Defect	Speech Defect	Other Important Information
°Brothers			
°Sisters			
Mat. Grandmother			
Mat. Grandfather			
Mat. Aunts			
Mat. Uncles			
Pat. Grandmother			
Pat. Grandfather			
Pat. Aunts			
Pat. Uncles			
Other persons living in home			

BIRTH HISTORY

Give age of the mother at the beginning of the pregnancy ....
Age of the father .... Number of months of pregnancy ....
Weight of child at birth .... Length of body at birth ....

Prenatal Conditions

    Give the approximate weight and height of the mother at the beginning of this pregnancy ....
    Was mother working during the pregnancy period? ....
        If so, what kind of work? .... How soon did she stop before the birth? ....
        How soon did she resume her activities after the birth? ....
    What was the condition of the mother's health during pregnancy? Good, fair, poor. Was mother able to eat regularly and retain the food? ....

Did mother have any severe shocks during pregnancy? _____
Injuries? _____
Was mother examined by a physician before and during pregnancy? ___
Was the pelvis measured? _____
What comments did the doctor make? _____
Will you furnish us with the name and address of the physician?
Name _____
Address _____
            Street   City   State

Birth and Postnatal Conditions

Number of hours of labor, including the time from the first pains
until the expulsion of the afterbirth _____
°At birth was the baby delivered feet first, head first, breech (hip)
first, or by Caesarean operation? _____
°Did delivery necessitate the use of instruments? _____
°Were there any injuries? _____ If so, where? _____
_____ Did baby have difficulty initiating
breathing? _____ If so, how was breathing started? _____
_____ How long was it before he started
breathing normally? _____ Did he cry as soon as he was
born? _____ Was it loud? _____ feeble? _____ Did he nurse as
soon as he was placed at the breast or did he need to be coaxed?
_____ How long did this condition last? _____
Did he move around much the first two or three days or was he
still and quiet? _____ Was his pulse strong,
weak, slow, fast, normal? _____
Was the soft spot on the top of the head soft and concave or
hard and bulging? _____
Did the baby have convulsions? _____ blueness of the
body, lips, or feet? _____ slow blood clotting
time? _____ slight bleeding about the nose and
mouth? _____ twitchings of the muscles of the
face? _____ Was he one of a pair of twins? _____
If so, was he the strong or weak one? _____
Did the head have an abnormal molding immediately after birth?
_____ Was mother attended by a doctor,
nurse, midwife, others? _____

DEVELOPMENTAL HISTORY

1. Was baby breast fed? _____ For how long? _____
2. Why was he weaned? _____
3. Was baby bottle fed? _____ For how long? _____
4. Did the bottle milk agree with him? _____

5. Were both fontanels closed before child was 20 months old?

_____

*6. Was the child's rate of growth seemingly normal?_____
If not, why not? _____

*7. Give age in months at which the following took place:
First tooth_____ Full set of teeth_____
Full set of second teeth _____ Creeping on all
fours_____ Sitting alone_____ Walking alone
_____ Feeding self _____ Got voluntary control of bowels_____ Got voluntary control of
bladder_____ Using spoon_____ Using any
object as tool_____
Do you have any other information with regard to the child's
development?_____

*8. The following is a list of common childhood diseases. Please
give age of child when disease occurred, whether it was serious
or mild, whether the child had a high fever, and any noticeable
effects which followed it:
Tonsillitis
Whooping cough
Pneumonia
Scarlet fever
Typhoid fever
Tuberculosis
Pleurisy
Chicken pox
Smallpox
Influenza
Diphtheria
Measles
Mumps
St. Vitus dance
Convulsions
Rickets
Enlarged glands
Heart trouble
Rheumatism
Thyroid disturbances
Nervous trouble
Infantile paralysis
Any others

9. Was child excessively spoiled and indulged because of his illness?

_____

*10. Has child ever been seriously injured? State nature, age at in-
jury, and effects _____
_____

11. Was the child: very active?................; fairly active?................; very inactive?................

12. Would you say that the child was slow, average, or rapid in his general development up to three years of age?................

Present Physical Condition of Child

°1. What is the child's weight................ and height................ at present time?

°2. Does the child have any physical deformities?................ What are they?................

3. Has the child had a physical examination lately?................ What were the main findings of his examination?................ Who was the physician?................

4. Is there any abnormality in the following:
   a. Size of tongue................
   b. Protrusion of upper or lower jaws................
   c. Arrangement of teeth................
   d. Palate................
   e. Nasal passages................

5. Has he ever had tonsils and adenoids removed?................ Tongue-tie clipped?................

6. Does the child have any defect in hearing?................ Seeing?................

7. Is the child usually in good health at the present time?................

----

8. Is he: very energetic?................; fairly energetic?................; not very energetic?................

Coordination

Check the following items according to whether the child shows inferior, average, or superior skill:

Gracefulness	Dancing	Skipping	Jumping
Throwing	Catching	Kicking	Sewing
Cutting	Drawing	Writing	

Mental and Educational Development

1. Has the child ever had a mental or intelligence test?................ What was the name of the test used?................

2. What was the IQ obtained, or general ranking?................

°3. If the child is in school, in what grade is he at present?................

°4. Are his marks above average, average, or below average?................

°5. Has the child ever failed a grade?_____ Has he ever skipped a grade?_____ Which one?_____

°6. What are the highest marks the child has ever received?_____ In what subjects?_____

°7. What are the poorest marks the child has ever received? _____ In what subjects? _____

8. Is the child frequently tardy?_____ Why?_____

9. Does the child play truant?_____

10. Has the child been absent from school very often?_____ If so, for what reason?_____

11. Has the child been punished by his teacher?_____ Why?_____

°12. Does the child like school?_____ If not, why not? _____

13. Which of his teachers does the child like most?_____ _____

14. Teacher's name_____ School_____

15. What other schools has the child attended?_____ When?_____

Handedness

1. Have the child's hands ever been bandaged, tied up, or restrained in any way?_____ For what reason and how long?_____

2. At what age did he show a definite tendency to favor one hand while eating?_____ Which hand?_____ Up to that age, did the child use either or both hands indiscriminately?_____

°3. Did anyone ever try to influence his handedness in order to change him from left to right or vice versa?_____ How?_____

4. What is the attitude of the father toward left-handedness?_____ _____

5. What is the attitude of the mother toward left-handedness?_____ _____

6. Did any injuries or illnesses ever change his handedness?_____ _____

°7. Has child ever written backward?_____

°8. Are there any activities which he can do better or as well with the usually nonpreferred hand? _____ What are they?_____

Play

1. Give names and ages of the three children with whom the child plays most often ....

....

....

°2. Is the child the follower or the leader? ....

3. Do they tease the child? ....

4. Do they fight with him? ....

5. Do they get along with him? .... Do any of them have speech defects? ....

6. What games does he prefer to play? ....

7. What toys does he prefer? ....

°8. Does he play alone as well as he does with other children? ....

....

9. Does he prefer to play alone? ....

°10. Which parent does the child prefer? .... Why?

°11. Which playmate does the child prefer? .... Why?

....

12. Who took care of the child when the mother was absent? ....

....

Language Development

°1. How many months old was the child when he began to say single words? ....; simple sentences and phrases? ....

2. What were the first single words spoken? ....

3. Give any other examples of the child's early speech with the approximate dates for each ....

....

4. What method was used in teaching the child to talk? ....

....

    a. Who did most of it? ....

   °b. Do you feel that the child was overstimulated or understimulated with respect to speech? ....

    c. Did he understand what was said to him before he had learned to talk? ....

   °d. Did anyone talk baby talk to child? ....
Who? ....

    e. Did anyone use **double-talking** to child? ....
Who? ....
(Double-talking is like this: We-we-will-will-go-go.)

f. Were the child's wants usually anticipated before he could communicate the need?..

g. Did the child gesture much in attempting to communicate?

....

h. Do you think that the child's present vocabulary is superior, average, or inferior to that of other children his age? ....

....

i. Did the child often surprise you by using large words? ....

....

j. Did the child habitually mispronounce certain words? ....

....

Give examples..

5. Were there any sounds that he could not say?....................
Which?..

*6. Did the child ever lisp?............ Describe........................

*7. Was the child taught to speak pieces?............ Was he often called upon to perform before strangers or friends of the family?..
What was his usual attitude toward such demands?..........

8. Has there ever been any tongue-tie?............ Cleft palate?............ Harelip?............

9. Was there any marked articulatory defect?........................

10. Describe the rate, intensity, and pitch of child's speech with respect to its being rapid-average-slow; loud-average-soft; high-average-low..

*11. Did the child ever tend to say words backward ("got for" instead of "forgot," etc.)?............ Give examples:

....

*12. Was the child generally retarded in speech development?..........

....

13. Was the child very talkative, average, or rather silent and quiet?..

14. Was any foreign language taught to the child or commonly spoken by his associates?..

Home

1. In what type of community is the home located: rural, town, city?..

2. Do the parents own or rent the home?........................

3. How many rooms in the house?..

4. Check the following items in possession of the family: car;

piano; radio; 100 or more books; daily newspaper; gas, oil, or
electric kitchen stove.

°5. Check the word which most nearly describes economic condition of
family: very poor, poor, comfortable circumstances, well-to-do.

6. Check phrase which most nearly describes father's attitude with
an "F," and phrase which describes mother's attitude with an
"M."

   a. Has no cultural interests (seems to live only to work and
   eat)._____

   b. Has slight interest in other people's experiences, likes radio,
   likes magazine stories, does some social visiting._____
   _____

   c. Has a hobby in some creative field (music, pictures, cabinet-
   making, gardening, reading, etc.)._____

   d. Takes a specialized interest in one of the arts: reads widely;
   is aware of other places and times; discriminating taste.
   _____

7. Is there family friction with regard to money matters, religion,
or anything else?_____ Is child aware of it?_____

8. Are both parents usually at home in the evening?_____

9. Does the child have plenty of playthings or amusements?_____
_____

10. Are the neighbors congenial?_____ Do the parents
like the neighbors?_____

11. Do the parents play with the children?_____

12. Has the child ever lived in another town?_____

°13. Of what things is the father proudest?_____

°14. Of what things is the mother proudest?_____

°15. What things have made the father unhappy?_____

°16. What things have made the mother unhappy?_____

°17. Of what things is the child proudest?_____

°18. What things have made the child unhappy?_____

°*Childhood Problems*

Following is a list of common childhood problems. Indicate how often
these problems occurred in this child by encircling the letter which most
clearly describes it. O indicates that it occurs often, S indicates seldom,
and N indicates never.

1. Nervousness	O S N	4. Bed wetting	O S N
2. Sleeplessness	O S N	5. Playing with sex organs	O S N
3. Nightmares	O S N	6. Walking in sleep	O S N

7.	Shyness	O	S	N	19.	Constipation	O	S	N
8.	Showing off	O	S	N	20.	Thumb sucking	O	S	N
9.	Refusal to obey	O	S	N	21.	Face twitching	O	S	N
10.	Rudeness	O	S	N	22.	Fainting	O	S	N
11.	Fighting	O	S	N	23.	Strong fears	O	S	N
12.	Jealousy	O	S	N	24.	Strong hates	O	S	N
13.	Selfishness	O	S	N	25.	Queer food habits	O	S	N
14.	Lying	O	S	N	26.	Temper tantrums	O	S	N
15.	Smoking	O	S	N	27.	Whining	O	S	N
16.	Tongue sucking	O	S	N	28.	Stealing	O	S	N
17.	Hurting pets	O	S	N	29.	Running away	O	S	N
18.	Setting fires	O	S	N	30.	Destructiveness	O	S	N

31. How did the child's associates (parents, etc.) react to these problems?_____

32. How is the child usually disciplined and who does it?_____

33. What types of discipline are most effective?_____
Least effective?_____

° *Adult Developmental History*

Vocational

1. What opportunities did the case have for earning money as a child?_____
2. Did he have an adequate allowance?_____
3. What positions have been held? Give salary, working conditions, length of time employed, reason for leaving._____

Educational

1. Preferred subjects in secondary schools and college._____
2. Subjects disliked._____
3. Attitudes toward instructors._____
4. Extra-curricular activities._____
5. Scholastic record._____
6. Reasons for quitting school._____
7. Conflicts with school authorities._____

Sexual experiences (Indicate type, frequency, and attitudes toward activity)

Social

1. Favorite associates. ....
2. Disliked associates. ....
3. Recreational activities. ....
4. Arrests, probations, commitments to institutions. ....
   ....

GLOSSARY

Abracadabra: A magical set of words or sounds used as an incantation.
Acalculia: Loss of ability in using mathematical symbols due to brain injury.
Acoustic: Pertaining to the perception of sound.
Adenoids: Growths of lymphoid tissue on the back wall of the throat (nasopharynx.)
Affricate: A consonantal sound beginning as a stop (plosive) but expelled as a fricative. The *ch* (tʃ) and the *j* (dʒ) sounds in the words *chain* and *jump* are affricates.
Agnosia: Loss of ability to interpret the meanings of sensory stimulation; due to brain injury; may be visual, auditory, or tactual.
Air wastage: The use of silent exhalation before or after phonation on a single breath.
Alexia: Difficulty in reading due to brain damage.
Allergy: Extreme sensitivity to certain proteins.
Alveolar: The ridges on the jaw bones beneath the gums. An alveolar sound is one in which the tongue makes contact with the upper gum ridge.
Anomia: Inability to remember familiar words due to brain injury.
Anoxia: Oxygen deficiency.
✓ *Anti-expectancy:* A group of devices used by the stutterer to distract himself from the expectation of stuttering.
Aphasia: Impairment in the use of meaningful symbols due to brain injury.
Aphonia: Loss of voice.
Approach-avoidance: Refers to conflicts produced when the person is beset by two opposing drives to do or not to do something.
Approximation: Behavior which comes closer to a standard or goal.
Apraxia: Loss of ability to make voluntary movements or to use tools meaningfully; due to brain injury.
Articulation: The utterance of the individual speech sounds.
✓ *Aspirate:* Breathy; the use of excessive initial air flow preceding phonation as in the *aspirate* attack.
Assimilation: A change in the characteristic of a speech sound due to the influence of adjacent sounds. In *assimilation nasality,* voiced sounds

followed or preceded by a nasal consonant tend to be excessively nasalized.

Asymmetry: Unequal proportionate size of the right and left halves of a structure.

Atrophy: A withering; a shrinking in size and decline in function of some bodily structure or organ.

√ *Athetosis:* One of the forms of cerebral palsy characterized by writhing, shaking, involuntary movements of the head, limbs, or the body.

Attack: The initiation of voice.

Auditory memory span: The ability to recall a series of test sounds, syllables, or words.

Autism: An emotional disturbance in children resulting in a detachment from their environmental surroundings; almost complete withdrawal from social interaction.

Avoidance: A device such as the use of a synonym or circumlocution to escape from having to speak a word upon which stuttering is anticipated; also a trick to escape from having to speak in a feared situation.

Babbling: A continuous free experimenting with speech sounds.

√ *Basal fluency level:* A period of communication in which no stuttering appears. See *desensitization therapy*.

Bicuspid: The fourth and fifth teeth, each of which has two cusps or points.

√ *Bifid:* Divided into two parts, as in a cleft or bifid uvula.

Binaural: Pertaining to both ears.

Bone conduction: The transmission of sound waves (speech) directly to the cochlea by means of the bones of the skull.

√ *Bradylalia:* Abnormally slow utterance.

C.A.T.: Children's Apperception Test, a projective test of personality.

Catharsis: The discharge of pent-up feelings.

Catastrophic response: A sudden change in behavior by the aphasic characterized by extreme irritability, flushing or fainting, withdrawal or random movements.

Cerebral palsy: A group of disorders due to brain injury in which the motor coordinations are especially affected. Most common forms are athetosis, spasticity, and ataxia.

Clavicular breathing: A form of shallow, gasping speech breathing in which the shoulder blades move with the short inhalations.

Cleft lip or palate: See Chapter Thirteen.

Cluttering: A disorder of time or rhythm characterized by unorganized, hasty spurts of speech often accompanied by slurred articulation.

Cochlea: The spiral shaped structure of the inner ear containing the end organs of the auditory nerve.

Cognate: Referring to pairs of sounds which are produced motorically in much the same way, one being voiced (sonant) and the other unvoiced (surd). Some cognates are *t* and *d*; *s* and *z*.

Commentary: The verbalization of what is being perceived as in self-talk or parallel talk.

Conductive hearing loss: Hearing loss due to failure of the bone levers in the middle ear to transmit sound vibrations to the cochlea.

Configurations: (in articulation therapy) Patterning of sounds in proper sequence.

Contact ulcers: A breakdown in the tissues of the vocal cords, usually near their posterior attachments to the arytenoid cartilages.

Continuant: A speech sound which can be prolonged without distortion; e.g., *s* or *f* or *u*.

√*Covert:* Hidden behavior; inner feelings, thoughts, reactions.

Creative dramatics: An improvised, unrehearsed playlet acted spontaneously by a group of children with the unobtrusive aid of an adult leader.

CV: A syllable containing the consonant-vowel sequence as in *see* or *toe* or *ka.*

CVC: A syllable containing the consonant-vowel-consonant sequence, as in the first syllable of the word *containing.*

Dental: Pertaining to the teeth. A dentalized *l* sound is made with the tonguetip on the upper teeth.

Deep testing: The exploration of an articulation case's ability to articulate a large number of words all of which include one specific sound to discover those in which that sound is spoken correctly.

Desensitization: The toughening of a person to stress; increasing the person's ability to confront his problem with less anxiety, guilt or hostility; a type of adaptation to stress therapy used for beginning stutterers. See Chapter Thirteen.

√*Diadochokinesis:* The maximum speed of a rhythmically repeated movement.

Differential diagnosis: The process of distinguishing one disorder from another.

Differentiation: The functional separation of a finer movement from a larger one with which it formerly coexisted.

Diphthong: Two adjacent vowels within the same syllable which blend together.

Distortion: The misarticulation of a standard sound in which the latter is replaced by a sound not normally used in the language. A lateral lisp is a distortion.

Dysarthria: Articulation disorders produced by peripheral or central nerve damage.

Dyslalia: Functional (nonorganic) disorders of articulation.

Dysphasia: The general term for aphasic problems.

Dysphemia: A poorly timed control mechanism for coordinating sequential utterance. It is variously conceived as being due to a constitutional and hereditary difference or to psychopathology. It reflects itself in stuttering and cluttering.

Dysphonias: Disorders of voice.

Ear-training: Therapy devoted to self-hearing of speech deviations and standard utterance.

Echolalia: The automatic involuntary repetition of heard phrases and sentences.

Echo speech: A technique in which the case is trained to repeat instantly what he is hearing, following almost simultaneously the utterance of another person. Also called "shadowing."

Egocentric: Self-centered; pertaining to the self and its display.

Ego strength: Morale or self-confidence.

Electroencephalogram: The record of brain waves of electrical potential. E.E.G. Used in diagnosing epilepsy, tumors, or other pathologies.

Embolism: A clogging of a blood vessel as by a clot.

Empathy: The conscious or unconscious imitation or identification of one person with the behavior or feelings of another.

Encephalitis: A disease characterized by inflammation or lesions of the brain.

Epiglottis: The shield-like cartilage that hovers over the front part of the larynx.

Epilepsy: A neurological disease characterized by convulsions and seizures.

Esophageal speech: Speech of laryngectomized persons produced by air pulses ejected from the esophagus.

Esophagus: The tube leading from the throat to the stomach.

Etiology: Causation.

Eunuchoid voice: A very high-pitched voice similar to that of a castrated male adult.

Expressive aphasia: The difficulty in sending meaningful messages, as in the speaking, writing, or gesturing difficulties of the aphasic. Executive aphasia.

Falsetto: Usually the upper and unnatural range of a male voice produced by a different type of laryngeal functioning.

Fauces: The rear side margins of the mouth cavity which separate the mouth from the pharynx.

Feedback: The backflow of information concerning the output of a motor system. Auditory feedback refers to self-hearing; kinesthetic feedback, to the self-perception of one's movements.

Fixation: In stuttering, the prolongation of a speech posture.

Flaccid: Passively uncontracted, limp.

Frenum: The white membrane below the tonguetip.

Fluency: Unhesitant speech.

Fricative: A speech sound produced by forcing the air stream through a constricted opening. The *f* and *v* sounds are fricatives. Sibilants are also fricatives.

Glide: A class of speech sounds in which the characteristic feature is produced by shifting from one posture to another. Examples are the *y* (j) in *you* (ju) and the *w* in we.

Glottal catch (or stop): A tiny cough-like sound produced by the sudden release of a pulse of voiced or unvoiced air from the vocal folds.

Glottal fry: A ticker-like continuous clicking sound produced by the vocal cords.

Glottis: The space between the vocal cords when they are not brought together.

Guttural voice: A low-pitched falsetto.

Hard contacts: Hypertensed fixed articulatory postures assumed by stutterers in attempting feared words.

Harelip: A cleft of the upper lip.

Hemorrhage: Bleeding.

Hyperactivity: Excessive and often random movements as often shown by a brain-injured child.

Hypernasality: Excessively nasal voice quality. Rhinolalia aperta.

Hyponasality: Lack of sufficient nasality, as in the denasal or adenoidal voice.

Identification: In articulation therapy, the techniques used to recognize the essential features of the correct sound or its error.

Idioglossia: Self-language with a vocabulary invented by the child.

Incidence: Frequency of occurrence.

Incisor: Any one of the four front teeth in the upper or lower jaws.

Infantile swallow: A form of swallowing in which the tongue is usually protruded between the teeth.

Inflection: A shift in pitch during the utterance of a syllable.

Interdental: Between the teeth. An interdental lisp would show itself in the substitution of the *th* for the *s* as in *thoup* for *soup*.

Interiorized stuttering: A form of stuttering behavior in which no visible contortions or audible abnormalities are shown but a hidden struggle usually in the larynx or breathing musculatures is present. Also characterized by clever disguise reactions.

Isolation techniques: Activities used to locate the defective sound in utterance.

Jargon: Continuous but unintelligible speech.

Kinesthesia: The perception of muscular contraction or movement.

Kinetic analysis: The analysis of error sounds in terms of their movement patterns.

Lalling: An articulatory disorder characterized by errors on sounds produced by lifting the tip of the tongue such as *l* and *r*.

Lambdacism: Defective *l* sounds.

Lateral: A sound such as the *l* in which the air flow courses around the side of the uplifted tongue. One variety of lateral lisp is so produced.

Laryngeal: Pertaining to the larynx.

Laryngectomy: The surgical removal of the larynx.

Larynx: The cartilaginous structure housing the vocal folds.

Laryngologist: A physician specializing in diseases and pathology of the larynx.

Lesion: A wound, broken tissue.

Lingual: Pertaining to the tongue. A lingual lisp is identical with an interdental lisp.

Lisp: An articulatory disorder characterized by defective sibiliant sounds such as the *s* and *z*.

Malocclusion: An abnormal bite.

Mandible: Lower jaw.

Maxilla: Upper jaw.

Medial: The occurrence of a sound within a word but not initiating or ending it.

Median: Midline, in the middle.

MMPI: Minnesota Multiphasic Personality Inventory, a test of personality problems.

Monaural: Hear with one ear.

Monitoring: Checking and controlling the output of speech.

Monopitch: Speaking in a very narrow pitch range, usually of 1-4 semitones.

Moto-kinesthetic method: A method for teaching sounds and words in which the therapist directs the movements of the tongue, jaw, and lips by touch and manipulation.

Mucosa: The mouth and throat linings which secrete mucus.

Multiple sclerosis: A progressive and deteriorating muscular disability produced by overgrowth of the connective tissue surrounding the nerve tracts.

Muscular dystrophy: A disease of unknown origin characterized by progressive deterioration in muscle functioning and also by withering of the muscles.

Mutism: Without speech. Voluntary mutism: refusal to speak.

Nares: Nostrils.

Nasal emission: Airflow through the nose.

Nasal lisp: The substituting of a snorted unvoiced *n* for the sibilant sounds.

Nasopharynx: That part of the throat, pharynx, above the level of the base of the uvula.

Negative practice: Deliberate practice of the error or abnormal behavior.

Nerve deafness: Loss of hearing due to inadequate functioning of the cochlea, auditory nerve, or hearing centers in the brain.

Nonfluency: Pause, hesitation, repetition, or other behavior which interrupts the normal flow of utterance.

Nucleus: A central core. Nucleus situations are those in which the case tries especially hard to monitor his speech so as to improve it. See Chapter Ten.

Obturator: An appliance used to close a cleft or gap.

Occluded lisp: The substitution of a *t* or a *ts* for the *s* or the *d* and *dz* for the *z*.

Omission: One of the four types of articulatory errors. The standard sound is replaced usually by a slight pause equal in duration to the sound omitted.

Operant conditioning: The differential reinforcement of desired responses.

Opposition breathing: Breathing in which the thorax (chest) and diaphragm work oppositely against each other in providing breath support for voice.

Optimal pitch level: The pitch range at which a given individual may phonate most efficiently.

Orthodontist: A dentist who specializes in repositioning of the teeth.

Oscillations: Rhythmic repetitive movements; repetitions of a sound, syllable, or posture.

Overt: Clearly visible or audible behavior.

Palpation: Examining by tapping or touching.

Parallel talk: A technique in which the therapist provides a running commentary on what the case is doing, perceiving, or probably feeling.

Paraphasia: Aphasic behavior characterized by jumbled inaccurate words. See Chapter Fourteen.

Perseveration: The automatic and often involuntary continuation of behavior.

Pharyngeal flap: A tissue bridge between the soft palate and the back wall of the throat.

Pharynx: The throat.

Phonation: Voice.

Phonemic: Refers to a group of very similar sounds represented by the same phonetic symbol.

Phonetic placement: A method for teaching a new sound by the use of diagrams, mirrors, or manipulation whereby the essential motor features of the sound are made clear.

Pitch breaks: Sudden abnormal shifts of pitch during speech.

Plosive: A speech sound characterized by the sudden release of a puff of air. Examples are *p, t, g.*

Polygraph: An instrument for recording breathing, heart beat, and other functions.

Preparatory set: An anticipatory readiness to perform an act.

Proboscis: Nose.

Prognosis: Prediction of progress.

Propositionality: The meaningfulness of a message or utterance. Its information content.

Proprioception: Sense information from muscles, joints or tendons.

Prosthodontist: A dental specialist who makes prostheses.

Prosthesis: An appliance used to compensate for a missing or paralyzed structure. See illustration in Chapter Thirteen.

Puberal: Pertaining to the period during which the secondary sexual characteristics begin to appear.

Pyknolepsy: A mild form of epilepsy characterized by stoppages in speech, among other things.

Receptive aphasia: Aphasia in which the major defects or impairments are in comprehending meanings.

Rhinolalia: Nasality.

Rhotacism: Articulatory errors on the *r* sounds.

Rorschach: An ink-blot test of personality.

Secondary stuttering: The fourth and terminal stage in the development of the disorder.

Self-talk: An audible commentary by the person describing what he is doing, perceiving, or feeling.

Semitone: A half-note, a half-step on the musical scale.

Septum: The partition between the right and left nasal cavities formed of bone and cartilage.

Shadowing: See echo talk.

Sibling: Brother or sister.

Sigmatism: Lisping.

Sonant: A voiced sound.

Spastic: (*noun*) An individual who shows one of the varieties of cerebral palsy. (*adjective*) Characterized by highly tensed contractions of muscle groups.

Spastic dysphonia: A voice disorder in which phonation is produced only with great effort and strain.

Stabilization: The process of making a response permanent and unfluctuating.

Stigma: A mark or sign of defect or disgrace.

Stop consonant: A sound characterized by a momentary blocking of airflow. Examples are the *k, d,* and *p.*

Strident lisp: Sibilants characterized by piercing, whistling sounds.

Strident voice: Harsh voice quality.

Surd: Unvoiced sound such as the *s* as opposed to its cognate *z* which is voiced or sonant.

Tempo: Rate of utterance.

Thorax: Chest.

Tooth prop: A small wooden or plastic peg to be held between the teeth.

Trauma: Shock or injury.

Tremor: A swift vibration of a muscle group.

Unilaterality: One handedness; preference for one hand as contrasted with ambidexterity.

Uvula: The hanging portion of the soft palate. The velar tail.

Velum: Soft palate.

Velo-pharyngeal closure: The more or less complete shutting off of the nasopharynx.

Ventricular phonation: Voice produced by the vibration of the false vocal folds.

Vocal fry: See glottal fry.

Vocal play: In the development of speech, the stage during which the child experiments with sounds and syllables.

Xanthippe: Why Socrates became a philosopher.

Index

Index

A

Abnormalities:
  breathing, in stuttering, 312, 314, 330, 339
  organic, 204-205, 417-420
Acalculia, 446
Adenoidal voice, 31
Agraphia, 120, 446
Airflow control, cleft-palate therapy, 432-438
Air pressure control, cleft-palate therapy, 431-438
Air wastage, 185
  with cleft palate, 433
Alexia, 120, 446
Alphabet of sound, in delayed speech therapy, 136
Alveolar process, 417-419
American Speech and Hearing Association, 457, 462
Ammons Picture Vocabulary Test, 111
Analysis of articulation disorders, 220-228
Analysis of voice disorders, 179-181
Anomia, 446
Antiexpectancy devices of stutterers, 342
Anxiety:
  and resistance to therapy, 58
  reactions to, 58-61
  in speech defectives, 57-61, 66-68
  in stutterers, 308-309, 313, 314
    desensitization to, in secondary therapy, 398-399
    development, 331-333
    effect on stuttering, 308-309, 340
    exploration, in secondary therapy, 392
    factor in therapy, 354-356, 381

reduction in early therapy, 361-365
varying reactions to, in secondary therapy, 402-403
Aphasia, 120-123, 445-455
  causes, 447
  in children, 32-33, 120-123
    characteristics, 120-122
    therapy, 123
  congenital, 121
  developmental, 120-121
  disorders, 445-447
  effect on speech, 5, 445-446
  emotional aspects, 8-9
  expressive, 32, 446
  prognosis, 447-448
  receptive, 32, 446
  symbolization disorder, 19, 32-33, 445-447
  therapy, 448-454
    body image integration, 454-455
    formulation, 452-454
    inhibition, 450
    memorization, 450-451
    organization, 452
    parallel talking, 448-449, 452-454
    scanning and concentrating, 451-452
    self-talk, 449, 452-454
    stimulation, 449
    symbolization translation, 450
Aphonia, 17, 168
  cause, 29
  hysterical, therapy, 187-188
  therapy, 187-188
Approach-avoidance conflict in stutterers, 334
Approach-avoidance theory of stuttering, 323
Approximation in secondary stuttering therapy, 403-408

Riper, Charles Van
Speech Correction